SECOND EDITION

Supporting Children with Communication Difficulties in Inclusive Settings

School-Based Language Intervention

D0080628

Linda McCormick
University of Hawaii

Diane Frome Loeb
University of Kansas

Richard L. Schiefelbusch
University of Kansas

Boston   New York   San Francisco
Mexico City   Montreal   Toronto   London   Madrid   Munich   Paris
Hong Kong   Singapore   Tokyo   Cape Town   Sydney

Executive Editor and Publisher: Stephen D. Dragin
Editorial Assistant: Barbara Strickland
Marketing Manager: Tara Whorf
Production Editor: Michael Granger
Editorial Production Service: Chestnut Hill Enterprises, Inc.
Composition Buyer: Linda Cox
Manufacturing Buyer: JoAnne Sweeney
Cover Administrator: Kristina Mose-Libon
Electronic Composition: Omegatype Typography, Inc.

For related titles and support materials, visit our online catalog at www.ablongman.com.

Between the time Website information is gathered and then published, it is not unusual for some sites to have closed. Also, the transcription of URLs can result in unintended typographical errors. The publisher would appreciate notification where these errors occur so that they may be corrected in subsequent editions.

Library of Congress Cataloging-in-Publication Data not available at time of publication.

ISBN 0-205-37954-0

Printed in the United States of America

10 9 8 7 6 5 4 3 2 1   08 07 06 04 03 02

CONTENTS

PART III

Like the first edition, this second edition translates our commitment to collaboration and meeting the needs of all children in general education classrooms and other inclusive settings into practical guidelines for teaching and intervention arrangements. Some speech and language pathologists (SLPs) and special education teachers may not currently be working together collaboratively in inclusive environments; this text points out the many opportunities for collaborative alliances. Ultimately, the success of inclusion for children with communication difficulties has less to do with the severity of the children's disability or disabilities than with whether teachers and SLPs are committed to working together to provide an environment that recognizes, supports, and enhances every child's strengths.

We are not arguing that every activity in the school day and all special assistance and support (e.g., remedial math, mobility training, computer activities) should be provided in the general education classroom. We are arguing that being culturally or developmentally "different" does not preclude belonging together in the same environments. Certainly, all children (those considered "typical" as well as those labeled as having a disability) need special help such as tutoring or extra drill at one time or another. They may need to leave the general education classroom to receive that assistance. Most important is for them to know that it is okay both to need and to receive extra help.

ORGANIZATION

The thirteen chapters are organized into three parts. In Part I, the first five chapters provide essential background information. Chapter 1 presents important terms and concepts and an overview of language acquisition. Chapter 2 presents the contributions of major researchers and theorists in language acquisition with a focus on the practical implications of their offerings. Chapter 3 describes characteristics of students with language and communication difficulties with extensive attention to the language difficulties of children with autism spectrum disorders. Chapter 4 presents practices for building effective partnerships with family members with an emphasis on working with families whose cultural backgrounds are different from those of the interventionists. Chapter 5 summarizes current legislative provisions that have implications for SLPs and special education teachers.

The chapters in Part II address assessment and intervention procedures. Chapter 6 describes formal and informal language assessment practices. Chapter 7 presents a rationale and procedures for ecological assessment and planning. Chapter 8 considers the focus of intervention, methods, and procedures for special instruction, the instructional environment, professional relationships and responsibilities, scheduling, and measurement and evaluation.

The five chapters in Part III deal with special populations. Chapter 9 describes language assessment and intervention with infants and toddlers. Chapter 10 presents strategies to encourage language and communication in inclusive preschool settings. This chapter includes a section on the language needs of culturally and linguistically diverse populations. Chapter 11 provides a more in-depth consideration of the needs of second-language learners. It describes procedures to facilitate the linguistic and academic achievement of bilingual/bicultural children with language difficulties. Chapter 12 describes procedures for meeting the special needs of students with severe disabilities, including autism. Finally, Chapter 13 provides an introduction to augmentative and alternative communication (AAC) with particular attention to the assessment and planning process.

ACKNOWLEDGMENTS

We wish to thank the reviewers: Patrick McCaffrey, California State University–Chico; Terry E. Spigner, University of Central Oklahoma; and Ruth H. Stonestreet, Valdosta State University. We would also like to thank the children and the families with whom we work. They deserve the most credit as our teachers.

Introduction to Language Acquisition

Linda McCormick

Long before they produce their first "baba," babies' minds are busy sorting out the sounds and shapes of words and sentences, communicating intentionally, repairing misunderstood messages, using others to accomplish goals, and participating in a variety of turn-taking routines that closely resemble language (Jusczyk, 1999). Not only are they learning what the words of their language sound like, they are sorting out what they mean, how to order them in a sentence, and how to make them agree grammatically. Most children have a vocabulary of fifty or more words, and many are producing short but intelligible sentences by age 2. By the time they enter preschool, they are understanding and using thousands of words and their tacit knowledge of grammar is already more sophisticated than the thickest style manual. They are already accomplished little conversationalists when they start kindergarten.

That children learn to talk even before they are out of diapers makes language learning seem easy. It isn't. Even for normally developing children, language acquisition is enormously challenging. For children with biological and/or environmental risk conditions, language acquisition may be impossible without special intervention/instruction.

The goal of this book is to provide a basic introduction to concepts and practices of language and communication intervention/instruction, with practical guidelines, strategies, and methods for inclusive settings. This first chapter presents key terms and concepts in linguistics, a discussion of the bases of normal language acquisition, and an overview of early language learning processes.

IMPORTANT TERMS AND CONSTRUCTS

Study in a new area is challenging because you must learn many new terms and you must learn new meanings for familiar terms. Of the two, learning new terms is often easier because all you have to do is learn the meaning of the new term and you have a new vocabulary item. Familiar terms with new meanings are more difficult because you must form new associations. Many of the terms in this first section are of the latter type; familiar terms for which you must learn more refined and specialized or different meanings. For example, you know the terms *language, speech,* and *communication,* but you may not know how the three concepts differ and how they relate to one another.

Speech

Speech is the oral modality for language, the expression of language with sounds. Other language modalities include manual signing and writing. Humans are not the only species to produce sounds, but we are the only species with the unique structure of the human vocal tract necessary to produce the variety and complexity of sounds that are required for speech. Speech production depends on precise physiological and neuromuscular coordination of respiration, phonation, resonance, and articulation. Respiration is the act of breathing; phonation is the production of sound by the larynx and vocal fold; resonance is the vibratory response that controls the quality of the sound wave; and articulation is use of the lips, tongue, teeth, and hard and soft palates to form speech sounds. Exhaled air from the lungs is modified by the vocal folds in the larynx and/or the structure of the mouth to produce speech sounds.

Speech is willed, planned, and programmed by the central nervous system—the brain, the spinal cord, and the peripheral nervous system, which includes the cranial and spinal nerves. The different parts of the nervous system are bound together by neurons to form a complex information exchange network that transmits motor impulses to and from the muscles of the speech mechanism.

Language

Languages are abstract systems with rules governing the sequencing of their basic units (sounds, morphemes, words, sentences) and rules governing meaning and use. Lahey (1988) defines *language* as "a code whereby ideas about the world are represented through a conventional system of arbitrary signals for communication" (p. 2). The term *code* is basic to defining language. Language is a code in the sense that it is not a direct representation of the world, but something with

which to *represent* ideas or concepts about the world. It is important to remember that these ideas and concepts (mental representations) are separate from the objects and events that they represent *and* from the words with which they are represented. Mental representations are inherent in people, *not* in words and not in what words represent.

When you know a language, you know its basic units (sounds, words) and the complex rules governing relationships among sounds, words, sentences, meaning, and use. The term *know* as used here, means 'are able to apply.' The unconscious knowledge that underlies our ability to produce and interpret utterances in a language is called *linguistic competence* (Chomsky, 1965). Linguistic competence is implicit knowledge that enables us to judge sentences as grammatical, ungrammatical, or ambiguous, and to generate sentences. The actual physical and psychological processes that we go through when we produce and interpret utterances—the expression of that unconscious knowledge—is *linguistic performance.*

Language has many subsystems or components. To know a language you must know its phonology, morphology, semantics, syntax, and pragmatics.

Phonology. Phonology is the study of the sound system of language but it is not the same thing as speech. Speech is what we are actually doing when we talk and listen. Phonology refers to the segments and rules (the mental or psychological processes) with which we organize our interpretation of speech. The phonological system of a language includes the sounds that are characteristic of that language, the rules governing their distribution and sequencing, and the stress and intonation patterns that accompany sounds. The task facing language learners is twofold: (1) how to recognize and produce the sounds of the language they are learning, and (2) how to combine the sounds into words and sentences with the proper intonation patterns.

Phonemes are the smallest units of sound that signal a difference of meaning in a word. The concept of the phoneme arose out of the awareness that the precise phonetic realization of a particular sound is not so important as its function within the sound system of a particular language. To demonstrate what a phoneme is, say the words *bat* and *pat* to yourself. Note that the only difference between the two words is the initial sound. The sounds /b/ and /p/ function to produce two different words, each with a different meaning. This difference in meaning is the reason that /b/ and /p/ are categorized as separate phonemes in English.

Every language uses a different assortment of phonemes, which combine to make syllables. For example, in English the consonant sound *b* and the vowel sound *a* are both phonemes, which combine for the syllable *ba,* as in *banana.* Adults find it difficult (sometimes impossible) to simply perceive, much less pronounce, the phonemes of a foreign language. However, infants can perceive the entire range of phonemes. By the time babies are 10 to 12 months of age, they have begun to focus on the distinction among phonemes of their native language and to ignore the differences among foreign sounds. As they get older they simply stop paying attention to foreign sounds and concentrate on learning the syllables and words of their native tongue.

Morphology. Morphology is the study of word formation. Words are made up of meaningful units called *morphemes*. A morpheme cannot be broken into smaller parts without violating the meaning or leaving meaningless remainders. Words consist of one or more morphemes. Examples of words that consist of a single morpheme are *cat, danger, toy,* and *big.* These are called *free morphemes:* they have meaning standing alone. Other morphemes, called *bound morphemes,* cannot function alone. They are always affixed to free morphemes as prefixes or suffixes. Examples include *-s, -er, re-,* and *un-.* There are two types of bound morphemes: inflectional morphemes (sometimes called grammatical morphemes) and derivational morphemes. Inflectional morphemes modify words to indicate such things as tense, person, number, case, and gender. There are a limited number of inflectional morphemes in English, and they are all suffixes. They are used to form plurals ("two boys"), possessives ("the boy's wagon"), third-person present tense ("she combs her hair"), past tense ("she combed her hair"), and word combinations.

The morphology of a language includes the rules governing how words are formed. Some morphemes, called *lexical morphemes,* have meaning in and of themselves; others, called *grammatical morphemes,* specify the relationship between one lexical morpheme and another. The distinction between lexical and grammatical morphemes is not well defined in linguistics. However, most linguists agree that lexical morphemes have a sense or meaning in and of themselves. Typical examples include nouns, verbs, and adjectives. Grammatical morphemes do not have a sense or meaning in and of themselves: they express some sort of relationship *between* lexical morphemes. Typical examples include prepositions, articles, and conjunctions.

Semantics. Semantics is the study of linguistic meaning. Semantic acquisition is the acquisition of vocabulary and meanings associated with words and word combinations. At the most basic level, semantics is the linguistic realization of what the speaker knows about the world—what people talk about. Semantics is concerned with relationships: (1) between words and meanings, (2) between words, (3) between word meanings and sentence meanings, and (4) between linguistic meaning and nonlinguistic reality.

With one exception, the relationship between a word and its meaning is arbitrary. The exception is onomatopoeic words. (An onomatopoeic word is formed by imitating the sound made by, or associated with, its referent.) That the piece of furniture you are sitting on is called a chair rather than a cup is an accident of linguistic history. Other languages, of course, have different words to represent the piece of furniture that English speakers call a chair. When thinking about words and their meanings, remember

1. the meaning of a word is a concept or an idea in the head of the speaker—the thing the word represents is the referent; and
2. words have an arbitrary relationship to the things they represent —they are elements of a code that have been arbitrarily assigned meanings.

The second type of relationship is the relationship *between* words. Words may have a synonymous, homonymous, or antonymous relationship with one another. Words that have the same meaning are synonymous (e.g., *sofa* and *couch*). Words that sound the same but have different meanings are homonymous with one another (e.g., *flower* and *flour*). Words that have opposite meanings are said to have an antonymous relationship (e.g., *tall* and *short*).

The third type of semantic relationship is between word meanings and sentence meanings. The meaning of a sentence is not the sum of the meanings of the words combined to form the sentence. If this were the case, then sentences that have the same words (i.e., "The girl loved the boy" and The boy loved the girl") would have the same meaning. Rather, the meaning of a sentence is determined by both the meaning of the words and word order. Making a sentence is something like building with blocks. The number of blocks in a set is limited, but there are unlimited possibilities for combining units to form different structures.

Finally, the fourth type of relationship is that between linguistic meaning and nonlinguistic meaning (cognitive knowledge). Cognitive knowledge is the structure we give to our experiences as we organize them into categories for efficient storage and retrieval. When words become linked with cognitive knowledge, the cognitive knowledge becomes semantic knowledge. Thus, semantic knowledge is a subset of cognitive knowledge.

Syntax. Syntax is the study of the structure of phrases, clauses, and sentences. The syntax of language contains rules for how to string words together to form phrases and sentences, what sentences are acceptable, and how to transform sentences into other sentences. Knowledge of the syntax of a language allows a speaker to generate an infinite number of new sentences and to recognize sentences that are not grammatically acceptable. For example, native speakers of English know immediately that one of these sentences is ungrammatical:

1. The waitress poured the coffee.
2. The poured coffee the waitress.

Now consider these sentences:

1. Visiting grandparents can be boring.
2. Jason gave his cousin a sock.

Both sentences are ambiguous. However, because you have linguistic competence in English, you are able to paraphrase them to eliminate the ambiguity. These examples illustrate the wealth of knowledge underlying the ability to form and understand sentences.

Pragmatics. Pragmatics is the study of how language is used to communicate within its situational context. The major concern in pragmatics is the effectiveness of language in achieving desired functions in social situations. Attitudes, personal history, the setting, the topic of conversation, and the details of the preceding discourse are among the social and contextual factors that determine how speakers cast their sentences (and how listeners interpret them).

There are three types of pragmatic knowledge and skills (Lahey, 1988). First is knowing how to use language forms and structures to accomplish certain personal and/or social goals and functions. An example of this type of pragmatic competence is persuading a person to act in a particular manner. Language can be used for an extraordinarily wide range of functions. A speaker's utterance can serve as a request for an object, or for information, attention, action, or acknowledgment: an utterance can also convey facts, attitudes, and beliefs, as well as promises and threats. These functions are called **speech acts.** A speech act is a speaker's goal or intent in using language. Speech acts have two facets: a **locutionary act** (the act of simply uttering a sentence from a language) and an **illocutionary act** (what the speaker *does* by uttering the sentence). Examples of illocutionary acts are stating, requesting, questioning, and promising.

A second type of pragmatic competence is knowing how to use information from the social context to determine what to say in order to achieve personal and social goals. Speakers must decide the appropriate form of a message to use in different contexts to accomplish whatever personal or social goals they are seeking. Adapting their messages requires them to make inferences about what the listener already knows (and does not already know). These judgments about the capacities and needs of listeners in different social contexts (i.e., what is assumed to be true) are called **presuppositions.**

Rules for engaging in social exchanges or conversational abilities constitute the third type of pragmatic competence. Among the most critical abilities is the ability to initiate, maintain, and terminate conversations. To initiate a conversation, the speaker must first solicit the potential conversational partner's attention. Then, to maintain a conversation, the speaker must know how to take turns, how to assert a position or opinion, and how to respond or react to what the listener has asserted. Finally, the speaker must know how to "sign off" the conversation in such a way that neither partner is left feeling abandoned. The rules for entering and initiating conversations, leaving or terminating conversations, taking turns, shifting topics, handling regressions, asking questions, and temporal spacing of pauses are called **conversational postulates.**

Communication

At the broadest level, communication is the exchange of ideas, information, thoughts, and feelings. Each person's role in the exchange is clearly defined (e.g., as either speaker or receiver) as the participants take turns sending and receiving messages. The communication process begins when a person has an idea or intention and wants to share it. The idea or intention is formulated into a message and then expressed to another person or persons. The other person or persons receives the message and reacts to or acknowledges it. Thus, the behavior of one participant is directed toward and affects the behavior and/or thoughts of a receiver (or receivers). Then the subsequent behavior and/or thoughts of the message sender are influenced by the response to the message. In any communication there is always a high probability that the message will be distorted because of the many possible message modalities and the many possible connotations and perceptions of the communication partners.

Communication does not necessarily require speech or language. Examples of nonlinguistic communication behaviors are gestures, posture, eye contact, facial expression, and head and body movement. Nonlinguistic communication modes may be used as the only method of communication or they may be used in conjunction with linguistically encoded messages. When they are used in conjunction with speech, there is a complex interrelationship between verbal and nonverbal behavior. Even the distance between participants provides information (Higginbotham & Yoder, 1982). Specifically, it sends a message about the level of interpersonal intimacy of the participants. In Western cultures, participants in a formal, public exchange typically maintain a distance of 12 feet or more. A distance of 4 to 12 feet is common for social–consultive exchanges, and a distance of 18 inches to 4 feet is usual for personal exchanges. Participants in intimate exchanges typically maintain a distance of direct contact to 18 inches.

There are numerous perspectives on communicative competence. The sociolinguistic perspective, which is heavily influenced by the early work of Hymes, emphasizes the appropriateness of communication with respect to the conversational parameters discussed above. Communicative competence is defined as the language user's "knowledge of sentences, not only as grammatical but also as appropriate" (Hymes, 1972, p. 277). It is "knowing when to speak and when not to speak, what to talk about with whom, when, where, and in what manner" (p. 277). Psychologists tend to emphasize the intelligibility of the communicative signal (the degree to which the message is conveyed or received), rather than appropriateness, as the most important aspect of communicative competence (Wang, Rose, & Maxwell, 1973). Psycholinguists are less concerned with appropriateness and more concerned with intention. They define communicative competence in terms of successful performance of speech acts (Searle, 1969). (Recall that a speech act is a speaker's goal or intent in using language.)

This section has considered basic concepts in linguistic theory. The next section reviews contributors to language acquisition. These contributors are organized under the broad headings: (a) biological preparation, (b) nurturance, (c) sensorimotor experiences, and (d) linguistic experiences.

THE BASES OF LANGUAGE ACQUISITION

The four sets of variables that have the most profound influence on language learning are (1) biological preparation, (2) successful nurturance (particularly social experiences), (3) sensorimotor experiences, and (4) linguistic experiences. The relative weight given to each of these factors depends on your theoretical biases regarding language acquisition. (Chapter 2 describes language acquisition theories.)

Biological Preparation

That all cultures have language and all humans learn to talk (unless limited by sensory, neuromuscular, or cognitive impairment) are the strongest evidence for the contention that language is a biologically determined capability. Infants arrive in this world with certain neuromotor capabilities, a supply of sensory and perceptual abilities, and a strong desire to interact with others. If provided with an appropriate variety of experiences, they will become competent communicators. The persistence and attentiveness with which they go about the momentous task of becoming communicators are testimony to what has been called the "motivational characteristic of infancy" (Hunt, 1965).

Neuromotor Potentialities. As noted above, speech is an enormously complex motor skill. It depends on coordination of the muscles of the vocal organs (tongue, lips, and vocal cords) and appropriate instructions from the brain. Impulses along the motor nerves set the vocal muscles into movement. This movement produces minute pressure changes in the surrounding air (sound waves). Over the past twenty years, neuroscientists have amassed a wealth of information about how the brain grows and how babies acquire language and other abilities. Babies are born with more than 100 billion brain cells, more than they will ever use. Some of these cells, called *neurons,* have already been hardwired to other cells. They control the baby's heartbeat, command its breathing, produce reflexes, and regulate other functions essential to survival. The remaining cells are waiting to be "hooked up." Which neurons connect and which connections will eventually wither and die from lack of use depends on the baby's experiences. Babies' early experiences depend on parents and other caregivers.

Lateralization is the specialization of the left or right hemisphere of the brain for different functions. Listening, understanding, talking, and reading each involve activities in specialized areas of the brain. Most adults (probably 70 to 95 percent of humans) have left hemisphere specialization for these abilities (regardless of what language they use). Infants and toddlers, however, deal with language in both hemispheres (Neville & Bavelier, 1999) until around the end of the third year. At that time, processing of words that serve special grammatical functions, such as prepositions, conjunctions, and articles, begins to shift into the left side. The two hemispheres assume different functions from then on. Both hemispheres know the meaning of many words, but the left hemisphere takes over responsibility for grammar. The right hemisphere continues to perform spatial tasks, such as following the trajectory of a baseball and predicting where it will land. It also attends to the emotional information contained in the cadence and pitch of speech.

This right-left division of labor maintains even when individuals use sign language. Corina, Bellugi, and Reilly (1999) studied deaf users of American Sign Language (ASL) who had suffered a stroke in specific areas of the brain. They found, predictably, that signers with damage to the right hemisphere had great difficulty with tasks involving spatial perception, such as copying a drawing of a geometric pattern. What *was* surprising, considering the fact that ASL relies on movements of the hands and body in space, was that right-hemisphere damage did not hinder ASL. In contrast, ASL users who had suffered damage to the left hemisphere found they could no longer express themselves in ASL *or* understand it. Some had trouble producing the specific facial expressions that convey grammatical information in ASL. This suggests that both speech (movements of the mouth to produce utterances) and sign language are processed in the left hemisphere.

The new brain research has shown us that the brain has a remarkable ability to change and adapt in response to experience. The neuroplasticity of the brain is most remarkable in the first ten years of life. During these years there appear to be times during which the brain is especially efficient at learning particular skills. These times are called critical windows of opportunity for learning or critical periods. The **critical-period hypothesis** posits that humans are most proficient at language learning between age 2 and puberty (Lenneberg, 1967). After that time, a child is no longer prepared to learn language because lateralization is complete.

Sensory and Perceptual Capabilities. Sensation refers to the process by which information about the environment is detected by the sensory receptors and transmitted to the brain. The sensory equipment of infants functions rather well from birth. They are capable of seeing, hearing, tasting, smelling, and responding to touch, temperature, and pain from the first day of life. Positive, nurturing experiences and an environment stimulating to the senses strengthens the neural connections in the developing brain.

Newborns clearly "sense" movement, colors, changes in brightness, and a variety of visual patterns, as long as these patterned stimuli are not too finely detailed and have a sufficient amount of light/dark contrast. They can follow slow-moving objects but lose the objects if they are more than eighteen inches away. By 2½ months they are spending approximately 35 percent of their waking hours visually scanning the environment with a definite preference for objects that move, objects with sharp contours, and objects with light-dark contrasts (Kagan, 1985). By seven months the infant has developed binocular vision.

That infants hear is attested to by the fact that they startle and turn away from loud noises and they often turn in the direction of soft sounds as if searching for the source. Young infants are particularly responsive to the sounds of a human voice. They stop crying, open their eyes, and begin to look around or to vocalize when they are spoken to. Auditory capabilities show significant improvement over the first 4 to 6 months.

Sensitivity to touch has not been studied as much as the other senses. Newborns show reflexive responses if touched on the cheeks (rooting reflex), palms (grasping reflex), or the soles of their feet (Babinski reflex). They are also quite sensitive to warmth, cold, and changes in temperature. They will refuse to suck if the milk in their bottles is too hot, and they will try to maintain their body heat by becoming more active should the temperature of a room suddenly drop.

Perception is the brain's categorization and interpretation of sensory input. Researchers have learned a great deal about the auditory perception of infants. Most importantly, they have learned that auditory perception, which can be thought of as *the path leading to language,* begins even before birth when the developing fetus is immersed in the muffled sound of its mother's voice in the womb (Kuhl & Meltzoff, 1997). Newborn babies discriminate and prefer their mothers' voices over those of their fathers or other women. Also, they discriminate and prefer the sound of their mothers' native language compared to a recording of another tongue. At first, infants respond only to the prosody and the cadence, rhythm, and pitch of their mothers' speech, not the words; but soon enough they home in on the actual sounds that are typical of their parents' language. By 4 months babies can discriminate between vowels and imitate the main features of the vowels.

Visual perception is rudimentary at birth but infants do seem to be able to distinguish between faces and other objects and they can focus on objects no farther than 13 inches away. (This is about the distance of a mother's face when she is breast-feeding or the face of a caregiver holding a bottle.) Between the ages of 2 and 12 months, infants' visual system is maturing rapidly, making increasingly complex visual discriminations possible. The ability to perceive faces and facial configurations seems to follow the same general course as the perception of other visual forms and patterns. Between 2 and 6 months, infants' visual capabilities make it possible for them to scan in a more systematic fashion and they begin to perceive a variety of forms. Forms that move (such as faces) are probably detected first, but 6- to 9-month-olds can even perceive the subjective contours of stationary objects.

Newborns' gustatory and olfactory abilities are more impressive. By three days after birth they can differentiate smells and tastes. Most prefer the sweetness of fruit (bananas and applesauce are first choices) over vegetables. (This comes as no surprise to parents who have been sprayed with rejected strained spinach or some other vegetable.) They are also capable of sensing and discriminating a variety of odors. They turn away with expressions of disgust in response to unpleasant smells such as vinegar, ammonia, or rotten eggs. Even more remarkably, breast-fed infants soon come to recognize their mothers by smell. Infants as young as 2 weeks of age can discriminate their own mother's body odors from those of other people, whereas babies who are bottle-fed cannot, possibly because they have less contact with their mothers' bare skin.

Interaction Propensities. Infants seem well prepared for social interactions, assuming certain kinds of environmental social supports. At birth, babies are responsive to all humans but they are especially and differentially responsive to their caregivers. Infants seem to know that they can create change in their environment with certain behaviors, and they have clear expectations for caregiver behavior patterns.

Parents (especially mothers) spend a great deal of time in face-to-face social interaction with their infants. Most of this time they are talking to the infant. This speech directed to children will be described below in the section on Linguistic Experiences. It was previously known as "motherese" but is now more appropriately called **parentese** or *child-directed speech* (CDS).

During the latter half of the first year, normally developing infants discover that their vocalizations and gestures affect their caregivers' responses in predictable ways. They use such behaviors as gaze, smiling, touch, and vocalization to motivate their caregivers to attend to them and to respond to their needs, and, in so doing, they actually prompt provision of the type of experiences that will assist the continuing growth of their language skills. There is a high level of mutual coordination and responsiveness between the partners, with the infant influencing the communication process and contributing to the interactions. Infants learn to be message senders as well as message receivers and to coordinate gaze, vocal, and gestural behavior into a fairly complex, patterned exchange that parallels the structure of a conversation.

Nurturance

Sameroff and Fiese (1988) describe the nurturing environment as one in which there is a "mutual dynamic regulation of the child's capacities to understand and [of] the experiences that are presented to be understood" (p. 10). Caregivers take advantage of social exchanges to help the infant learn (1) the rules of turn-taking, (2) the meaning of particular gestures, (3) imitation of sounds and gestures, and (4) mutuality. Development of shared meanings, shared intentions, shared codes of conduct, sensorimotor concepts, and symbolic representation will eventually emerge from these attainments.

Caregivers treat babies as if they are intentional communicators long before they actually are. At the same time, they never seem to lose sight of the infant's language and communication limitations. They temporarily support the infant's emerging skills and abilities in much the same way that a temporary framework supports builders and materials when a building is being erected, regulating presentation of both linguistic and nonlinguistic stimuli. The term for this dynamic regulation that goes on between the infant and caregivers in a nurturing environment is *scaffolding*.

Vygotsky (1978) and others (Rogoff, 1990; Rogoff & Wertsch, 1984) offer a theory of learning based on the scaffolding and joint attentional focus (when adults describe aspects of the environment that capture the baby's attention). Children develop and internalize new capacities during these interactions; they make the leap from lower to higher cognitive processes. Vygotsky's term for the dynamic zone of sensitivity in which learning and cognitive development occur is the **zone of proximal development** (or ZPD). The ZPD can be thought of as the difference between the developmental level of the child when independently engaged in problem solving and the child's competence when guided by caregivers or in collaboration with more capable peers. Vygotsky argued that the primary concern of assessment should be the ZPD, not what children can do by themselves or already know but what they can do with the help of another person—thus, what they have the potential to learn.

Nurturance is the context in which infants acquire the social knowledge essential for language (Dore, 1986; Rice, 1984; Snow, 1984). They learn two important truths from play and routine interactions with caregivers: (1) that communication exchanges have a predictable structure, and (2) that others are responsive to their signals. They begin to use vocal and gestural signals to intentionally influence the attention and actions of their partners. As they eventually take full advantage of their power to direct others, infants learn the directive function of language. Nurturance is mediating and regulating the pace at which new stimuli are imposed on the child. Nurturing caregiver–child contexts in which there is dynamic regulation of stimuli include caregiving rituals such as feeding, dressing, and diapering, and play interactions such as pat-a-cake and peekaboo.

Play with caregivers is a learning context that serves a cognitive, social, and integrative function in development. The function of play is to exercise and develop manipulative and interactional strategies that can later be integrated into more sophisticated task-oriented sequences. Caregiver–child exchanges have a highly structured pattern, with rules that teach the infant about communication. Around the middle of the first year, turn-taking games, such as pat-a-cake and peekaboo dominate. The caregiver starts the game and initially takes both roles with the infant as the amused audience. Over time, the infant's behavior gradually changes from observer to initiator of actions. By 5 to 9 months of age, he has learned to be a partner in the exchange process. Shortly thereafter, object play increases, with infant and caregiver participating in ritualized give-and-take of objects. What is important about these games with respect to nurturance is the shared meaningful communication at a completely nonverbal level.

Piaget (1952) discussed play in the sensorimotor period as setting the stage for practice and mastery of emerging cognitive skills. Because play centers on the children's interests, it permits them to reenact environmental experiences and to construct rich fantasy worlds for themselves. The earliest forms of pretend play begin around 11 to 13 months. Like language, pretend play is initially very dependent on the "here and now." Infants pretend to engage in familiar activities such as eating, sleeping, or drinking from a cup. Such play in a nurturing environment teaches young children to regulate emotional arousal and "read" the emotions of others in ways that will later facilitate interactions with peers.

Sensorimotor Experiences

Piaget's (1952) developmental theory continues to spawn a great deal of conjecture about the association between cognitive changes (specifically those in the sensorimotor period) and the emergence of intentional communication. Infants pass through a series of predictable stages in the construction of their knowledge of the world and some language achievements seem to be associated with the achievements of these stages. This association has been documented in children who are developing at a normal rate (Corrigan, 1978) *and* children with disabilities (Mundy, Seibert, & Hogan, 1984). However, there is a big difference between associations and causal relationships. There is a lack of hard evidence that language development is *contingent* on mastery of any specific subset of cognitive abilities as was once argued (Lenneberg, 1967). Rather, cognitive development and language development appear to proceed on parallel and closely related courses. The observation that mastery of certain cognitive and language abilities often seem to coincide may be explained by the simple assertion that children learn the words they need for whatever they are interested in at that point.

From birth to age 2, the infant's sensory and motor behaviors undergo significant integration, refinement, and reorganization, permitting the development of increasingly more complex cognitive abilities. This is the beginning of "knowing." "Knowing" in the sensorimotor sense of the term begins with reflexes that are present at birth and ultimately leads to the ability to use mental images for problem solving. Children construct their understanding of the world by acting on the world, both physically and mentally (Piaget, 1952). Like tireless little scientists, they explore, hypothesize, test, and evaluate. Acquisition of sensorimotor abilities affords children the critical skills necessary for achieving higher-level thought processes that, in turn, will enable them to share a subset of basic meanings with caregivers and to grasp the relationship of words to meaning.

Piaget uses the term *schemata* (the singular is *schema*) to describe the models, or mental structures, that humans create to represent, organize, and interpret their experiences. Schemata are patterns of thought or action similar in many respects to what we think of as a concept or strategy. Their knowledge of the world, their schemata, changes as children organize and reorganize their existing knowledge and adapt to new experiences. Among the most important things they learn are that the world is a permanent place with predictable effects and that there are any number of means for controlling the events that occur around them.

According to Piaget (1952), the basic processes of cognitive development, or ways of learning, stay essentially the same from birth through adulthood. What differs across stages are the products—the knowing. Both the content and the structure of cognitive functioning become progressively more complex (qualitatively different) as the child moves through the four broad stages of cognitive development: sensorimotor, preoperational, concrete operational, and formal operational. Piaget believed that all cognitive structures are created through the operation of two inborn intellectual functions. He called these basic processes of cognitive development **organization** and **adaptation.**

Organization is the process by which existing schemata are combined into new and more complex intellectual structures. It is the tendency to reduce, systemize, and categorize the environment into cohesive, orderly, and ultimately more manageable proportions. Learning comes about through progressive, qualitative organization and reorganization of actions and perceptions. To get a feeling for organization, think about an infant whose primary means of exploring the environment is by looking and grasping. Initially, each functions independently; the infant can grasp an object or she can look at it, but she cannot manage both at the same time. As the weeks pass, she organizes these two actions into a pattern, evidenced by the fact that she is now able to look at what she grasps and grasp what she is looking at. The result of this organization of initially unrelated schemata into a complex structure is visually directed reaching.

The goal of organization is to further the adaptive function, the second key process. **Adaptation,** adjusting to the demands of the environment, has two complementary and mutually dependent aspects, **assimilation** and **accommodation.** Assimilation is the process by which new information and new experiences are incorporated into the organism's existing cognitive schemata. Because not all stimuli will fit into existing structures, the cognitive structures must be adapted. For example, the young child who sees a cow for the first time will try to assimilate it into one of his existing schemata for four-legged animals. He may think of it as a "doggie." He notices, however, that this creature is very big and the sound it makes is different from that of a dog. If the child recognizes that the creature is not a dog and is interested in understanding and naming it, he will have to modify his schema to include a new category of four-legged animals. This is the accommodation process, modifying existing cognitive structures in accordance with new information. Assimilation and accommodation never occur in isolation. They are two sides of the same coin, complementary aspects of all intellectual acts.

Equilibrium is a state of balance between the existing cognitive structures and the environment, a more complex and sophisticated repertoire. It comes about as the result of accommodation and assimilation. Four-month-old Jessica's experiences with a small teddy bear, an object she had never seen before, provide an example of equilibrium. Initially she applies her limited "learning strategies" to this strange new "thing." She grasps it by one ear, mouths it, hits it, and shakes it vigorously. Then she throws it on the floor. The new "thing" has two properties that are new to Jessica: softness and furriness. After a few experiences with the teddy bear, she begins to attend to these properties; she begins to cuddle and rub the bear. Apparently Jessica is learning something from this new object. The new experience and the new information have been incorporated into existing schemata for toys (assimilation) and her existing schemata have changed as a function of the new information (accommodation). What has been accomplished is equilibrium (also sometimes called equilibration). In other words, learning has occurred.

Between the ages of 18 and 24 months, infants progress from sensorimotor intelligence, which is reflexive, self-centered, and disorganized, to concepts that are sophisticated, refined, well-organized, and adapted to the demands of the environment. A substage is never skipped: the sequence is stable. However, some infants progress more rapidly than others. By the end of the sensorimotor stage (18 to 24 months), the young child has constructed the following broad concepts: (1) object permanence, (2) schemes for relating to objects, (3) spatial relationships, (4) means-end understanding, (5) causality, and (6) imitation.

Object permanence is understanding that objects continue to exist even when not immediately perceptible. It is knowing that people, places, and things exist independently of one's own perceptions. Object permanence begins with the ability to visually fixate on an object (animate or inanimate) and then track its disappearances and appearances. In early infancy, before infants have the notion of object permanence, the disappearance of an object causes no more than a fleeting glance in the direction where it disappeared. Infants act as though the object does not exist unless they can see it. By the end of the first year, however, infants begin to show searching behaviors that are appropriate to the recovery of a desired object (if they observed the object's disappearance). More prolonged search will indicate that children have some mental representation of the object. Mental representation is considered to be the crowning achievement of the sensorimotor period, possibly related to a spurt in vocabulary growth at the end of the second year. Representational thought continues to develop as children become increasingly able to deal with complex relationships that are not directly perceptible in the environment. Table 1.1 summarizes development of object permanence and the object concept (schemes for relating to objects).

TABLE 1.1   Representative sensorimotor behaviors: Object permanence and schemes for relating to objects

Stage (Ages)	Object Permanence	Schemes for Relating to Objects
Stage 1: (0–1 month) Reflexive	Continuously practices reflexes No active search for objects that drop out of view Demonstrates some visual pursuit when lying on back	No discernable separation of self from objects
Stage 2: (1–4 months) Primary Circular Reactions	Gradually coordinates sensory schemes—vision and hearing, sucking and grasping, and vision and grasping Able to visually follow a slowly moving object through a 180-degree arc in a smooth tracking response Very little, if any, visual or manual search for a vanished object—"out of sight is out of mind" Lingers with a brief glance at the point where a slowly moving object disappears	Shows incidental object use in the process of practicing different behaviors such as grasping and looking Mouths some objects Holds and briefly inspects various objects
Stage 3: (4–8 months) Secondary Circular Reactions	Visually anticipates the future position of a moving object Continues manual search for an object if grasping movements are interrupted while in process Recognizes and obtains an object that is partially hidden Behaves as if an object no longer exists when it is completely covered or drops out of sight	Shows systematic object use in practicing different behaviors Bangs objects together Shakes a rattle, bell, and other objects Visually inspects an object while tactually exploring it Displays other differentiated actions with objects, including crumpling (of paper), sliding (of toys on surface), tearing, stretching, rubbing, mouthing
Stage 4: (8–12 months) Coordination of Secondary Reactions	Looks for an object after it has vanished behind a screen and reliably retrieves it Reacts with only mild surprise or puzzlement when object retrieved differs from the one hidden Continues searching for an object at point A (where it is usually found) even after watching it being hidden at location B	Demonstrates new actions on objects resulting from (related to) object properties Intentionally drops and throws objects Uses objects in a socially relevant manner Combines functional relationships, such as placing cup in saucer, to some extent

(continued)

TABLE 1.1   Representative sensorimotor behaviors: Object permanence and schemes for relating to objects (*continued*)

Stage (Ages)	Object Permanence	Schemes for Relating to Objects
Stage 5: (12–18 months) Tertiary Circular Reactions	When the hiding is visible, infant will search in the place where it was last seen (even with 3 screens) Not successful at retrieving objects if hiding is not visible because infant cannot yet "think" where an object might be	Varies action on objects to "experiment" with different effects (such as dropping objects to study their trajectory) Links more objects in functional relationships: Puts cup in saucer, pretends to drink from cup, slides brush or comb over his hair
Stage 6: (18–24 months) Invention of New Means through Mental combinations	Systematically searches for an object that has undergone as many as 3 invisible displacements— searches each hiding place (sometimes in reverse order)	Demonstrates understanding of the functions and social meanings of a large number of objects: Holds telephone to ear and vocalizes, tries to put shoes and socks on, names familiar objects

The phrase **schemes for relating to objects** refers to the infant's ability to perform specific actions or action sequences consistently and habitually on a variety of objects. The scheme itself is the mental organization of the overt actions. These object-specific action patterns are possible because of cognitive capacity. Initially, schemes for relating to objects are more like reflexes than voluntary behavior. They represent a kind of action-based scientific method that the infant uses to learn about objects. At first, all objects elicit the same action schemes (sucking, grasping, shaking), which are part of the infant's reflexive repertoire. For example, the young infant who sucks everything that finds its way into her mouth would be said to have a sucking scheme. Initially she is indiscriminate, but in time she will develop the ability to discriminate "suckables" and apply this action scheme only to these particular objects. Gradually, all schemes become differentiated and are applied according to object properties.

The phrase **spatial relationships** refers to understanding of two related concepts: (1) an object's position in space, and (2) how objects relate to one another. Development of the awareness of spatial relationships begins with visual tracking of moving objects. Soon after, the infant begins to act on objects as though they have a given location and to rotate them in relation to perceived spatial orientation. For example, if presented with a bottle with the nipple turned away, the infant will turn the nipple toward her and begin to suck it. Finally the infant gives evidence of mental representation of the spatial relationship between two objects (without testing the relationship with her own body). When a child unhesitatingly goes around a hedge to retrieve a ball, rather than first trying to go through the hedge, he is demonstrating understanding of spatial relationships.

Means-end understanding is the ability to separate problem-solving processes from problem-solving goals. It begins early (1 to 4 months) with simple reflexive responses to external stimuli. In the next few months these behaviors become less reflexive. Through repeated experiences with positive consequences the infant discovers predictable behavior sequences. He discovers, for example, that if he hits the top of the jack-in-the-box toy the clown pops out. By the first half of the second year, the infant has begun to vary the components of behavior sequences in a systematic fashion in order to observe changes in the outcomes. By the middle of the second year the infant understands that problems can be solved mentally so that a goal can be attained by methods other than trial-and-error.

Causality is closely related to the means-end concept. It is the ability to anticipate what consequences will follow from a certain cause or, conversely, what cause is likely to produce a particular consequence. Infants learn about causality when they accidentally create pleasurable effects through such behaviors as hand waving and kicking. Once they learn that they can cause effects and thus control their environment effectively through systematic application of certain motor behaviors, they begin to use more complex control behaviors. As experiences with pleasurable effects increase, infants begin to anticipate results and events and they begin to search for activating or causal mechanisms to produce the anticipated pleasurable outcomes.

The one-year-old is aware only of causal relations that have some personal consequence for her (e.g., crying causes mother to pay attention). Somewhere around 18 months she becomes aware of causal relations involving other people and objects and she realizes that her behavior can be affected by, as well as affect, other people and things in the environment. By age two, children are able to classify many of their own behaviors and the behaviors of others in terms of the consequences they produce. Table 1.2 presents some parallels between development of means-end and causality concepts and the emergence of communicative functions.

Imitation is performance of a response that matches, or approximates, the behavior of a model. Piaget recognized the adaptive significance of imitation. At the very least, imitation requires the ability to pay careful attention to, and precisely copy the topographical features of, a behavior produced by another, immediately after the model. Table 1.3 summarizes the development of imitation in the sensorimotor period. Infants use imitation to add new behaviors to their repertoire. In the early months, they can imitate only actions that are already in their repertoire but by their second year they can accommodate

TABLE 1.2   Parallels between means-end and causality development and emergence of communicative functions

Sensorimotor Stage (Ages)	Means-End Behavior and Causality Development	Interaction-Communication Strategies
Stage 1: (0–1 month) Reflexive Reactions	Repeats/practices reflexes No understanding of causal relationships	Perlocutionary acts Quiets and responds to human voice
Stage 2: (1–4 months) Primary Circular Reactions	No differentiation of self and moving objects Immediately repeats behaviors that have accidentally produced interesting results (e.g., attempting to keep a mobile in motion)	Perlocutionary (unintentional) acts Smiles and coos in response to adult smiling and/or vocalization Shows anticipation when about to be picked up Emits distinguishable cries for anger, hunger, pain
Stage 3: (4–8 months) Secondary Circular Reactions	Uses such behavior as consistent vocalization, kicking, waving as if attempting to "cause" continuation of an interesting sight	Perlocutionary acts Shows enjoyment when played with Vocalizes states such as pleasure, satisfaction, anger Follows adult gaze (if adult breaks eye contact to look elsewhere) "Recognizes" caregiver Performs joint action "rituals" with caregiver (turn-taking routines)
Stage 4: (8–12 months) Coordination of Secondary Circular Reactions	Intentional, goal-directed behavior apparent in releasing or pushing aside one object to grasp another, pulling a support to obtain desired toy Appreciation of causality outside the self demonstrated by pushing the adult's hand to continue an interesting sensory effect, anticipating the occurrence of events from signs (e.g., crying when mother gets her coat out)	Perlocutionary acts Extends arms to be picked up Withdraws from approach of a stranger Reacts negatively when a toy is taken away Waves "bye-bye" Shows affection to parents and other adults Looks at caregiver's face when receiving an object as if to acknowledge receipt Plays peekaboo, hiding face for another to watch
Stage 5: (12–18 months) Tertiary Circular Reactions	Experiments with means and ends as if to see what will happen Demonstrates considerable interest in novelty for its own sake	Illocutionary acts Tries to turn doorknobs as a request to "go outside" Uses gestures such as pointing to direct adult attention

TABLE 1.2   Parallels between means-end and causality development and emergence of communicative functions (*continued*)

Sensorimotor Stage (Ages)	Means-End Behavior and Causality Development	Interaction-Communication Strategies
Stage 5: (12–18 months) Tertiary Circular Reactions	Uses an attached string or stick to obtain a desired toy without demonstration (even if toy is not in direct view) Hands a mechanical toy to an adult to be reactivated Shows object to others to instigate social interaction	Hands book to adult to request reading of a story Pulls adult to view certain situations or a new location Shows/displays/points out objects to others to elicit attention and social interaction
Stage 6: (18–24 months) Invention of New Means through Mental Combinations	Ability to use mental problem solving (mental foresight of effects) Immediately looks for causes of own actions Able to infer a cause, given only its effect, or foresee an effect, given a cause	Locutionary acts Asks for desired object (with conventional symbol) Uses words to make wants/desires known Names objects in the presence of others Says "What's that?" for adult attention

their behavior to imitate novel actions (called *coordinating secondary schemes*). Imitation continues to become even more efficient until the latter part of their second year, when infants demonstrate **delayed or deferred imitation,** a clear indication of mental representation.

While imitation cannot account fully for language acquisition, it undoubtedly plays some role in the process. Vocal and gestural imitation have been positively correlated with language level (Snow, 1989).

In summary, we have seen how infants progress, in two short years, from being totally reflexive and largely immobile to becoming planful thinkers who can move about on their own and communicate many of their intentions—a truly remarkable achievement. During the preconceptual period (2 to 4 years of age) children become increasingly proficient at constructing and using mental symbols to think about objects, situations, and events (called *symbolic thought* or *mental representation*) and using words to make reference to objects, persons, and events.

Linguistic Experiences

Teaching language seems to be as natural for adults as learning and using language is for babies. Adults in all cultures spend a great deal of time talking to infants in face-to-face social interaction. Most interesting

TABLE 1.3   Development of sensorimotor imitation

Stage (Ages)	Type of Imitation	Characteristics
Stage 1: (0–1 month)	Vocal contagion	Infant is incapable of "true" imitation, but acts that appear to be imitative do occur. One crying newborn is likely to stimulate the other infants to cry. Piaget describes this phenomenon as the triggering of existing response patterns through external stimulation.
Stage 2: (1–4 months)	Mutual imitation	The infant will often repeat a habitual response (gesture or vocal) if someone has immediately mimicked the production. Reproductions are limited and are only gross approximations of the model.
Stage 3: (4–8 months)	Systematic imitation	Since the child is now able to coordinate vision and prehension, she can imitate many more acts. She can now imitate movements, such as opening and closing the fist, but cannot imitate acts, such as opening and closing the eyes, that she cannot see herself performing. The child apparently needs a visual impression that matches that which she has seen the model create in order to duplicate the model. Also, the child will imitate only those sounds and movements that are already in her repertoire. Thus, imitation at this stage is less a learning strategy than a strategy to prolong or continue those events the child finds meaningful.
Stage 4: (8–12 months)	Imitation of new behaviors	The ability to imitate movements that she cannot see herself, and to produce and imitate some acts that are not already known, emerge simultaneously. Imitation undergoes a transition from being a means for continuing interesting events to being a means for learning new ones. However, only actions and vocalizations similar to those in the child's repertoire are imitated.
Stage 5: (12–18 months)	Expanded imitation of new behaviors	Reproductions of new models are immediate, deliberate, and usually quite accurate. Imitation is used in a trial-and-error fashion to discover the properties of objects. Novel vocalizations will be imitated repeatedly as if to perfect the reproduction.
Stage 6: (18–24 months)	Deferred (or representative) imitation	Imitation no longer requires that the model be immediately present. The child is now capable of mental representation and long-term memory for what was modeled. She is also capable of imitating complex new acts and objects as well as persons.

is that they unconsciously and automatically modify their speech when they speak to babies, continuously adjusting its phonologic, semantic, syntactic, and pragmatic characteristics. This singsong type of exaggerated speech was previously called "motherese," but is now called **parentese** or *child-directed speech* (CDS).

Parentese is like a tutorial that teaches infants the phonetic elements of their parents' language. It has a melody that gets the baby's attention and exaggerated prosodic patterns to help the infant become aware of a message's communicative intent. There are fewer *different* words and they are used less often. As the child gets more competent adults tend to use more modifiers and more questions. They repeat what the young child does not seem to understand and they talk only about the "here and now" (those aspects of the world that are present in the immediate environment). Another especially valuable feature of parentese is the running commentaries on what children are doing when they are engaged with objects and events that interest them. When children are attending to an object or activity, particularly during picture-book reading activities, caregivers play a "naming game." In the case of pictures, caregivers name the object or action that is depicted. Their language directed to the child is marked by brevity, concreteness, and few pronouns and contractions.

Analysis of the less complex linguistic style that parents use with children suggests that they are guided by three assumptions: (1) that some words are easier for children to understand and pronounce than others, (2) that some words are more useful for children than others, and (3) that some words and word endings should be omitted and others should be avoided (because they are difficult to understand). Caregivers seem to be aware of the role that modeling and imitation play in language learning. They model words and sentences for the child to reproduce and then specifically direct the child to imitate ("Say _____"). However, not all young children use imitation as a learning strategy and those who do imitate do so selectively (Bloom, Hood, & Lightbown, 1974). They tend to imitate only those words and phrases that they are in the process of learning: they do not imitate words and syntactic structures that are either very familiar or very unfamiliar. Children are most likely to imitate an adult utterance that is a repetition or expansion of their own language efforts. With increasing language competence, children's imitation of adult utterances decreases.

Adults use both expansion and extension with young children. **Expansion** is responding to the child's utterance with a more sophisticated version of the utterance while preserving the word order of the child's utterance. For example, if the child says "Daddy bye-bye," the adult expansion might be "Yes, Daddy is going bye-bye." A substantial percentage of the speech directed to children is expansions. Expansions let children know that they have been understood. Very often, when adults imitate and expand children's utterances, children imitate the expansions. **Extension** is responding with a comment that adds information to the topic established by the child. For example, an extension of the "Daddy bye-bye" utterance could be "Yes, Daddy is going to the store to get some milk."

Adults begin asking questions of infants when they are as young as 3 months of age. They also, of course, supply the answers. The questions that caregivers ask infants demonstrate that they have precise understanding of the infant's knowledge and his language abilities. Caregivers rephrase and "break down" the structure of a question if the child does not respond to the original form.

Adults also use many fill-ins in their speech directed to children. For example, they may say "This is a _____," and pause for the child to supply the final element. If the child does not respond or responds incorrectly, the adult will usually provide a prompt or cue ("This is a b_____") or a model ("You can say 'baby,' This is a 'baby' "). What seems uppermost in the mind of adults is maintaining the interaction at a level that allows the child to participate and keep the conversation going.

Linguists have a long way to go before they can say exactly how a child goes from babbling to banter or how the brain transforms vague thoughts into concrete words that sometimes fly out of our mouths before we can stop them. We do know that speech addressed to children plays an important role in this process. There is evidence that how much their mothers talk to them may, in fact, determine the size of toddlers' vocabularies (Huttenlocher, Haight, Bryk, Seltzer, & Lysons, 1991). At 20 months, children of talkative mothers had 131 more words in their vocabularies than children whose mothers were more taciturn (disinclined to talk). By age 2, the gap had widened to 295 words.

Parking a toddler in front of the television will not contribute to vocabulary growth. Children need real human interaction and they need it early. It is the only way they can learn words and then to attach meaning to words. Hearing more than one language in infancy is even better. This makes it easier for a child to hear the distinctions between phonemes of more than one language later on.

OVERVIEW OF EARLY LANGUAGE ACQUISITION

The routines of play and daily caregiving provide the contexts for early language learning. Through participation in these routines infants learn about the persons, objects, and events in their environment. They also learn about their language. While they do not *always* guess correctly when organizing their mental representations of the world, and the "tags" they attach to their mental representations are not always correct, by the latter half of their second year young children are on their way to becoming competent in their native language.

The following propositions are basic to the language learning process. We know that

- humans have at least some innate structure for acquiring language;
- language learning requires substantially more than simple imitation;
- language is acquired in stages;
- the child infers systems of rules;
- humans have mental abilities intended solely for the purpose of learning and using language.

Otherwise, it would not be possible for young children to acquire the phonology, morphology, syntax, semantics, and pragmatics of their native language in such a short time. Even before they start kindergarten, young children have learned (1) sounds and sound patterns, (2) words and word combinations, (3) sentence variations, (4) conversational abilities, and (5) social functions. The remainder of this chapter will provide an overview of these major achievements in the language acquisition process. We deal solely with the acquisition of English but the principles typically apply, when they are relevant, to the acquisition of other first languages as well.

Sounds and Sound Patterns

Infants seem to be born with the capacity to discriminate the phonetic contrasts of any of the world's languages. Over time, with exposure to their own language, they focus on the contrasts that are relevant for their language and they lose the ability to perceive certain contrasts not found in their language. Infants must also learn to recognize sequences of sounds if they are to eventually learn words. The first sound sequence infants learn to recognize is probably their name. Infants as young as four-and-a-half months give evidence that they prefer the sound of their names over other words with similar stress patterns (Mandel, Jusczyk, & Pisoni, 1994).

Regardless of the linguistic community into which they are born, all infants seem to pass through the same stages of sound production. From the moment of their first cry, infants begin learning precise control of their lips, tongue, and hard and soft palates, and how to coordinate their respiration, phonation, and resonance for speech. This earliest state of sound production is characterized by a majority of reflexive vocalizations, such as fussing and crying, and sounds like coughing, burping, and sneezing. Around the third and fourth months, cooing and babbling monologues become more frequent, and sound use more varied (laughter and chuckling). Very loud and very soft sounds (yells and whispers) and some rudimentary syllables are produced between 4 and 6 months. Babbling sounds begin to resemble the consonants and vowels of adult speech in the child's culture. Deafness does not have detrimental effects on speech production until after babbling has begun. However, as babbling increases there begins to be a noticeable difference in the sounds made by hearing and deaf children.

Between 6 to 10 months, infants sound like they are actually trying to produce words. Babbling changes to experimentation with consonant–vowel syllable sequences (e.g., "da-da-da") with adultlike timing. The repetitive syllable production that characterizes the infant's speech during this period is called **reduplicative babbling.** This sound pattern makes up about half of babies' noncrying sounds from about 6 to 12 months of age (Mitchell & Kent, 1990).

At around 9 to 12 months, infants begin to produce strings of sounds and syllables with a rich variety of stress and intonational patterns. They begin to use imitation to expand and modify their repertoire of speech sounds but initially imitate only those sounds they have already produced spontaneously on their own. This stage is characterized by strings of sounds and syllables called **conversational babbling,** or jargon, which are produced with adultlike stress and intonation patterns. Early words tend to use the sounds that the child preferred in babbling (the sounds that the baby has under voluntary control). Infants producing conversational babbling give the impression of trying to carry on a conversation. They use gestures, context, and intonation as if conveying meaning but, in fact, the sounds they are using are not yet attached to meanings.

Pronunciations of first words vary. Some words may be perfect according to adult standards while others are difficult to understand. Some of the sound sequences produced at this stage are not based on adult words. These are called **vocables** or *phonetically consistent forms* (PCFs) (Dore, Franklin, Miller, & Ramer, 1976). Infants may develop as many as a dozen vocables (and use them consistently) before producing their first words. An example of a PCF would be the use of *b* for *ball*.

Children learning languages (e.g., Spanish, Finnish, and Japanese) that have very few one-syllable words may have different strategies and patterns from children learning English, which has many monosyllables. The frequency of different sounds in their native language may also affect acquisition: Infants learning languages that have more /l/s tend to learn them earlier than do children learning English (Pye, Ingram, & List, 1987).

Children learning English must learn to correctly articulate twenty-five consonants and twenty-one vowels and diphthongs, and they must learn to produce these sounds individually and then combine a variety of sounds in a word. There is enormous variability among children with the age of acquisition for some sounds varying as much as three years. By age 3, most children can produce all of the vowel sounds and nearly all consonant sounds (though not with total accuracy in all words). As the normative data previously presented indicate, even at 4 and 5 there will be some consonants that are in error. The acquisition process continues well into early elementary school as children continue to work on mastery of a complete repertoire of speech sounds and two sets of rules: the rules that govern the position of sounds in words, **distributional rules,** and the rules for sequencing these sounds, **sequential rules.**

Words and Word Combinations

By 13 to 15 months, most infants have acquired ten words. First words, produced around the end of the first year, are typically a combination of lexical, vocal, and gestural forms. The majority of these words are names for favorite toys or foods, family members, or pets. Action words such as *up* and *bye-bye,* modifiers such as *pretty,* and grammatical function words such as *what* are also represented in this first vocabulary, but much less frequently. These single words are typically used for different functions: requesting, commenting, and inquiring (as well as naming). Early vocabulary growth is slow, with short periods of time when the child does not add any new words and may even stop producing some of the words in his initial vocabulary. This is usually due to changing interests and improved production capabilities. Although there is wide individual variation, it is not uncommon for a child's receptive vocabulary to be as much as four times the size of the expressive vocabulary in the first half of the second year. Some meanings will be similar to adult meanings, but most will be very restricted compared to adult definitions.

Vocabulary growth accelerates as the child nears a fifty-word vocabulary. For many children, the composition of the second set of forty words, typically acquired by 18 to 20 months, is two-thirds nouns. Action words account for less than 20 percent of the total (Benedict, 1979; Nelson, 1973). In Nelson's listing of the nominals used by the eighteen children in her study, there was no noun that was used by all of the children. Children learn names for different objects and events because they encounter different objects and events. The fact that very few words were shared by even half the children is impressive evidence for the influence of environmental differences.

One commonality among all children is that they learn names for things that move or can be acted on. Early vocabulary lists rarely include such words as *stove, lamp, tub, sofa* and the like because these objects are not acted on by the young child in any significant way. Instead, we find many words for food and drink, animal names, clothing, and toys, objects children directly experience or objects that move. Another variable is pronunciation: Children learn words that contain sounds they can produce.

As discussed earlier in this chapter, children are capable of representational thought by age 2, in preparation for the more advanced cognitive period that Piaget calls *preoperational thought.* They know that object existence is absolute—that objects exist and continue to exist even when not immediately visible—and that different objects have different perceptual and functional properties. Similarly, they know (1) that "things" can cease to exist and then recur, (2) that people (including themselves) can relate to objects in certain prescribed ways (e.g., owning them, locating and relocating them), and (3) that objects also relate to themselves and each other in a relatively consistent manner. Their single-word utterances reflect this growing knowledge of the world. Most early single-word utterances can be classified as either substantive or relational. **Substantive words** refer to specific entities or classes of entities that have certain shared perceptual or functional features. The words *cup, bottle, mama, doggie,* and *ball* are substantive words. When children begin combining words into two-word combinations, they classify substantive words on the basis of action. Words are classified as agents (the source of action) or objects (the recipient of action).

Relational words make reference across entities. They refer to dynamic relations that an entity shares with itself or with other entities. In relation to itself, an entity can exist or not exist, disappear and reappear. An example is "all gone," which can apply to an empty bowl or a vacant doghouse. Other entities may share static states such as possession and attribution, dynamic states (actions), or locations. Relational meanings transcend the individual objects involved. Use of relational words is evidence that the child is able to conceptualize and encode the dynamic state of the entity separately from the entity itself.

The years from 2 to 6 are marked by changes in the *kinds* of words children use. As noted above, a substantial proportion of a child's first fifty words are nouns and verbs, with labels for objects that move or can be acted on and action verbs appearing most frequently. Around 18 to 20 months, modifiers (*hot, big*) and function words (*no, more*) begin to appear. Expressions for temporal relations (*then, after, before*), causality (*if, because*), and quantity (*many, few, three*) appear much later. At around age 2, children begin to recognize that a pronoun can refer to an already established referent and to use some pronouns correctly. Their first pronouns signal notice, such as *this* and *that* (e.g., *That* a birdie). The pronoun *it* also appears early, usually in the subject position (e.g., *It* a swing). When children begin to combine words, the pronouns *one, some,* and *other* begin to occur. Person pronouns appear after age 2½. Subjective case pronouns (*I, you, they, he/she, we*) are acquired first; objective case pronouns are acquired somewhat later. Other pronouns emerge much later, with order of acquisition varying across children.

Around the age of 2, the child begins to form two-word utterances and after that they gradually increase until age 3 when the majority of utterances are three-word. The most notable change during this multiword stage is the appearance of **grammatical morphemes.** (Recall that grammatical morphemes are morphemes that specify the relationship between lexical morphemes [morphemes that have meaning in and of themselves].) The acquisition of grammatical morphemes is gradual and lengthy, beginning at around 27 months or when the mean length of the child's utterances is about 2.0. (The concept of mean length of utterance is explained in the next section.) Although they do not carry independent meaning, grammatical morphemes (also called morphological inflections) subtly affect the meaning of sentences. Brown's (1973) study of the mastery of grammatical morphemes found that the rate of development varies but the order of acquisition (as listed below) is fairly predictable.

1. *-ing* marking the present progressive tense (children first use this *without* an auxiliary verb). Example: I running.
2. *in* and *on* used in locative state utterances. Example: Cookie *in* there. Ball *on* bed.
3. *-s* marking the regular noun plural (and some irregular forms). Example: My doll*s*.
4. some past tense irregular verbs such as *went* and *came*. Example: She *went*.
5. *-s* marking the noun possessive. Example: Daddy*'s* shoe.
6. uncontractible copula forms of *to be: am, is, are, was,* and *were.* (The contractible forms are acquired much later.) Example: He *was* good.
7. use of *a* and *the* to distinguish between definite and indefinite referents. Example: That *a* doggie.
8. -ed marking the regular past tense. Example: She cook*ed*.
9. —s ending on third-person regular verbs. Example: He move*s*.
10. third-person irregular verb forms. Examples: *is, has, does.*
11. uncontractible auxiliary forms of *be* verbs preceding another verb: *am, is, are, were,* and *was.*
12. contractible copula verbs. Example: It*'s* my book.
13. contractible auxiliary verbs. Example: He*'s* reading a book.

While there are not definitive data on the acquisition of grammatical morphemes in all languages, what data there are suggest that grammatical morphemes are acquired in similar ways and at about the same stage of development in different languages (Pizzuto & Caselli, 1991). This evidence lends strong support to the notion that the cognitive relationship between the semantic and syntactic complexity of the earliest morphemes is the key to developmental order. Forms that are semantically and syntactically easier tend to be learned and produced earlier.

The multiword utterances that are evident as early as 16 months are more properly termed successive single-word utterances than short sentences in that children use two words together (separate one-word utterances) to comment on two aspects of an ongoing event. These utterances are evidence that they are beginning to perceive relations among persons and objects though they do not yet have sufficient language skills to express these relationships. The next step after successive single-word utterances is encoding of semantic relations in multiword utterances, a major contributor to increased length of utterances. These multiword utterances, in which the meaning depends on relationships *between* or *among* the words rather than the meanings of the individual words, are called **semantic relations** (sometimes, semantic–syntactic relations). Think of them as "meaning relations." For example, when Brendyn holds up his shoe after searching for and finding it under the bed and says "Brendyn shoe," he is expressing a possessor–possession relationship. (Semantic relations are discussed below and semantic relations analysis is described in Chapter 6.)

A second factor accounting for increased length of utterances is **concatenation.** Concatenation is chaining together several two-term semantic relations. It is evident shortly after children begin producing single two-term semantic relations. For example, the agent–action relation *baby eat* and the action–object relation *eat cookie* might be combined and the redundant term omitted, to yield *Baby eat cookie*.

A third factor accounting for increased sentence length is expansion. Once children are understanding and expressing semantic relations, they begin to expand simple terms in these relations by adding modifiers and auxiliaries. These expanded constructions give the listener more accurate and precise information. The 3-year-olds who produce these expanded constructions are generally expressing the same intentions they expressed earlier with two or three words, but the addition of modifiers and auxiliaries makes it easier for listeners to interpret what they are saying without having to depend on contextual information. The child who said "more juice" at 18 months and "want more juice" at 24 months, now at 30 months may say "want more apple juice."

A fourth factor in increasing the length of utterances is the emergence of grammatical morphemes at around age 2 or 2½. (Acquisition of grammatical morphemes was described previously.)

Expressing Meanings

Children have a range and variety of experiences with objects, action, and events in their physical and social worlds. These experiences are the source and the content for their concepts about objects, actions, and events (their nonlinguistic knowledge). Because the vast majority of these experiences also involve language, children have myriad opportunities to experience co-occurrences of words and phrases and their particular referents. Once concepts and ideas about the world become linked to, and expressed (and understood) through language, they are classified as linguistic knowledge—more specifically, semantic knowledge.

Children progress steadily and gradually toward adultlike meanings. Based on analysis of data from his cross-cultural study of language acquisition, Slobin (1971) put it this way: "New forms first express old functions, and new functions are first expressed by old forms" (p. 184). In other words, children first use new words and phrases to express well-established (familiar) meanings and they use familiar words to express newly constructed meanings. They try out either a new form or a new meaning, but not both. An example illustrates this premise. Slobin quotes his 3-year-old daughter as saying "Anything is not to break—just glasses and plates" (1971, p. 186). She has arrived at a new and complex (for a 3-year-old) idea: That only glasses and plates are breakable. However, she lacked the words to express this idea properly so she did the best she could with the words in her repertoire (with amusing results).

When you think about meaning in language you probably think about word meaning. A second type of meaning that has been noted several times throughout this chapter is relational meaning. Relational meaning maps the relationships among objects, actions, and events. Relational meaning can be encoded with a single word, but it is often difficult for the listener to interpret the intended meaning when only a single word is used. Consider the word *more,* for example. If a child with an empty cup and an empty plate simply says, "more" and does not point to or otherwise indicate the cup, or dish, or a food item, there will be some question as to the intent of the utterance. However, if the word is combined with a gesture or a second word, then the intent is clear. When a child uses a single word like *more* to communicate a meaning that an adult would say with a sentence (e.g., "I'd like more juice"), the one-word utterance is said to be **holophrastic.**

Recall from the earlier discussion that earliest relational meanings, called **semantic relations,** are combinations of two or more words to convey more and different meaning than any one of the words used alone could convey. Semantic relations incorporate two types of meaning: the meaning of the individual words plus the meaning implicit in the way the words are ordered. Encoding of semantic relations begins around 18 months. It is evidence of two things: (1) that the child's awareness and understanding of different types of nonlinguistic relationships has expanded, and (2) that the child now has some understanding of how to express nonlinguistic knowledge through language. The problem is that the former exceeds the latter: The range and variety of ideas and relational concepts children have acquired by this age generally exceed their expressive abilities. Thus, they are frequently in the position of having to use the same word or words to express more than one meaning. Those who are trying to understand the

Sentence Variations

In the early stages of language learning, as mean length of utterance (MLU) increases the complexity of children's utterances also increases. This relationship between length and linguistic complexity seems to maintain until the child attains an MLU of approximately 4.0. MLU is computed by counting the morphemes in 50 (or 100) utterances from a spontaneous speech sample and then dividing by 50 (or 100). (Detailed guidelines for MLU computation are provided in Chapter 6.) By the time that children attain an MLU of 2.5 (at around 2½ years of age) and have begun to master grammatical morphemes, the next major accomplishment is learning about and producing different types of sentences, such as negatives, questions, and imperatives.

NEGATIVE SENTENCES.   There are three periods in learning to produce negative sentences (Bellugi, 1967). In the first stage, at about age 2, children form negative sentences by attaching *no* or *not* in the initial position to a simple declarative sentence. They form sentences like "Not more juice" (said while holding up an empty cup) and "No can make it" (said while trying to force a wooden puzzle piece into the puzzle). The negative function used most often is *nonexistence* (e.g., *no cookie,* indicating the cookie is not in his pocket), but *rejection* (e.g., *not meat,* said while pushing the spoon away), and *denial* (e.g., *not my bear,* said when offered someone else's bear) also appear. While children may initially express all three negative functions in the same way—by tacking on *no* or *not*—the different meanings are generally quite clear.

In the second period, children place the negative word next to the main verb within the sentence (e.g., "I *no* sleep," or "Mommy *no* go car"). Finally, in the third period, when children are around 42 to 48 months, their negative sentences approximate the adult form. By this age they have an extensive repertoire of negative possibilities. They use *can, does, do, did, will,* and *be* with *not* in uncontracted form. (Initially they use them in the present tense.) The negative element is consistently incorporated into the sentence. This progression in the acquisition of negatives is logical. The child's early positive utterances form a nucleus to which the child appends a negative, sometimes at the beginning and other times at the end. Then, as would be expected once child begins to analyze utterances into subject and predicate, the negative item appears between them (as in adult grammar).

QUESTIONS.   Children do not learn to ask some types of questions until they have learned to answer questions of the same kind. For example, they typically do not ask *why* questions until they are able to answer *why* questions. Ervin-Tripp (1970) studied the sequence in which five children responded to different questions after the age of

21 months. First they respond to these *wh-* questions, in this order: (1) *where*, (2) *what*, (3) *whose*, and (4) *who*. *Why, how,* and *when* were responded to somewhat later.

Klima and Bellugi (1966) described three stages in the development of question-asking skills:

Stage 1:
At about 24 to 28 months (MLU around 2.0), young children begin to use a few *wh-* words (*what* and *where*). Most questions at this age are like statements with a rising intonation. The reason these particular *wh-* words appear early is that they relate to the immediate environment. Their use helps the child to (1) gain labels, and (2) locate lost objects. Another possible explanation for the early appearance of *what* and *where* could be that they are words that caregivers use frequently. Finally, a third possible explanation would be that *what* and *where* are learned first because they are related to two of the earliest semantic categories—nomination and location.

Stage 2:
At about 26 to 32 months (MLU around 2.5), young children begin to use the *wh-* forms, *why, where,* and *what,* to introduce statements. They might say "Why you go?" and "Where my coat?" These sentences have a subject and a predicate but auxiliaries are notably absent. At this stage, questions of the *yes–no* type are still statements with a rising intonation. Mistaking one form of *wh-* question for another is common and continues until around age 3. Younger children (between about 20 and 28 months) will typically treat most *wh-*questions as *where* questions. Older 2-year-olds often answer *why* questions as if they were *what* questions.

Stage 3:
At about 33 to 36 months (MLU around 3.0), young children produce inverted *yes/no*-type questions. Shortly thereafter they use inverted *wh-* forms. A variation at this stage is use of the carrier phrase *do you know* to introduce many questions.

Thus, the order of use of *wh-* forms is *what, where, who, when, why, how.* By about age 4, children have learned most of the necessary auxiliary verbs and pronouns and how to use the adult question form.

IMPERATIVE SENTENCES.   Imperative sentences request, demand, ask, or command the listener to perform an action. Most imperative sentences have no overt grammatical subject and the verb is uninflected (e.g., "Give me the paper"). Children between the ages of 19 to 26 months (MLU around 1.75) produce forms (often accompanied by gestures) that serve an imperative or directive function. However, imperative sentences do not appear until around 31 months. By 35 months (MLU of 3.0), children have begun to use modal auxiliaries (e.g., *can, could, will*) in embedded imperatives (e.g., "Could you give me a cookie"). Production of the latter imperatives suggests that the child is beginning to understand the importance of modifying directives according to the status of the listener.

Conversational Abilities

The basic ingredients of conversation—turn-taking and reciprocity—are observable in early caregiver–infant caregiving and play routines (e.g., feeding, diaper changing, "peekaboo" games). Both the infant and the adult are active participants in these exchanges: There are clearly rules for each turn and expectations for particular words and actions within the action sequences. However, adult–child exchanges continue to be heavily dependent on adult scaffolding until well into the child's preschool years. The adult provides the exchange frames in which the child is to produce appropriate responses, and selects and phrases questions carefully so that the child's response options are very clear (e.g., "the big one or the little one?").

While children as young as 2 years old are quite good at introducing new topics, they typically do not sustain a topic beyond one or two turns. Moreover, because they have not yet learned about linguistic contingency or contextual contingency, their responses may be unrelated to their partner's comment. Linguistic and contextual contingency develop slowly. Even at age 3½, only about 50 percent of children's utterances demonstrate contingency (Bloom, Rocissano, & Hood, 1976; Garvey, 1977).

Children as young as age 2 make distinctions in their speech on the basis of whom they are addressing. Their use of significantly more imperatives when addressing their mothers than when talking to their fathers is evidence that they are aware of social relationship variables such as power and familiarity. They already know to use polite request forms when addressing visitors, rather than the type of direct orders addressed to siblings. Other instrumental language strategies, such as gaining a listener's attention and providing explanations or justifications when making requests, are evident at about age 4.

Children learn discourse and conversational skills in the context of social relationships—first with caregivers and later, when they start school, in interactions with a broader social community. Conversational and discourse skills that are fairly well developed by school age include:

- **ability to sustain simple three-term *contingent queries*** in which there is a comment, a request for clarification, and a clarifying response;
- **ability to participate in conversations** by introducing a topic, sustaining it through several turns, and then closing or switching topics;
- **speech adjustments** (e.g., elaboration) for listeners with different and/or less sophisticated language abilities;

- **elimination of redundant information** in recognition of the listener's knowledge about the topic (based on understanding that information shared with a partner does not need to be repeated);
- **ability to take the perspective of the listener** as evidenced by proper use of deictic terms (*here, there, this, that,* and personal pronouns).
- **effective use of instrumental language** (to get a listener to co-operate with or carry out a goal), suggesting understanding of social relationship variables.

Social Functions

By 12 months of age, most infants have learned to use their vocal and gestural abilities to intentionally engage their social environments. Their predisposition for social interaction is a powerful motivator for imitation of, interactions with, and eventually sharing their feelings, experiences, and thoughts with other human beings. So much so that much of the infant's early language is directed toward maintaining contact with, and regulating the behavior of, others. These early social intentions have been described by a number of researchers (e.g., Bates, 1976; Halliday, 1975). Children gradually progress from reflexive, nonintentional communication to expression of intentions in a conventional manner. Development proceeds through three stages that Bates (1976) labeled the **perlocutionary stage,** the **illocutionary stage,** and the **locutionary stage.** Initially, in the perlocutionary stage, the infant's behaviors are undifferentiated and not intentionally communicative. Adults infer the meaning. Then, in the illocutionary stage, the child begins to use conventional gestures and vocalizations to intentionally affect the behavior of others. Finally, in the locutionary stage, the child uses words to convey intentions. Table 1.5 summarizes the development of language use skills from birth to age 3.

There are numerous taxonomies listing the range of communicative intentions that develop prior to age 2 (e.g., Roth & Spekman, 1984). Most include at least the following early communicative intentions:

- **Seeking attention.** Infants use gestures and speech (e.g., "look") to solicit and maintain attention.
- **Requesting.** Infants use gestures and vocalizations to get desired objects, to command the action of others, and to solicit information.
- **Protesting.** Infants use gestures and speech to command cessation of, and to resist, undesired actions and to reject offered objects or events.

TABLE 1.5   Emergence of language use

Age Range	Characteristics
0–1 month	Regards faces momentarily Quiets in response to voice Eyes follow a moving person Cries in reaction to physiological distress
1–4 months	Smiles/coos in response to voice and smile Becomes "excited" when caregiver approaches Quiets upon seeing or hearing caregiver Shows anticipatory response upon seeing bottle Shows anticipation when about to be picked up Shows awareness of strange situations or strange person
4–8 months	Increases activity at the sight of a desired toy or caregiver Initiates mutual interactional dialogues with caregivers Cries and shows other indications of distress when caregiver leaves the room Smiles, head movements, and gestures in interactional dialogues with caregivers Turn-taking in play and other interactional dialogues Deliberate imitation of movements and vocalizations Vocalizes to accompany different attitudes (pleasure/displeasure, satisfaction/anger, eagerness) Responds differentially to interactional partners
8–12 months	Vocalizes deliberately to initiate interpersonal interactions Shouts to attract attention, listens, then shouts again Shakes head for "no" Gives affection to caregivers and other familiar adults Waves "bye-bye" Repeats a behavior if people laugh at it Expresses anger and distress if a toy is taken away Looks at caregiver's face when receiving an object (as if to acknowledge receipt)
12–18 months	Indicates wants by gesturing and vocalizing Hands mechanical toy to an adult to "request" reactivation Shows and offers objects to "request" social interactions Tries to turn the doorknob and looks at adult to "request" outside play Uses gestures, such as pointing, to direct adult attention Hands book to adult to "request" a story Pulls adult to certain locations to "request" attention to an object or event Gestures and vocalizes loudly to "request" desired objects and events
18–24 months	Gestures and vocalizes loudly to "request" proximity of caregiver or familiar adult Uses words to request desired objects and events Names objects spontaneously in the presence of others Vocalizes immediately following the utterances of another

TABLE 1.5   Emergence of language use (*continued*)

Age Range	Characteristics
2–3 years	Talks about objects and events that are not immediately present Initiates spontaneous vocal interactions Adds information to the prior utterances of communication partner Uses an increasing number of utterances that serve interpersonal functions (i.e., calling attention to self or objects and events, regulating the behavior of others, obtaining desired objects and services, participating in social interaction rituals, commenting about objects and events)

- **Commenting.** Infants use gestures and speech to call attention to, describe, and label objects and events.
- **Greeting.** Infants use gestures (typically waving) and speech to participate in such rituals as greeting and taking leave.
- **Answering.** Infants respond to requests for information.

Throughout the infancy and early childhood period, caregivers and other adults treat children as effective communicators, and eventually they do become very skilled conversationalists. By kindergarten (and often before), they are ready for the rhymes, songs, and word games so important to engagement in social and instructional activities. Also, by school age they are ready for what Owens (1988), with tongue in cheek, calls "those special oaths and incantations passed along on the 'underground' from child to child" (p. 321).

SUMMARY

Although socialization alone does not fully account for language acquisition, there seems little question that children's early socialization experiences drive the language learning process. Children learn language by using it to communicate within a social context. Ultimately, our understanding of children's difficulties with language and communication and the impact these difficulties have on children's lives hinge on our understanding of the nature of language and communication and the early socialization process.

This chapter has reviewed the terms and concepts most relevant for understanding the research on the normal development of linguistic skills. This research helps us understand how, why, and when children learn language. The variables that have the most profound influence on language learning and use were also discussed. Finally, the chapter has provided an overview of children's major accomplishments in the areas of language and communication prior to beginning kindergarten.

DISCUSSION QUESTIONS

1. What if you were told that you could only develop speech, language, or communication (not all three), which one would you choose? Why? What do you think life is like for a person who cannot use speech? What is life like without language? What would life be like without communication?

2. Discuss how the basic requirements for speech, language, and communication differ.

3. Discuss what "knowing" a language means. What do you know when you "know" a language?

4. Imagine yourself talking to a group of expectant parents about language development. What would you want to tell them about the four sets of variables that influence language learning and their role in optimizing these?

REFERENCES

Bates, E. (1976). *Language and content.* New York: Academic Press.

Bellugi, U. (1967). *The acquisition of negation.* Unpublished doctoral dissertation, Harvard University.

Benedict, H. (1979). Early lexical development: Comprehension and production. *Journal of Child Language, 6,* 183–200.

Bloom, L. (1970). *Language development: Form and function in emerging grammars.* Cambridge, MA: MIT Press.

Bloom, L. (1973). *One word at a time: The use of single-word utterances before syntax.* The Hague: Mouton.

Bloom, L., Hood, L., & Lightbown, P. (1974). Imitation in language development: If, when and why. *Cognitive Psychology, 6,* 380–420.

Bloom, L., Rocissano, L., & Hood, L. (1976). Adult–child discourse: Developmental interaction between information processing and linguistic interaction. *Cognitive Psychology, 8,* 521–552.

Brown, R. (1973). *A first language: The early stages.* Cambridge, MA: Harvard University Press.

Chomsky, N. (1965). *Aspects of the theory of syntax.* Cambridge, MA: MIT Press.

Corrigan, R. (1978). Language development as related to stage six object permanence development. *Journal of Child Language, 5,* 175–190.

Corina, D., Bellugi, U., & Reilly, J. (1999). Neuropsychological studies of linguistic and affective facial expressions in deaf signers. *Language and Speech, 42,* 307–332.

Dore, J. (1986). The development of conversational competence. In R. Schiefelbusch (Ed.), *Language competence: Assessment and intervention* (pp. 3–59). San Diego: College Hill Press.

Dore, J., Franklin, M., Miller, R., & Ramer, A. (1976). Transitional phenomena in early language acquisition. *Journal of Child Language, 3,* 13–28.

Ervin-Tripp, S. (1970). Discourse agreement: How children answer questions. In J. Hayes (Eds.), *Cognition and the development of language* (296–308). New York: Wiley.

Garvey, C. (1977). *Play.* Cambridge, MA: Harvard University Press.

Halliday, M. A. K. (1975). Learning how to mean. In E. Lenneberg & E. Lenneberg (Eds.), *Foundations of language development* (Vol. 1, pp. 17–32). New York: Academic Press.

Higginbotham, D., & Yoder, D. (1982). Communication within natural conversational interaction: Implications for severely communicatively impaired persons. *Topics in Language Disorders, 2,* 1–19.

Hunt, J. McV. (1965). Intrinsic motivation and its role in psychological development. In D. Levine (Ed.), *Nebraska symposium on motivation* (pp. 283–310). Lincoln: University of Nebraska Press.

Huttenlocher, J., Haight, W., Bryk, A., Seltzer, M., & Lysons, T. (1991). Early vocabulary growth: Relation to language input and gender. *Developmental Psychology, 27,* 236–248.

Hymes, D. (1972). On communicative competence. In J. B.Pride & J. Holmes (Eds.), *Sociolinguistics* (pp. 96–120). Harmondswoth, England: Penguin.

Jusczyk, P. W.(1999). How infants begin to extract words from speech. *Trends in Cognitive Science, 3,* 323–328.

Kagan, J. (1985, May). *Early novelty preferences and later intelligence.* Paper presented at the meeting of the Society for Research in Child Development, Toronto.

Klima, E. S., & Bellugi, U. (1966). Syntactic regularities in the speech of children. In J. Lyons & R. J.Wales (Eds.), *Psycholinguistic papers.* Edinburgh: Edinburgh University Press.

Kuhl, P. K., & Meltzoff, A. N.(1997). Evolution, nativism, and learning in the development of language and speech. In M. Gopnik (Ed.), *The inheritance and innateness of grammars* (pp. 7–44). New York: Oxford University Press.

Lahey, M. (1988). *Language disorders and language development.* New York: Macmillan.

Lenneberg, E. H.(1967). *Biological foundations of language.* New York: Wiley.

Mandel, D. R., Jusczyk, P. W., & Pisoni, D. B.(1994). *Do 4½ month olds know their own names?* Paper presented at the 127th meeting of the Acoustical Society of America, Cambridge, MA.

Mitchell, P. R., & Kent, R. D.(1990). Phonetic variation in multisyllable babbling. *Journal of Child Language, 17,* 247–265.

Mundy, R., Seibert, J., & Hogan, A. (1984). Relationship between sensorimotor and early communication abilities in developmentally delayed children. *Merrill-Palmer Quarterly, 30,* 33–48.

Nelson, K. (1973). Structure and strategy in learning to talk. *Monographs of the Society for Researching Child Development, 38,* 1–2.

Neville, H. J., & Bavelier, D. (1999). Specificity and plasticity in neurocognitive development in humans. In M. Gazzaniga (Ed.), *The new cognitive neurosciences* (pp. 83–98). Cambridge, MA: MIT Press.

Owens, R. E.(1988). *Language development: An introduction* (2nd ed.). Columbus, OH: Merrill.

Piaget, J. (1952). *The origins of intelligence in children* (Margaret Cook, Trans.). New York: International Universities Press.

Pizzuto, E., & Caselli, M. C.(1991). *The acquisition of Italian morphology in a cross-linguistic perspective: Implications for models of language development.* Paper presented at the workshop on Cross-Linguistic and Cross-Populations Contributions to Theory in Language Acquisition, The Hebrew University, Jerusalem, Israel.

Pye, C., Ingram, D., & List, H. (1987). A comparison of initial consonant acquisition in English and Quiche. In K. E. Nelson & A. Van Kleeck (Eds.), *Children's language* (Vol. 6, pp. 175–190). Hillsdale, NJ: Lawrence Erlbaum.

Rice, M. (1984). Cognitive aspects of communicative development. In R. L. Schiefelbusch & J. Pickar (Eds.), *Communicative competence: Acquisition and intervention* (pp. 141–190). Baltimore: University Park Press.

Rogoff, B. (1990). *Apprenticeship in thinking: Cognitive development in social context.* New York: Oxford University Press.

Rogoff, B., & Wertsch, J. V.(1984). *Children's learning in the "zone of proximal development."* San Francisco: Jossey-Bass.

Roth, R., & Spekman, N. (1984). Assessing the pragmatic abilities of children: Part 1: Organizational framework and assessment parameters. *Journal of Speech and Hearing Disorders, 49,* 2–11.

Sameroff, A. J., & Fiese, B. H.(1988). The context of language development. In R. L. Schiefelbusch & L. L. Lloyd (Eds.), *Language perspectives* (pp. 3–20). Austin, TX: PRO-ED.

Schlesinger, I. (1971). Production of utterances and language acquisition. In D. Slobin (Ed.), *The ontogenesis of grammar* (pp. 39–64). New York: Academic Press.

Searle, J. (1969). *Speech acts.* London: Cambridge University Press.

Slobin, D. (1971). *Psycholinguistics.* Glenview, IL: Scott, Foresman.

Snow, C. E. (1984). Parent–child interaction and the development of communicative ability. In R. L.Schiefelbusch & J. Pickar (Eds.), *The acquisition of communicative competence* (pp. 69–108). Baltimore: University Park Press.

Snow, C. E. (1989). The use of imitation. In G. E.Spiedel & K. E. Nelson (Eds.), *The many faces of imitation in language learning* (pp. 103–129). New York: Springer-Verlag.

Vygotsky, L. (1978). *Mind in society: The development of higher psychological processes.* Cambridge, MA: Harvard University Press.

Wang, M., Rose, S., & Maxwell, J. (1973). *The development of language and communication skills tasks.* Pittsburgh, PA: University of Pittsburgh, Learning Research and Development Center.

CHAPTER 2

Language Theory and Practice

Diane Frome Loeb

Accurate diagnosis and intervention with children who display language disorders requires knowledge of the course of typical language development. Oftentimes, specific targets for intervention are determined by the developmental sequence observed in typical language development. In addition, the language interventionist also must be knowledgeable about the current theoretical views that attempt to explain how language is learned or acquired. Most individuals have some ideas about how they think language develops. For example, some believe that children learn language in direct response to their caregivers' input. Others believe that children may be born with certain capacities that mature over time, with input playing a minor role. One's own theoretical beliefs will influence the definition of language impairment, the selection of children seen for language intervention, intervention techniques, creativity and flexibility, and quality control (Brinton & Fujiki, 1989; Friel-Patti, 1994; Johnston, 1983).

A theory is an orderly set of statements that explains and predicts behavior and is subject to scientific verification for continued existence (Berk, 1989). In contrast, a model is a working system based on theoretical assumptions. A theory of language development will need to be specific enough to lead to predictions and empirical tests, yet broad enough to encompass the variation seen in all the world's languages. It will detail the processes or mechanisms that drive language learning across the life span. Further, it should provide insight as to why some children are slow at learning language and why some children are precocious in their language skills. A theory of language development needs to inform us about the role of the input from caregivers and the role of the child, and specify the role of maturation. Lastly, it should consider those areas of development that are likely to influence learning—such as motivation and reinforcement—in a way that meaningfully connects teaching with learning (Kwiatkowski &

Shriberg, 1993). Unfortunately, such a theory does not yet exist. Current theories have been criticized as being too narrow or too broad or lacking in instructional function (Kamhi, 1993). Given these shortcomings, why should language interventionists or other professionals be informed about theory and utilize their theory of choice as the underlying foundation for intervention? Probably the best reason to base one's intervention on theory is because it sets a framework for proposing and testing hypotheses about a child's problem with language learning. It can be unique to the child's difficulties, yet broad enough to account for robustness of language learning in the general population. It allows for a systematic, rather than haphazard, way of approaching a problem. The alternative to using theory to guide one's assessment and intervention is to "do what works" based on previous experience. This alternative is less desirable for one compelling reason—language learning is a robust phenomenon across nonimpaired populations and, as such, should have mechanisms and principles associated with it that are applicable to all children.

The purpose of this chapter is to show how current theories of language development inform both assessment and intervention. In order to understand some of the current ideas and controversies, we need to revisit the history of theoretical accounts. Most of this chapter will be dedicated to theories that are currently influencing practices in early language intervention.

HISTORICAL TRENDS IN THEORY

The writings of Piaget (1954), Skinner (1957), and Chomsky (1957) gave rise to a rich history of events for language theory. Each theorist had his own perspective on how children learn language, especially in regard to the influence of the environment or the resources that the child brought to the task of learning. The extent that language and cognition were involved with one another and whether one system drove the other was a topic for debate. A final difference was that the theories of Piaget and Skinner centered around ideas about learning in general, whereas Chomsky's theory was specific to language acquisition.

Piaget (1954) believed that a child's cognitive abilities guided the acquisition of language. Language was not seen as a separate ability, but as one of several cognitive achievements. Further, language was not considered innate; however, the cognitive ability to develop language was innate (i.e., given at birth). The interaction between cognition and environmental factors gave rise to language. The child was seen as an active learner in understanding the world around him or her. According to Piagetian theory, true language may occur only after the child can represent ideas symbolically. The child needs to attain sensorimotor development Stage 6 of object permanence (around 18 months of age) before symbolic representation may be achieved. Thus, the child needs to be able to understand that objects exist when they are displaced or no longer present before he or she can produce true language. Symbolic play, or the ability to make one object represent another during play, should be used before words are used as symbols. Further, means-end behavior, which occurs around the second year of life, reflects a child's knowledge of ways to achieve goals. Because language is a tool that can be used to accomplish a goal, it is thought that means-end behavior is needed before a child can use language for different communicative intents and word combinations.

Skinner's (1957) operant learning theory, known as behaviorism, maintained that language learning occurred because of environmental influences. Verbal behavior was the gradual accumulation of vocal symbols and sequences of symbols learned through imitation, practice, and selective reinforcement. Skinner proposed that verbal behavior was similar to other types of learned behavior. Whereas other behaviors were subject to control by a variety of events, Skinner defined verbal behavior as "reinforced through the mediation of other persons" (p. 2). He argued that the distinctive characteristic of verbal behavior (as opposed to other behavior) is the nature of the consequences that come to control it. Skinner's operant theory emphasized the role of parents in modeling and reinforcing grammatical sentences. Language was learned through environmental contingencies and was not innate. The child's role was that of a passive participant, a clean slate on which to be drawn.

Chomsky (1957) proposed a theory of grammar in which the child is born with a language acquisition device that develops gradually over time. Referred to as the Standard Theory of Grammar, this theory allowed for elaborate explanations for how grammar was represented abstractly (as displayed by tree diagrams, phrase structure, and transformational rules). Chomsky's first version of his theory is well known for its claims that language is an infinite set of sentences that are rule-governed. That is, the number of sentences that we can produce is endless and we are able to generate sentences that we have never heard before. As speakers of a language, we have an innate knowledge of language, or language competence, that allows us to recognize if sentences are ill-formed. This competence is revealed when we can determine if a sentence is grammatical or ungrammatical regardless of whether it is a novel sentence. Chomsky characterized syntax as an autonomous system and rejected claims that language was a behavioral learning event or a by-product of cognitive achievement."

The language intervention programs used by language interventionists in the fifties, sixties, and seventies reflected these theoretical orientations. Many programs emphasized the importance of the behavioral paradigm and relied on imitation, shaping, and drill-oriented procedures. Other programs focused on cognitive precursors and correlates. Still others focused on training sentence structures. Much of the early intervention was trainer-oriented (Fey, 1986) in that the clinician controlled what children would learn, how they would learn it, and under which conditions mastery would be shown.

By the 1970s, interest in cognitive abilities and their relation with language dominated the field. Several researchers in the seventies supported the view that words are simply mapped onto sensorimotor concepts. This maxim of the cognitive view of language learning states simply that children talk when they have something to talk about, and they talk about what they understand. Language is an expression of developing conceptual knowledge. Cromer (1974) called this the *cognitive hypothesis;* Schlesinger (1977) referred to it as *cognitive determinism*. Further empirical data in the 1980s have to some extent supported the claim of a relationship between some cognitive and language skills. For instance, early symbolic play and first word usage have been found to be correlated. Likewise, higher means-end behavior and symbolic play are correlated with emerging word combinations. Finally, object permanence seems related to types of words used that refer to the disappearance or absence of objects, *allgone, find,* and *more* (Gopnik & Meltzoff, 1987). One of the major problems with interpreting these studies is that a finding of a significant correlation indicates that the variables of interest are related in some fashion. It does not measure cause, or indicate whether one is a precursor and one is not. One can only infer that these abilities are related or occur together in time. This is the homologous view of the language/cognition debate, in which cognition and language are seen as parallel paths versus one path occurring before the other (Bates, Benigni, Bretherton, Camaioni, & Volterra, 1977; Brown, 1973).

Bandura's theory of social learning was also proposed during this period. His theory emphasized the importance of social interaction to language learning (Bandura, 1966; Bandura & Harris, 1966). The child brought to the task of language learning the internal cognitive variables that interacted with the environment. The extent of learning was related to four interrelated variables: attention, retention, motor reproduction, and motivation. A process called "abstract modeling" was a key component to learning in this theory. Abstract modeling is when the child observes various situations and the verbalizations that accompany the situations. Although imitation may be helpful, it is not required. The child extracts regularities from these situations and generates a rule-based system as a result of these observations. Intervention programs using Bandura's theoretical framework of modeling language targets have been successful in facilitating change in language abilities (Leonard, 1975).

Language intervention in the 1970s continued to utilize behavioral theory methods; however, other theories that emphasized the child as an active learner of language became increasingly popular. Researchers heightened our awareness of the important contributions of pragmatics and social interaction to the process of language learning and these tenets were adopted to make language intervention more naturalistic and functionally-oriented (Bates, 1976; Bruner, 1983; Dore, 1979). Language intervention programs frequently adopted Bloom & Lahey's (1978) psycholinguistic model of form, content, and use. Thus, emphasis was given to semantic and pragmatic aspects of language, as well as syntax, phonology, and morphology.

During the 1980s, theory building efforts escalated in multiple areas. Learnability issues, or models that explicitly describe how the child comes to learn language in a brief period of time, were proposed (Pinker, 1984, 1989; Wexler & Culicover, 1980). Linguistic theory was revitalized with the introduction of Chomsky's (1981) book, *Lectures on Government and Binding,* and Hyams' work in parameter theory (Hyams, 1986). Computer simulation of human language learning was detailed and implemented (MacWhinney, 1987; Rumelhardt & McClelland, 1986). Cognitive development through event learning influenced clinicians to use more scripted events in their intervention (Nelson, 1986). Theorists in the area of social interaction proposed new ideas that reshaped previous views (Bates & MacWhinney, 1988; Nelson, 1987). Behavioral theory continued to be used but in combination with more natural consequences, such as those seen in Milieu Teaching and Enhanced Milieu Teaching (Kaiser, Yoder, & Keetz, 1992; Warren & Kaiser, 1986). Lastly, a learning theory that stresses the importance of social interaction, Vygotskian theory, has been applied by special educators and language interventionists. In the nineties, cognitive science has offered a new version of how working memory and language are related (Gathercole & Baddeley, 1993). The Principles and Parameter Theory has been modified by the addition of the Minimalist Program (Chomsky, 1995).

Language intervention in the eighties through the early twenty-first century has been dominated by social interaction approaches to language learning. Behavioral theory utilized within appropriate pragmatic contexts continues to be used within Milieu Teaching and Enhanced Milieu Teaching (Hemmeter & Kaiser, 1994; Kaiser & Hester, 1994). In addition, there have been a few efforts toward incorporating linguistic theory with assessment and intervention (Connell, 1990; Loeb & Armstrong, 2001; Loeb & Mikesic, 1992; Rice, Wexler, & Cleave, 1995; Wilson, 1994; Wilson & Pascoe, 1997). The remainder of this chapter will focus on two theoretical orientations that continue to influence research and clinical practice: social interactionist theory and linguistic theory.

CURRENT TRENDS IN THEORY

Social-Interactionist Theoretical Approaches

According to the social interactionist theory, several factors are interrelated in the acquisition of language. These factors are social, linguistic, maturational, and cognitive in nature. All of these factors interact with and modify one another. This view maintains that language is learned primarily through social interactions. Language is taught by parents and caregivers. It is learned through child-oriented talk such as parentese, recasts, and expansions. The child is an active participant in learning and, to some extent, guides the learning if caregivers are receptive to his or her cues.

A major criticism aimed at proponents of social interactionist theory is that it is difficult to determine which features of interaction are necessary for language acquisition. There is evidence that some elements of parentese are related to language development (Cross, 1978). When children are between 18 and 24 months of age and their caregivers provide expansions of their utterances (i.e., repeat part or all of the utterance and add information to it), these children are more linguistically advanced and have greater sentence lengths compared to other children. However, it is unclear if this type of language facilitation is a necessary part of language learning. The lack of parentese in other languages raises the question of whether specially tailored interaction is required for language acquisition (Bernstein-Ratner & Pye, 1984; Schieffelin, 1985). Another important criticism is that the theory lacks necessary and sufficient specificity in describing the internal process by which language is acquired.

Several theories and models of language learning assume that social interaction drives the process of language learning. Four viewpoints that accept this assumption of the importance of social interaction will be discussed: the Interactive Model (Tannock & Girolametto, 1992); Functional Theory (Bates & MacWhinney, 1982); the Rare Event Cognitive Comparison Theory (Nelson, 1987, 1989); and Vygotskian theory (Vygotsky, 1978).

Interactive Model

The interactive model is built on the premise that the child's active involvement in social interactions with peers and caregivers is crucial for language development. Not only does the child have to be an active participant in communication exchanges, but these interactions need to be reciprocal in nature and frequently occurring. Interactions that occur as a result of the child's behavior or interests may be especially valuable to language learning. Importantly, in order to effectively facilitate language learning, caregivers need to have a style of interacting that is a good match with the child's abilities and that is responsive to the child's interests. Thus, two key factors of this model are: (1) child engagement (or involvement) in the activity, and (2) caregiver responsiveness to the child's interaction participation.

There are three aspects of the interactive model that differ from other language intervention approaches. First, learning is child-oriented. As such, no communication targets are selected for teaching. This means that the child is not required to produce certain target forms or functions. Second, there is no use of operant training by the caregivers. For example, there is no shaping or differential reinforcement relied on. Third, the caregiver is encouraged to use the techniques at all times of the day, not only at a specified period each day or in a specified setting.

APPLICATION TO LANGUAGE IMPAIRMENT. Tannock & Girolametto (1992) suggest that the ability of children with language impairment to assimilate and organize information may be a trouble source. As a result, social interactions with these children may require special adjustments. They have identified three intervention techniques based on the assumptions of the interactive model and evaluated parents' use of these techniques and the child's progress within a parent–child intervention program. These intervention techniques included child-oriented techniques, interaction-promoting techniques, and language-modeling techniques.

- Child-Oriented Techniques: The purpose of child-oriented techniques is to provide children with opportunities for joint attention largely by responding to them at their level and following their lead in play. The children guide the interaction, and the caregiver needs to be sensitive and responsive to their cues and signals. Child-oriented techniques are believed to make the input to children more salient. In order to be child-oriented, caregivers need to respond to what the children are interested in and participate in a way that puts them at the same level as the children (i.e., physical level, play level, and interest level).
- Interaction-Promoting Techniques: The goal of interaction-promoting techniques is to get children actively engaged in the interaction, not only as responders, but as initiators. The inclusion of both responding and initiating leads to enhancing the children's ability to take turns within an interaction. The caregivers learn to take one turn at a time, use waiting techniques to allow time for the children to respond, signal for turns, and decrease their directiveness. By decreasing directives (i.e., telling someone what to do) caregivers reduce the amount of responses, thus evening out the turn-taking events of initiating and responding.
- Language-Modeling Techniques: The purpose of language-modeling techniques is to help organize the linguistic input in a way that facilitates the children's induction of form, content, and use.

Caregivers are encouraged to talk about what the children are doing (description) and talk about what they are doing (self-talk) using short, simple sentences, expanding on the children's previous sentence, and repeating sentences in a meaningful context. The timing of the caregiver input is important in that it should occur after the children's production or at the time of joint attention.

Tannock & Girolametto (1992) found that the parent-training language intervention program was effective in modifying the caregiver styles that led to more positive and responsive interactions with children. Contrary to clinical and theoretical beliefs, there was little evidence that increasing parental responsiveness enhanced children's learning of *new* language skills. However, this type of program may be most effective in facilitating a child's *existing* language behaviors. However, in further studies, Girolemetto, Verbey, & Tannock (1994) learned that the previously described parent-implemented language intervention was successful in helping children acquire the beginning steps in joint engagement (i.e., joint attention and joint action). More recent studies indicate that using language intervention techniques associated with the interactive model have led to successful facilitation of phonological, lexical, and early grammatical development in toddlers with expressive language delays (Girolametto, Pearce, & Weitzman, 1996, 1997).

Functional Theory

Functional theory seeks to explain the child's use of language (or functions) as well as the forms of a given language. The strongest version of the functional theory says that grammatical forms are determined and maintained by communicative functions and processing constraints (Bates & MacWhinney, 1988). According to functional theory, children do not start with an adult grammar that unfolds over time. Rather, their major task is to induce the relationship between form, content, and use. This results in the acquisition of putting together the form of a word with its meaning and use (i.e., form-function mappings). Form refers to surface word order patterns and morphological markings, whereas function refers to underlying meanings or meaningful relations. Functionalists believe that grammatical surface forms arise from semantic and pragmatic functions and that children learn language through communicative interactions. In addition, the existing state of their knowledge influences the course of development. It is not necessary that language be taught formally, because learning experiences occur in the natural contexts of interaction.

The competition model is a detailed model of the acquisition component of functional theory (MacWhinney, 1987). It has a number of assumptions that are noteworthy. First, it adopts the idea of gradualism. Gradualism means that children work through correct and incorrect hypotheses about language over time and do not begin with an adultlike grammar. Second, this model of language learning is lexically-driven. That is, learning takes place at the level of the lexicon or word. It works from the bottom upward and is influenced by the "cues" in a child's given language. Cues are those events that provide evidence to children about their native language. For example, word order is a strong and reliable cue in English, whereas in Italian it is less predictable. Cue extraction, or deriving the cues from one's native language, is an active undertaking for children. Cues that are highly available (i.e., there when needed) and highly reliable (i.e., readily lead to a correct interpretation) will emerge from occasional exposure. If cues are not highly available or reliable, the child will work to increase his or her exposure to these cues.

As with functional theory, mapping occurs between the functional and the formal levels of language. However, this does not mean that there is a one-to-one relationship between form and function. Many functions can map with many forms. In the sentence "He is a great dad," at the functional level *he* is the agent or topic, at the formal level it has subject case marking and is marked for verb agreement. Form and function mapping is accomplished through cue validity. Cue validity is how available and reliable a cue is in a language. For example, in English, the cue of preverbal positioning in English for the assignment of the noun phrase as the subject has high cue validity. It is almost always available and almost always reliable. Cue validity of verb agreement is low in English, because it is only available when there is competition between two nouns and those nouns differ in number. Importantly, the major determinant of the order of acquisition and the strength of a cue is related to cue validity. Thus, the characteristics of a given language determine if certain structures are acquired early or late in that language.

The competition model utilizes the neural network model used in the information-processing accounts of learning. Thus, as lexical items are encountered in the input, the neuronal associations of these items are strengthened. There are constraints to learning, particularly when various semantic and pragmatic cues compete with one another. This competition is an occurrence of one event set against another. The "Principle of Competition" is that a given language will not allow a situation in which two different forms express exactly the same meanings (e.g., "goed" vs. "went"). This principle must be intact for children to learn language. A competition is resolved by building up strengths of association in one lexical item versus another. As the activation of one item increases, its competitor decreases. Again, the strength of a cue is determined by the characteristics of the child's native language.

APPLICATION TO LANGUAGE IMPAIRMENT. MacWhinney (1989) suggests a number of problems that could occur in normal processing and learning that might result in impairment. These problems are related to "cue cost," that is, problems with processing information in the speech signal, memory, attention, speed or accuracy of lexical access, and insufficient feedback or problems processing feedback. Mild problems in any of these areas would slow the rate of learning. Severe problems are hypothesized to result in major disruptions in language learning. According to functional theory, language is teachable if the teacher understands the principles of competition and the need to reinforce structures and functions. Competition will change depending on the input the child hears. The child who receives input for one competing form will decrease the activation for the other competing form.

Another important aspect of the language learning environment is that language learning should take place in meaningful contexts in order to enhance shared meaning and referential forms. Thus, frequent models should be presented in meaningful contexts. Children will learn language through positive instances. Recasts and expansions can be used to facilitate correct learning should the child produce an error. Recasts are types of utterances in which the meaning of a child's utterance is maintained, but the new adult utterance has a different linguistic structure, for example, if a child says "Mommy go bye bye," and the adult responds by saying, "Yes, mommy will go bye bye." Finally, one can increase the child's attention to aspects of the sentence by increasing saliency. This increased saliency or heightening of certain aspects of the speech signal assists the understanding of form relationships.

Rare Event Cognitive Comparison Theory

Nelson (1987) proposes that children are active language learners who possess a powerful processing mechanism responsible for the development of language. The model of this theory claims that children have a rare event learning mechanism (hereafter RELM). This rare event mechanism is available to children at around Brown's Stage II or III of language development, and the mechanism gains strength as children's language, cognitive skills, and age advance through the first four years of life. The learning mechanism is composed of the following components: selective attention, selective comparison, selective storage and retrieval, and hypothesis monitoring abilities. However, it is only on rare occasions that children go through the process of selectively attending and formulating new structural hypotheses about language. The rare event processing mechanism itself is driven by cognitive forces, rather than being a specific language learning device. Further, children's interactions (self and other-directed) and their ability to identify mismatches in the input will direct learning.

Children need to interact with proficient language users with whom there is an emotional, social, motivational, and communicative commitment. They develop "hot spots" or focal areas of attention that indicate where they are working at a particular point in development. Such hot spots may arise because of some especially salient event or they may be a result of the child's current language system. Regardless, hot spots are areas undergoing intensive structural analysis. Selective attention, storage and retrieval, comparison, and hypothesis testing are dedicated to areas indicated as hot spots.

As an example, a child may learn modal auxiliaries (e.g., *will*) by selectively attending to a small sampling of input during a conversational exchange. Imagine that the input sentence ("I will sing") is a mismatch with one already stored in the child's long-term memory (e.g., "I sing"). The child then compares the new input sentence to sentences that have been tagged in long-term memory and comes up with a hypothesis about the structure that is being learned. The mismatches and the child's analysis combined make the "rare event." It is this latter type of abstraction (i.e., the process of noting a discrepancy, selectively retrieving and storing information, comparing and then hypothesizing new structures) that is crucial and driven by general cognitive abstraction processes. The child's hypothesis is then monitored with future input. The child keeps this newly learned language structure or rule if it is supported by the input. This type of cycle continues until the child has figured out his or her language system. Because hot spots differ from child to child, they nicely capture the range of individual differences observed in the process of language learning. In fact, different children receiving similar input can be working on different hot spots.

The benefit that children receive from interactions cannot be overstated. It is suggested that they may benefit optimally from certain types of conversational exchange, particularly if they are producing their highest level of complexity and the conversational partner is producing a simple recast at a slightly higher level of complexity. Research has found beneficial effects for the use of recasts in children with typical development. Specifically, Baker & Nelson (1984) found that, between 22 and 27 months, syntactic growth is greater in a group of children whose mothers used a high percentage of topic continuations and simple recasts (i.e., a change in only one sentence element, such as subject or verb).

APPLICATION TO LANGUAGE IMPAIRMENT. Much of the application of the RELM has been to evaluate the effects of recasts on language change in children with typical development (Baker & Nelson, 1984; Nelson, 1977). RELM assumes that children's eventual language ability will be a reflection of their interaction opportunities, differing levels of capability of the processing mechanism, and their motivation and emotional influence on the communicative exchange. Oftentimes, language assessment will involve collecting an audio- or videotape sample of caregiver–child or sibling–child interaction. According to the RELM one cannot simply evaluate and tally the child's and the partner's utterances separately. Instead, the interaction between partners needs to be evaluated in context with an understanding of how one's utterance is influencing another. Another factor that may influence the course of language development is the child's past experiences or abilities in abstracting new language structures. Because the system strengthens and guides itself, the child who has been successful at language learning will continue to be successful. The child who has not been successful at this process will experience problems in the future. Early intervention helps to deter this course of development.

According to Nelson, children with language impairments should benefit from recasts if their processing systems are similar to those or children developing language normally. Critically, the child's components of the rare event processing mechanism (i.e., selective attention, storage and retrieval, comparison, abstraction, and monitoring) need to be intact. An intervention assumption is that the frequency with which a child hears a language target is not as important as the way in which it is presented. That is, it would be more beneficial for the child to hear particular structures in recasts versus a more structured, drill-type activity. However, once a child has hypothesized a new structure, frequent exposures to the structure may be helpful to confirm his or her hypothesis.

Regarding intervention targets, it may not be apparent what a child's current hot spot is. Thus, activities that follow the child's lead may be most effective. This leads to the question of "Can hot spots be created?" The experimental data from children with language impairment provides an affirmative answer to this question. Camarata and Nelson (1992) and Camarata, Nelson, & Camarata (1994) selected linguistic targets to use in recasts for four children with specific language impairments. They randomly assigned the children language targets (areas of language to learn) taking into account their stage of language development. They found that the children learned the targeted structures with fewer presentations compared to a condition in which they were asked to imitate structures. However, they also found that the success of the recast intervention depended on the linguistic structure itself. That is, some structures were learned more readily than others. These studies provide evidence that the conversational-recast approach is an efficacious way to provide language intervention. However, it is not clear what type of recasts assist the child's developing language. Further studies of the effects of recasts for children with specific language impairment (SLI) have indicated that these children and typically developing children did not benefit from fronted auxiliary verb recasts to facilitate the production of new forms such as the auxiliary *be* or the modal *will* (Fey & Loeb, 2002). In addition, it may be that children with SLI may need more recasts than children with typical language development to benefit from them (Fey, Krulik, Loeb, & Proctor-Williams, 1999).

Finally, children will not fully benefit from conversation if they are not active participants. According to Nelson, when children elicit information it may be an especially good indicator of the areas they are working on. However, some children who are less willing to participate, or who are frequently off topic during conversation, may need specific assistance in becoming more involved with conversational partners prior to the onset of an intervention program designed to emphasize recasts of their utterances.

Vygotskian Theory

Vygotskian Theory is based on the work of a Russian psychologist who sought to explain the process of learning within the context of social interaction. Vygotsky (1978) proposed that psychological functioning, including language, is learned through social interactions with a more capable member of society. Children are seen as active participants in learning assisted by an adult or more competent peer. There are two planes on which development occurs: (1) the social plane (interpsychological category), and (2) the psychological plane (intrapsychological category). The social plane occurs between people and is termed "other-regulated." In contrast, the psychological plane occurs within oneself and is referred to as "self-regulated." The task of learning involves moving from "other-regulated" to "self-regulated" problem solving.

An important aspect of Vygotskian theory is the notion of the Zone of Proximal Development (ZPD). The ZPD is the "distance between the actual developmental level determined by independent problem solving and the level of potential development as determined through problem solving under adult guidance or in collaboration with more capable peer" (Vygotsky, 1978, p. 86). There are four stages of the ZPD (Table 2.1). The child's developmental task is to move from "other" to "self-regulated" behavior. In Stage I, the child's performance is assisted by more capable others. Van Kleeck & Richardson (1993) describe the process of learning in Stage I as involving "scaffolding" (Bruner, 1983) whereby adults assist the child with cues in event scripts (i.e., familiar routines) (Nelson, 1986). The child's communication helps to determine the level of the cues given by the adult. In Stage II, performance is assisted by the child. Self-directed speech is an important occurrence at this stage, because the child directs learning with speech directed toward oneself. Although assistance is not given at this stage, children have not fully learned the ability or task. Stage III is characterized by performance that has become automatic on the part of the child. At this stage no "self" or "other" regulation is needed or occurs. If the child encounters assistance, it is disruptive. At the final stage, Stage IV, performance becomes deautomatized and the child may once again go through earlier stages. The process is recursive in that it can occur over and over again. The child may return to self-regulating and, perhaps, other-regulation as needed. These stages of learning occur for adults as well as children in each new thing learned (Tharp & Gallimore, 1988). A good way to understand these stages is to apply them to your own learning situations. Think back to the first time you had to prepare a lesson plan or transcribe a tape. At first, you needed the assistance of a more capable person and progressed to being able to do it by yourself. Finally, the procedure became automatic for you. However, when a new problem arose in planning or transcription that was not solvable through old, established methods, you may have had to seek the help of a more capable peer once again or do outside reading on your own.

TABLE 2.1   Four Stages of the Zone of Proximal Development

Stage I	Capable other provides assistance to child using scaffolding within routines. During this stage motivation to participate may be facilitated by the more capable other (i.e., entices the child to participate). For example, a parent provides models of vocabulary during a routine such as dinnertime. The caregiver arranges the environment and monitors the child's responses to the input.
Stage II	Child assists self. Self-directed speech. For example, the child initiates own production of vocabulary words associated with dinnertime. Child internally monitors own language.
Stage III	Child automatized performance. No self- or other-regulation. For example, the child easily uses vocabulary associated with dinnertime without needing to monitor self or have assistance from others.
Stage IV	Child de-automatizes performance. This is when he or she may go back through earlier stages if needed. For example, the child attempts to use dinnertime vocabulary during pretend play and uses mother's phrasing or tone of voice to support his or her own context for the vocabulary. De-automatization may also occur when outside stress factors or new conditions occur, for example, when a child's milk is put in a different cup.

RECURSIVE

APPLICATION TO LANGUAGE IMPAIRMENT.   Within the last few years, Vygostkian theory has become increasingly prominent in its application to children with language impairment (Bain & Olswang, 1995; Olswang & Bain; 1991; Olswang, Bain, & Johnson, 1992; van Kleeck & Richardson, 1993). Prior to that, it had been applied to individuals with mental retardation (Feuerstein, 1979) and in reading and learning disabilities (Braun, Rennie, & Gordon, 1987). Assumptions associated with this approach are that children can learn from a more competent peer or adult, that learning takes place within a social context, and that children move gradually toward increasing ability depending on their zone of proximal development.

Integral to this theory's application to language impairment is the concept of "dynamic assessment." Dynamic assessment involves determining where a child is functioning with support from others such as cues, models, or prompts. A child's dynamic performance in a given task is compared to his or her static performance, which is the child's performance independent of assistance. The distance between these two, the static and the dynamic assessment, is the child's zone of proximal development for a given area (Olswang & Bain, 1991; Olswang, Bain, & Johnson, 1992).

Olswang & Bain argue that dynamic assessment may be used to determine whether a child may benefit from language intervention. They describe three possible child profiles in which the ZPD differs. For the first child, there is no difference between the actual and potential performance, or no ZPD. For the second child, the difference is quite large, with the child responding greatly to assistance. The third child would be the one who makes some minimal gains with assistance. Olswang & Bain suggest that the third child would be the best candidate for language intervention. The first child may not be ready to learn and the second child may be in the process of accomplishing the task independently. Data from two small groups of children, one learning single words (Olswang & Bain, 1991) and one learning two-term semantic relations (Olswang, Bain, & Johnson, 1992) support these predictions. In another study, Bain & Olswang (1995) found dynamic assessment to be a valuable tool for determining the readiness of children with specific expressive language impairment at the early word combination stage. They found that the children who were ready for immediate change responded to less cuing from adults (i.e., cues such as imitation, indirect models, sentence completion, etc.). In contrast, the children who were not as ready for change needed more supportive cuing. Dynamic assessment may also be a helpful tool for reducing cultural bias in standardized testing. Pena, Iglesias, and Lidz (2001) found that dynamic assessment procedures were better than static testing procedures for determining if a language difference or a language disorder is present in preschoolers from diverse cultural backgrounds.

With respect to language intervention, language interventionists could facilitate language within familiar events that involve social interaction appropriate to a child's ZPD until a given ability is learned. Early language interventionists must be aware when assistance is at too high or too low a level for a given skill and adjust their assistance as needed. Otherwise, the children's progress may be hindered. Thus, one must be knowledgeable about the area targeted for intervention in order to track a child's developmental progress.

Finally, van Kleeck and Richardson (1993) suggest that, when a language interventionist uses the Vygotskian framework, errors that the child produces should be viewed differently than the traditional view of errors (i.e., something to be "corrected"). Errors are no longer seen as things that need fixing in the child's repertoire, but are part of the process of learning. These errors give clues as to where the child is functioning on the developmental path. As such, errors are responded to differently depending on the child's stage of ZPD.

Linguistic Theory

Since its introduction in 1957, Chomsky's theory of language acquisition has undergone several major revisions. Earlier versions of linguistic theory were too powerful in that they could generate unrealistic patterns of language. In the 1980s and 1990s the Government and Binding Theory and then the Principles and Parameters Theory (PPT) were explanations for grammatical representation. A new addition to the PPT is the Minimalist Program (Chomsky, 1995). The minimalist program attempts to reduce to a minimum the number of necessary steps to generate a grammar. The PPT Minimalist Program focuses on how language is constrained to assure that it is learnable. The grammar is constrained through innately given principles and through limited evidence from the environment.

According to the PPT Minimalist Program, all children at birth possess an innate Universal Grammar (UG). The UG is genetically determined, and is separate from general cognitive processes and pragmatic competence. That is, it is modular in nature. The UG consists of a set of principles that apply across languages as well as parameters that are "set" on the basis of language from the child's environment. The UG has four levels of representation: the d-structure, s-structure, phonetic form (PF), and the logical form (LF). The d-structure consists of categorical rules and the lexicon. Categorical rules are sentence formulation rules that generate abstract syntactic structures. The lexicon assigns abstract syntactic and morphophonological details to each lexical items. The lexicon is a dictionary in the mind that encodes each word's grammatical features. Each word has semantic, grammatical and phonetic features. There are two sets of grammatical categories in the lexicon: the lexical categories and the functional categories. The lexical categories consist of noun, verb, prepositions, and adjectives.

The functional categories consist of determiners, inflectional morphemes, and complementizers. The next level of representation is the s-structure, which is derived from the d-structure. The next two levels are phonetic form and logical form. The phonetic form is an abstract characterization of sound, including phonological rules. The logical form is an abstract characterization of interpretation. Although meaning is generated at the d- and s-structure levels, other rules are necessary to avoid ambiguity of interpretation. The language faculty consists of a cognitive system and a performance system. The cognitive system stores information and interacts with the phonetic and logical form levels. The performance system accesses stored information and uses this information for perception and production.

Both principles and parameters influence language acquisition. Principles, in general, constrain or limit representation. Such constraints are needed because without them children would utter incorrect sentences and could not learn language as quickly as they do on the basis of limited positive evidence. Although the principles are innate, they are believed to develop or mature over time. In contrast to principles, parameters are those components of grammar that can be changed or "set" to one of two values. The initial or "unmarked" setting is what every child is born with. However, if the child's native language is inconsistent with this setting of the parameter, the parameter can change to the "marked" setting. Typically, a parameter is reset once the child realizes certain "triggering" data. Triggering data are specific input that children can analyze from the language they hear in their native language that will cause a change in their grammar. Triggering data are parameter specific. That is, the type of linguistic input that will change a parameter setting will depend on the characteristics of the parameter itself.

A change in the setting of a parameter can result in changes throughout the entire grammar. After all the parameters of a language have been set, the child will be producing language comparable to competent adult speakers. Thus, the principles of UG are innate, yet some structural variations across languages are possible through parameter setting. At this point, it is unclear how many or what parameters might exist. However, three parameters have been extensively written about and applied to language impairment. One parameter, the null subject parameter, accounts for the variations seen across languages with the optional use of subjects in sentences (Hyams,1989). For example, some languages, such as Spanish, allow subjects to be omitted. In contrast, English does not allow optional subjects. English requires that the subject be present. English-speaking children have been noted to omit subjects in early language development. These subjectless sentences are observed in sentences such as "ride bike," "throw ball," and so on. In order to trigger a resetting of the null subject parameter, the child will need to receive input data consistent with the correct setting.

Wexler (1994a) has proposed two other parameters that are responsible for setting the word order of a language: the Specifier-Head parameter and the Complement-Head parameter. In English, specifiers or subjects occur before the head, whereas complements occur after the head of a phrase. For instance, in the phrase "Stan watched the football game," *watched* is the head of the Verb Phrase; it is preceded by *Stan,* the specifier, and *football game* is the object or complement. Children learning English will need to set these parameters to complement final and specifier first in order to use and understand English word order. Wilson & Fox (1994) suggest that sentences contrasting subjects of sentences, direct objects of sentences, and reversible sentences may reset these parameters.

Several criticisms have been aimed at the linguistic approach to language learning. Issues of debate rest largely on the extent to which children are active participants, how much of the grammar is innate, and the role of the environment. For instance, other theories do not accept the idea that children are endowed with innate grammatical categories. Further, the emphasis on grammar and the lack of attention to areas related to the influence of pragmatic variables on language acquisition have often been criticized. Finally, the modular process of grammar is unacceptable for those who firmly believe that cognitive processes drive the process of language learning.

APPLICATION TO LANGUAGE IMPAIRMENT.   The PPT Minimalist Program is applicable to language impairment in many ways. One avenue that has been explored involves looking for differences in the underlying structural representations between children with normal language and those with language impairment. Preliminary results indicate that the tremendous morphological and syntactic problems exhibited by children with specific language impairment (SLI) may be explained by evaluating functional categories in the underlying grammar (Leonard, 1995; Rice & Oetting, 1993). Rice et al. (1995) provide data that support the idea that children with SLI are like their typical peers with the exception that they extend the amount of time that they do not mark verbs for finiteness. In English, verbs appear in either finite or nonfinite contexts. Finite forms are marked for tense and agreement and appear in main clauses. Finiteness also can be marked by *be* and *do* forms. For example, a child who says "I walked fast" is marking finiteness with the *-ed* on the verb *walk*. However, in the sentence "I wanted to go there," the verb *wanted* is marked for finiteness, but the verb *go* is in a nonfinite context and, as such, does not receive morphological marking. Wexler (1994b) claims that English-speaking children with typical language development go through a period of time when they treat verbs as nonfinite and optionally mark finiteness. That is, they will omit *-ed,* third person singular *-s,* and copula and auxiliary forms. Rice and her colleagues have found this period of optionally marking finiteness to be extended in children with SLI. They refer to this phenomenon as the period of the extended optional infinitive. Importantly, this finding suggests that many morphological and syntactic problems are related to one underlying problem: not marking verbs for finiteness. Implications for assessment are clear. Children with language impairment should receive a thorough evaluation of their finite verb morphology (Goffman & Leonard, 2000). If finite verb morphology is problematic, intervention strategies might be introduced that contrast finite and nonfinite verbs (Leonard, 1998).

Application of the PPT Minimalist Program to language impairment also results in a different way of thinking about the language learning problem. Connell (1990) suggests that the label of "language disorder" would not be a "delay" or a "simpler" language if a Principles and Parameters perspective were to be adopted by language interventionists. Instead, children with language impairment would be viewed as having the "wrong" or an "intermediate" grammar that is not the same as the adult language. This reconceptualization of the language learning problem would also have ramifications for intervention. The goal of language intervention would be to stimulate the child to choose the "right," or "input," language. In inclusive service delivery, the "right" or "input" language could be presented through specific language models provided by the teacher or language interventionist that would be believed to reset a given parameter. The following section provides specific types of language models that might serve as "triggers" to switch a parameter. These language models with specific grammatical contrasts could be presented during play time, reading in a large group, or during individualized language art instruction.

As previously mentioned, many children with language impairment display a marked difficulty in learning morphology and syntax. Wilson and Fox (1994) suggest "that treatment for problems with the grammar module should be directed specifically to this area and not addressed indirectly through pragmatics" (p. 1). Areas of intervention that focus on parameters are especially appealing because changes within one aspect of a parameter may alter other parts of a child's grammar. Thus, if a child with language impairment were experiencing difficulty due to some delay or impairment of the parameter process, then subsequent facilitation of a given parameter may result in widespread changes in the grammar. Under this framework a child cannot be taught a missing structure that he or she is not ready to learn if the parameter has not been reset to the right setting. Instead, the clinician would direct the learner's attention to "trigger" information that would reset a parameter, thereby making possible a change in the grammar. To do so, precise input information would be needed in order for the child to reset the parameter. Also, the clinician would need to highlight and emphasize those aspects of the input that contain trigger material and de-emphasize those that do not. Following parameter setting, the language interventionist should provide information that gives the child many examples of the form and meaning to be learned.

It is not yet apparent whether children with language impairment have difficulties with parameter setting. Loeb and Leonard (1988) found that children with SLI did not display a "delay" in resetting the null subject parameter. The profiles of these children were not consistent with a child's grammar at an unmarked setting. However, Connell's (1990) training study with children with language impairment that was aimed at resetting the null subject parameter led to a number of the predicted positive changes in these children's language. His triggering data included making the subject of the sentence more salient. This was accomplished through left-dislocated topics. For example, in pointing to a picture that had two boys, one of whom was petting a deer, the clinician would point to the boy doing the petting and say, "Him, he is petting the fawn." Connell suggests that the increased saliency of the subject resulted in the children's increased correct use of pronoun case marking, copula, auxiliary, third person singular -s, and question inversion.

Another attempt to trigger changes in the null subject parameter contrasted verb inflections in the language models provided to children with language impairment (Loeb & Mikesic, 1992). The child who received the input that contrasted verbs with bare stems (*walk*) with verbs without bare stems (*walking*) made the most progress in pronoun subject case marking and verb morphology related to the null subject parameter.

Wilson (1994) and Wilson & Fox (1994) propose yet another intervention program aimed at resetting a parameter. Their approach provides contrasts as triggers for the child's Complement-Head parameter and the Specifier-Head parameter. For instance, the child needs to hear sentence contrasting objects to make the complement final position in English salient ("The girl ate the cookie" vs. "The girl ate the cake"). Presentations of contrasting subjects focuses the child's attention on the Subject-Verb order of English needed for the Specifier-Head parameter ("The boy chased the cat" vs. "The girl chased the cat"). Finally, reversible sentences are suggested as helpful for both parameters ("The girl kissed the boy" vs. "The boy kissed the girl"). Importantly, they suggest that such an intervention program should occur before the child begins to combine words. Unlike current procedures, which often wait until the child is much older, this approach focuses on grammar early in development. Loeb and Armstrong (2001) utilized a modified version of Wilson and Fox's suggestions for resetting the SVO parameter during play with children displaying expressive language delays and with a history of expressive language delays and were successful in increasing SVO structures and mean length of utterance. Further examination of this parameter and other parameters in children with language impairment should shed some light on the nature of the child's problem as well as chart the course for intervention.

SUMMARY

All of the theories and models discussed in this chapter are continually undergoing change as new ideas and new data influence their direction. As the reader may have surmised, there are many areas of similarities and important differences between the theories presented (Table 2.2). While areas of difference are often the focus of heated debate, researchers and theoreticians agree that the end goal is an explanation of language development. The influence of these theories on how we understand the underlying difficulties and how we work with children exhibiting language problems cannot be overstated. Without such theories we have to resort to treating symptoms without understanding the underlying system. Although there is not a single theory at this time that can explain fully the development of language, existing theories allow language interventionists to make hypotheses about expected change following language facilitation or triggering.

In a direct service delivery model, language interventionists apply the assumptions associated with their theory of language acquisition (i.e., behavioralism, linguistic theory, social interactive model, etc.) to the children with whom they work. When language interventionists work with a parent, a child-care provider, or a teacher as a consultant or team member, theory continues to be important. The team approach requires that those working together share a common theory (Coufal, 1993). The language interventionist and team members will need to discuss how they think language is learned and examine their assessment and intervention approaches for evidence of a shared theory. When a shared theory is not achieved, it is likely that the intervention will vary depending on who provides the services. For instance, a teacher who strongly believes in behavioralism teamed with a language interventionist who is oriented toward social-interactionism will approach intervention differently. The teacher will emphasize the need for the child to respond, particularly through imitation, whereas the language interventionist will be satisfied with frequent models of the appropriate target without an overt response from the child. Spontaneous use of the target by the child will suffice. Although it is not always possible for all team members to agree on a theory of language development, it is important that the team be able to discuss their differences and understand the impact of those differences on the course of assessment and intervention. Importantly, the exact role that theory will play when working with children with language impairment will vary depending on the interventionist's knowledge of the theory, the theory's breadth of application, and the extent to which we understand what has gone differently in children with language impairment in their course of development. As Nittrouer (1999) eloquently states in

TABLE 2.2   Comparison and Summary of Theoretical Assumptions

Question	Interactive Model	Functional Theory
How is language learned?	Through social interactions with caregiver	Through child hypothesis-testing via interactions with their language environment
What is the mechanism by which language is acquired?	Not specified, however, repeated exposures to joint attention episodes in daily routines is important	Cue validity: cue reliability and cue availability
Why do errors in typical development occur?	Child has difficulty organizing and assimilating information from context.	Cue costs Competition
What is the theory's application to Language impairment?	Increase child engagement and caregiver responsiveness to improve child's ability to assimilate and organize contextual information	Meaningful context for intervention, frequent models using recasts and expansions: all designed to increase saliency of cues.

her discussion of the need for clinicians to carefully evaluate the underlying theory associated with their intervention choices, "Every clinician must be a theorist; otherwise we will never know if we are doing the best we can for our clients" (p. 938).

DISCUSSION QUESTIONS

1. Divide the class into various theories associated with social-interactionist approaches, for example: Interactive Model, Vygotskian, RELM, and Functionalism. Have each group present its view on the following topics:
   a. What is the role of imitation?
   b. What is the role of reinforcement?
   c. What is the most crucial aspect of this approach?
   d. What might be the source of a language learning impairment?

TABLE 2.2   Comparison and Summary of Theoretical Assumptions (*continued*)

Rare Event Cognitive Comparison Theory	Vygostky	PPT Minimalist Program
Through the interactions of cognitive abilities and social communication	Through social contexts with a more capable peer	Through innate universal principles and by setting parameters to be consistent with one's environment
A rare event that occurs once the child selectively attends, stores, compares, retrieves, and makes hypothesizes about input.	The social plane and the psychological plane ZPD	Universal Grammar which is an autonomous system of principles and parameters
Problems with attending, storage, comparing, retrieving, or hypothesis-testing	It is part of the process of learning.	Problems with the principles that constrain representation, setting a parameter, mapping from one level of representation to another, or an extended period of optional infinitive
Provide models in contingent, recasts; emphasizes need for early intervention; importance of evaluating language production within context	Dynamic assessment using zpd tells of child's readiness for learning or if a language difference or language disorder exists.	Reset parameters: trigger data important to consider

Based in part on Houston (1972).

2. Ask class members to devise a ten-item questionnaire that would distinguish between a person who is a social interactionist or a person who has a linguistic perspective on language development. Have the students administer their questionnaire to either a classmate or a layperson outside of class. Ask the students to summarize the results and discuss them in class.

3. Divide the class into various theoretical groups. Give them a brief case study of a child referred with a suspected language impairment. Discuss how each theoretical group would approach assessment and intervention differently.

4. Select ten vocabulary words, one morphosyntactic goal, and one pragmatic goal that you might work on with a hypothetical child. How would a social interactionist approach these specific intervention targets compared to a linguist?

5. Divide the class into two groups. Have one group argue why theory is important to assessment and intervention and one group argue why it is not important.
6. Divide your class into small groups of four to five members. Assign roles such as teacher, SLP, psychologist, social worker, special educator, parent, and principal to each member of each group. Give each person a theoretical position (behaviorist, social-interactionist, linguist) and have him or her discuss his or her view of language development within the framework of his or her theoretical perspective with one another. Have the groups note where differences of opinion occur and how it might affect the group's ability to collaborate.

REFERENCES

Bain, B. A., & Olswang, L. B. (1995). Examining readiness for learning two-word utterances by children with specific expressive language impairment: Dynamic assessment validation. *American Journal of Speech-Language Pathology: A Journal of Clinical Practice, 4,* 81–91.

Baker, N., & Nelson, K. (1984). Recasting and related conversational techniques for triggering syntactic advances by young children. *First Language, 5,* 3–22.

Bandura, A. (1966). *Social learning theory.* Englewood Cliffs, NJ: Prentice-Hall.

Bandura, A., & Harris, M. (1966). Modifications of syntactic style. *Journal of Exceptional Child Psychology, 4,* 341–352.

Bates, E. (1976). *Language and context: Studies in the acquisition of pragmatics.* New York: Academic Press.

Bates, E., Benigni, L., Bretherton, I., Camaioni, L., & Volterra, V. (1977). From gesture to first word: On cognitive and social prerequisites. In M. Lewis and L. Rosenblum (Eds.), *Interaction, conversation, and prerequisites.* New York: Wiley.

Bates, E., & MacWhinney, B. (1982). A functionalist approach to grammar. In E. Wanner and L. Gleitman (Eds.), *Language acquisition: The state of the art* (pp. 173–218). Cambridge: Cambridge University Press.

Bates, E., & MacWhinney, B. (1988). What is functionalism? *Papers and Reports on Child Language Development, 27,* 137–152.

Berk, L. (1989). *Child development.* Boston: Allyn & Bacon.

Bernstein-Ratner, N., & Pye, C. (1984). Higher pitch in BT is not universal: Acoustic evidence from Quiche Mayan. *Journal of Child Language, 11,* 515–522.

Bloom, L., & Lahey, M. (1978). *Language development and language disorders.* New York: Wiley.

Braun, C., Rennie, B., & Gordon, C. (1987). An examination of contexts for reading assessment. *Journal of Educational Research, 80,* 283–289.

Brinton, B., & Fujiki, M. (1989). *Conversational management with language-impaired children.* Rockville, MD: Aspen.

Brown, R. (1973). *A first language: The early stages*. Cambridge, MA: Harvard University Press.

Bruner, J. (1983). *Child's talk*. New York: W. W. Norton

Camarata, S., & Nelson, K. (1992). Treatment efficiency as a function of target selection in the remediation of child language disorders. *Clinical Linguistics & Phonetics, 6,* 167-178.

Camarata, S., Nelson, K., & Camarata, M. (1994). Comparison of conversational-recasting and imitative procedures for training grammatical structures in children with specific language impairment. *Journal of Speech and Hearing Research, 37,* 1414–1423.

Chomsky, N. (1957). *Syntactic structures*. The Hague: Mouton.

Chomsky, N. (1981). *Lectures on government and binding*. Dordrecht: Foris.

Chomsky, N. (1995). *The minimalist program*. Cambridge, MA: MIT Press.

Connell, P. (1990). Linguistic foundations of clinical language teaching: Grammar. *Journal of Speech-Language Pathology and Audiology, 14,* 25–49.

Coufal, K. (1993). Collaborative consultation for speech-language pathologists. Topics in *Language Disorders, 14,* 1–14.

Cromer, R. (1974). The development of language and cognition: The cognitive hypothesis. In B. Foss (Ed.), *New perspectives in child development* (pp. 19–47). New York: Penguin.

Cross, G. (1978). Mothers' speech and its association with rate of linguistic development in young children. In N. Waterson & C. Snow (Eds.), *The development of communication* (pp. 199–216). New York: Wiley.

Dore, J. (1979). What's so conceptual about the acquisition of linguistic structures? *Journal of Child Language, 6,* 129–138.

Feuerstein, R. (1979). *The dynamic assessment of retarded performers*. Baltimore: University Park Press.

Fey, M. E. (1986). *Language intervention with young children*. Boston: College-Hill Press.

Fey, M. E., Krulik, T. E., Loeb, D. F., & Proctor-Williams, K. (1999). Sentence recast use by parents of children with typical language and children with specific language impairment. *American Journal of Speech-Language Pathology, 8,* 273–286.

Fey, M. E., & Loeb, D. F. (2002). An evaluation of the facilitative effects of inverted yes-no questions on the acquisition of auxiliary verbs. *Journal of Speech, Language, and Hearing Research, 45,* 160–174.

Friel-Patti, S. (1994). Commitment to theory. *American Journal of Speech-Language Pathology: A Journal of Clinical Practice, 3,* 30–34.

Gathercole, S. E., & Baddeley, A. D. (1993). *Working memory and language*. Hillsdale, NJ: Lawrence Erlbaum.

Girolametto, L., Pearce, P. S., & Weitzman, E. (1996). Interactive focused stimulation for toddlers with expressive language delays. *Journal of Speech, Language, and Hearing Research, 39,* 1274–1283.

Girolametto, L., Pearce, P. S., & Weitzman, E. (1997). Effects of lexical intervention on the phonology of late talkers. *Journal of Speech, Language, and Hearing Research, 40,* 338–348.

Girolametto, L., Verbey, M., & Tannock, R. (1994). Improving joint engagement in parent-child interaction: An intervention study. *Journal of Early Intervention, 18,* 155–167.

Goffman, L., & Leonard, J. (2000). Growth of language skills in preschool children with specific language impairment: Implications for assessment and intervention. *American Journal of Speech-Language Pathology, 9,* 151–161.

Gopnik, A., & Meltzoff, A. (1987). Early semantic developments and their relationship to object permanence, means-ends understanding, and categorization. In K. Nelson & A. van Kleeck (Eds.), *Children's language* (Vol. 6, pp. 191–212). Hillsdale, NJ: Lawrence Erlbaum.

Hemmeter, M., & Kaiser, A. (1994). Enhanced milieu teaching: Effects of parent-implemented language intervention. *Journal of Early Intervention, 18,* 269–289.

Houston, S. (1972). *A survey of psycholinguistics.* The Hague: Mouton.

Hyams, N. (1986). *Language acquisition and the theory of parameters.* Dordrecht: D. Reidel.

Hyams, N. (1989). The null subject parameter in language acquisition. In O. Jaeggli & K. Safir (Eds.), *The null subject parameter* (pp. 215–238). Dordrecht: Kluwer Academic.

Johnston, J. (1983). What is language intervention? The role of theory. In J. Miller, D. Yoder, & R. Schiefelbusch (Eds.), *Contemporary issues in language intervention.* Rockville, MD: American Speech-Language-Hearing Association.

Kaiser, A., & Hester, P. (1994). Generalized effects of enhanced milieu teaching. *Journal of Speech and Hearing Research, 37,* 1320–1340.

Kaiser, A., Yoder, P., & Keetz, A. (1992). Evaluating milieu teaching. In S. Warren & J. Reichle (Eds.), *Causes and effects in communication and language intervention* (pp. 9–48). Baltimore: Brookes.

Kamhi, A. (1993). Some problems with the marriage between theory and clinical practice. *Language, Speech, and Hearing Services in Schools, 24,* 57–60.

Kwiatkowski, J., & Shriberg, L. (1993). Speech normalization in developmental phonological disorders: A retrospective study of capability-focus theory. *Language, Speech, and Hearing Services in Schools, 24,* 10–18.

Leonard, L. (1975). Modeling as a clinical procedure in language training. *Language, Speech, and Hearing Services in Schools, 6,* 72–85.

Leonard, L. (1995). Functional categories in the grammars of children with specific language impairment. *Journal of Speech and Hearing Research, 38,* 1270–1283.

Leonard, L. (1998). *Specific language impairment in children.* Cambridge, MA: MIT Press.

Loeb, D., & Armstrong, N. (2001). Case studies on the efficacy of expansions and subject-verb-object models in early language acquisition. *Child Language Teaching and Therapy, 17,* 35–54.

Loeb, D., & Leonard, L. (1988). Specific language impairment and parameter theory. *Clinical Linguistics and Phonetics, 2,* 317–327.

Loeb, D., & Mikesic, E. (1992). Facilitating change in specifically language-impaired children's grammar. Poster presented at the American Speech, Language, and Hearing Convention, San Antonio.

MacWhinney, B. (1987). The competition model. In B. MacWhinney (Ed.), *Mechanisms of language acquisition*. Hillsdale, NJ: Lawrence Erlbaum.

MacWhinney, B. (1989). Competition and teachability. In M. Rice & R. Schiefelbusch (Eds.), *The teachability of language* (pp. 63–104). Baltimore: Brookes.

Nelson, K. (1977). Facilitating children's syntax acquisition. *Developmental Psychology, 13,* 101–107.

Nelson, K. (1986). *Event knowledge: Structure and function in development*. Hillsdale, NJ: Lawrence Erlbaum.

Nelson, K. (1987). Some observations from the perspective of the rare event cognitive comparison theory of language acquisition. In K. Nelson & A. van Kleeck (Eds.), *Children's language* (Vol. 6, pp. 289–332). Hillsdale, NJ: Lawrence Erlbaum.

Nelson, K. (1989). Strategies for first language teaching. In M. Rice & R. Schiefelbusch (Eds.), *The teachability of language* (pp. 263–310). Baltimore: Brookes.

Nittrouer, S. (1999). Do processing deficits cause phonological processing problems? *Journal of Speech, Language and Hearing Research, 40,* 925–942.

Olswang, L., & Bain, B. (1991). When to recommend intervention. *Language, Speech, and Hearing Services in Schools, 22,* 255–263.

Olswang, L., Bain, B., & Johnson, G. (1992). Using dynamic assessment with children with language disorders. In S. Warren & J. Reichle (Eds.), *Causes and effects in communication and language intervention* (pp. 187–216). Baltimore: Brooks.

Pena, E., Iglesias, A., Lidz, C. S. (2001). Reducing test bias through dynamic assessment of children's word learning ability. *American Journal of Speech-Language Pathology, 10,* 138–154.

Piaget, J. (1954). *The construction of reality in the child*. New York: Basic Books.

Pinker, S. (1984). *Language learnability and language development*. Cambridge, MA: Harvard University Press.

Pinker, S. (1989). *Learnability and cognition*. Cambridge, MA: MIT Press.

Rice, M., & Oetting, J. (1993). Morphological deficits of children with SLI: Evaluation of number marking and agreement. *Journal of Speech and Hearing Research, 36,* 1249–1257.

Rice, M., Wexler, K., & Cleave, P. (1995). Specific language impairment as a period of extended optional infinitive. *Journal of Speech and Hearing Research, 38,* 850–863.

Rumelhardt, D., & McClelland, J. (1986). On learning the past tense of English verbs. In J. McClelland, D. Rumelhart, & the PDP Research Group (Eds.), *Parallel distributed processing* (Vol. 2, pp. 216–271). Cambridge, MA: MIT Press.

Schieffelin, B. (1985). The acquisition of Kaluli. In D. Slobin (Ed.), *The crosslinguistic study of language, Volume 1: The data*. Hillsdale, NJ: Lawrence Erlbaum.

Schlesinger, I. (1977). Production of utterances and language acquisition. In D. Slobin (Ed.), *The ontogenesis of grammar*. New York: Academic Press.

Skinner, B. F. (1957). *Verbal behavior*. New York: Apppleton-Century-Crofts.

Tannock, R., & Girolametto, L. (1992). Reassessing parent-focused language intervention programs. In S. Warren & J. Reichle (Eds.), *Causes and effects in communication and language intervention* (pp. 49–80). Baltimore: Brookes.

Tharp, R., & Gallimore, R. (1988). *Rousing minds to life: Teaching, learning, and schooling in social context*. Cambridge, England: Cambridge University Press.

van Kleeck, A., & Richardson, A. (1993). What's in an error? Using children's wrong responses as language teaching opportunities. *National Student Speech-Language-Hearing Association, 20,* 9–21.

Vygotsky, L. (1978). *Mind in society: The development of higher psychological processes*. Cambridge, MA: Harvard University Press.

Warren, S., & Kaiser, A. (1986). Incidental language teaching: A critical review. *Journal of Speech and Hearing Disorders, 51,* 291–299.

Wexler, K. (1994a). Triggers and parameter setting. Paper presented at the Linguistic, Cognitive Science, & Childhood Language Disorders Conference, City University of New York, April.

Wexler, K. (1994b). Optional infinitives. In D. Lightfoot & N. Hornstein (Eds.), *Verb movement*. New York: Cambridge University Press.

Wexler, K., & Culicover, P. (1980). *Formal principles of language acquisition*. Cambridge, MA: MIT Press.

Wilson, M. S. (1994). Early language intervention: Implications of the principles and parameters model. Presentation at the American Speech-Language-Hearing Association Annual Convention. New Orleans, LA.

Wilson, M. S., & Fox, B. J. (1994). *Simple sentence structure*. Winooski, VT: Laureate Learning Systems.

Wilson, M. S., & Pascoe, J. P. (1997, November). Chomsky's minimalist program and its implications for early language intervention. Seminar presented at the American Speech-Language-Hearing Convention, Boston.

CHAPTER 3

Characteristics of Students with Language and Communication Difficulties

Linda McCormick and Diane Frome Loeb

Every society has long-established standards to which the vast majority of people in that society conform. People tend to look the way they are expected to look, behave the way they are expected to behave, learn the way they are expected to learn, and communicate the way they are expected to communicate. Those who deviate substantially from society's physical, social, and intellectual expectations, whether because of biological or environmental factors, or both, are given labels. The labels (e.g., *physically disabled, emotionally disturbed, learning disabled, sensory impaired*) are *presumed* to reflect the problem produced by the deviation from "normal" expectations. Efforts are then made to determine the cause of the problem. These efforts are based on the assumption that once a cause for the problem can be determined it will be possible to prescribe an intervention that will eliminate, or at least lessen, the deviation.

Unfortunately, pinpointing the specific cause of a disability is extremely difficult (and sometimes impossible). The reason that attempts to determine etiology are rarely productive is that causality is multifaceted and complex. Moreover, even when there is some certainty as to causality, there is not always a cause-and-effect relationship between the nature of the problem and its effect on development and behavior. While it can help us understand what the child is experiencing, putting a label on a child's difficulties does not translate to a prescription for appropriate and effective instructional and intervention services.

Children's individual differences override many, if not most, characteristics associated with a disability diagnosis. Children who share the same disability label may differ from one another as much as they differ from children with another label (or no label at all). Thus, they have very different instructional and intervention needs.

There *is* value in knowing the factors necessary for "normal" development. Information about these factors helps us understand developmental delays, deviation, and dysfunction. The following are necessary for normal development of speech, language, and communication (Miller, 1983):

Neurological factors
Cognitive development
Information processing (e.g., attention, discrimination, memory)
Motor output capabilities (neuromuscular control/coordination)
Social–emotional development and motivation

Structural and physiological factors
Sensory acuity (auditory, visual, tactile, gustatory, olfactory)
Oromuscular capabilities
Speech transmission mechanisms

Environmental factors
Social–cultural variables (socioeconomic level, language culture)
Experiences (caregiver–child interactions, linguistic input, responsiveness)
Physical context (availability of toys, pictures, manipulable objects)

A delay, disruption, or dysfunction in any of the above factors will contribute to speech, language, and/or communication difficulties. Because of their interrelatedness, the child's difficulties will be compounded when there is delay or dysfunction in more than one area. For example, the child with a visual impairment who experiences delayed social development (because she is not able to see and interpret social cues) and delayed physical development (because of restricted mobility) can be expected to have problems with the rate and course of early language development. Ultimately, how much of an effect any one or combination of these factors has on development of speech, language, and communication abilities will depend on (1) the degree of the deficit, (2) the type of deficit (e.g., structural and physiological factors may have more detrimental effects than environmental factors), (3) the age at which the problem occurs, (4) when the problem is identified, and (5) the quality of intervention efforts.

DESCRIPTIVE CLASSIFICATION OF LANGUAGE DIFFICULTIES

There are a number of possible descriptive classification systems for language and communication difficulties. One would be classification according to whether the difficulties are with receptive language or expressive language. Another would be according to the aspect of language that is affected (phonology, morphology, semantics, syntax, or pragmatics). The latter option is not as straightforward as it sounds because children who have problems with one aspect of language generally experience some type of deficiency in one or more of the others. At the same time, there is usually one aspect with which the child has greater problems.

Phonological Disorders

Speech and hearing professionals now use the label *phonological disorders* for problems that were previously termed *functional articulation disorders*. Phonological disorders are common in children with language difficulties. They are usually articulation problems that have no known or obvious organic, neurological, or physical correlates. They may be due to speech-motor difficulties or to difficulties related to phonological organization. Leonard (1990) provides these examples to illustrate the two types of phonological disorders. The child whose phonological problems are associated with speech-motor difficulties might say "gup" for *cup* and "doo" for *two,* demonstrating an inability to coordinate the timing of voicing so that it begins after the release of the consonant. The child whose phonological problems are associated with lack of phonological organization might say "tee" for see and "tack" for *sack,* while at the same time he is capable of producing [s] (e.g., says "soo" for *shoe* and "sip" for *chip*).

Phonological deficits are frequently observed in children who are experiencing reading and learning difficulties. They may demonstrate the following phonological deficits: (1) delayed acquisition of a mature phonological system for speech production; (2) inferior perception and/or production of complex phonemic configurations; (3) inefficient use of phonological codes in short-term memory; and (4) impaired phonological sensitivity (Gerber, 1993). The last, impaired phonological sensitivity, may interfere with establishing phoneme–grapheme correspondences for reading and spelling.

Morphological Difficulties

Recall from Chapter 1 that morphological inflections (also called *grammatical morphemes* or *grammatical markers*) are inflections on nouns, verbs, and adjectives that signal different kinds of meanings; for example, adding the morpheme -*s* to dog signals plurality. Children with learning disabilities often have difficulties with morphological inflections. They seem to have problems with verb tense, plurality, and possession (Leonard, 1990; Siegel & Ryan, 1984) and morphological rules (e.g., Vogel, 1977). Learning the rules for words such as auxiliaries, modals, prepositions, and conjunctions is also a problem (Wiig, 1990). Five-year-old Taylor is an example of a child with morphological difficulties: He omits *-ing* and confuses *a, an,* and *the,* and he is inconsistent in the use of suffixes indicating possession, gender, and number in nouns. Children with autism also experience difficulties with morphology, especially with pronouns and verb endings. The morphological difficulties of children with mental retardation fall under the heading of delay: School-age children typically demonstrate morphological abilities similar to those of younger children.

Semantic Difficulties

Children and adolescents identified as language disordered, learning disabled, dyslexic, and aphasic very often have language difficulties associated with semantics. Most evident are problems with word finding: the ability to generate a specific word that is evoked by a situation, stimulus, sentence context, or conversation (Gerber, 1993; Leonard, 1990; Nippold, 1992). Tests of comprehension and their productive vocabularies indicate that word knowledge is restricted, literal, and concrete (Gerber, 1993). Students with semantic difficulties also demonstrate (1) restrictions in word meanings, (2) difficulties with multiple word meanings, (3) excessive use of nonspecific terms (e.g., *thing* and *stuff*), and indefinite reference (e.g., *that* and *there*), and (4) difficulties with comprehension of certain conjunctions (e.g., *but, or, of, then, either, neither*) and relational terms (e.g., *in front of, more/less, before/after*). Children with mental retardation experience difficulties with verb tense markers, possession, and pronouns.

Syntax Difficulties

Children with syntactic difficulties are experiencing problems acquiring the rules that govern word order and other aspects of grammar such as subject–verb agreement, as evidenced by their problems processing sentences, even relatively simple ones. They typically produce shorter and less elaborated sentences than their peers, often failing to fully encode all possible relevant information. They also use fewer cohesive conjunctions than their peers without disabilities, and there is less variation in the types of conjunctions they use. They make many errors of omission, reversal, and substitution in sentence repetition tasks and sentence completion tasks (Synder & Downey, 1991).

Children with autism often construct sentences with superficial form, disregarding underlying meaning. Their sentences are similar to those of younger peers. Children with language learning difficulties have difficulty learning different sentence forms. The sequence of sentence development of children with mental retardation is delayed but typical. They use shorter, less complex sentences with fewer subject elaborations and fewer relative clauses. In most cases, the sentences of children with traumatic brain injury are lengthy and fragmented, making it very difficult to understand what they are trying to communicate.

Pragmatic Difficulties

Because pragmatic skills are those skills that allow the child to use language as a social tool (i.e., communication functions, appropriate turn-taking, ability to adapt to the context), difficulties in this area interfere with interpersonal communication. Many children with disabilities have poor social interaction and poor communication skills. They typically have problems related to listener needs (what and how much information they need to provide to their listeners). They do not seem to know (1) when to make eye contact, (2) how close it is permissible to stand when talking to another person, (3) when to request clarification of information (e.g., "Can you tell me again what you mean?"), (4) how to interpret direct and indirect requests, or (5) how to introduce topics.

Not unexpectedly, considering the social deficits associated with autism, children with that diagnosis have a multitude of pragmatic difficulties (e.g., Mundy, Sigman, & Kasari, 1990). Deficits in the ability to interpret affective states, an important foundation for communication and language development, are especially pronounced.

DISABILITY CLASSIFICATION

Although classification according to the aspects of behavior with which the child is having difficulty provides more information that is useful for planning and implementing intervention, it is not the prevalent method of classification. The most common means of grouping children with special needs is according to disability. However, grouping according to disability is not helpful for planning intervention and/or instruction. It makes some unfounded assumptions: (1) that there are specific factors that have caused the disability; (2) that these factors can be identified; and (3) that all children with the same disability will benefit from the same intervention and/or instructional techniques.

The reason that the practice of grouping students by disability continues is that it is tied to our system for distributing state and federal funds. How many special education dollars a state or district receives depends on the number of children determined eligible for and provided with special services. The only way students with special needs can receive individualized instructional activities and related services is meeting the eligibility criteria for one of the disabilities categories specified in the Individuals with Disabilities Education Act (IDEA):

- visual impairment
- hearing impairment
- orthopedic impairment
- other health impairment
- mental retardation
- specific learning disabilities
- emotional disturbance
- speech or language impairment
- traumatic brain injury
- autism
- deaf-blindness
- deafness
- multiple disabilities
- developmental delay

Developmental delay is an additional category for children ages 3 to 9 who demonstrate delays in physical, cognitive, communication, emotional, social, and/or adaptive development and, because of these delays, need special education and related services. This category is available at the discretion of the state and local education agency.

Most of the disability categories include students with language and communication disorders. The only time that these difficulties are considered to be a primary disability is students in *the speech or language impairment* category. For students in the other categories, language and communication are a secondary disability (when they are present). Interestingly, identification of the etiology of language and communication disorders is most likely when they are secondary to another disability. Even then, however, when a presumed cause of the disorder can be specified, it is rarely possible to predict the precise nature and severity of the disorder. Children in the same disability group sometimes demonstrate very different language difficulties: In fact, the language and communication difficulties in one category may be more similar to those of children in one or another of the other categories.

The remainder of this chapter considers *possible* causal factors, general characteristics, and language characteristics of students in the IDEA disability categories that have language components. As noted above, in the ideal world, children would be grouped for instruction according to descriptive, instructionally relevant variables. In the real world, children are categorized according to the IDEA definitions. Therefore, it is critical for all school personnel to know these definitions and criteria for determining eligibility for special education and related services. The IDEA categories are grouped under these headings: (1) learning difficulties; (2) motor disabilities; (3) sensory impairments; (4) behavior disorders and autism; and (5) cognitive deficits.

Learning Difficulties

Among the labels used to refer to children with learning difficulties are (1) learning disabilities, (2) attention deficit disorder, and (3) specific language impairment. The common denominator across these subcategories is that, despite intelligence scores within the normal range, these children do not seem to learn in the same way or as efficiently as their peers. Because of their academic, social, and communication difficulties, they have many problems in school settings.

Learning Disabilities

Arguments about definition have been almost continuous since the inception of the field of learning disabilities (LD). The oldest and most well-known definition was developed in 1967 by the National Advisory Committee on Handicapped Children. That definition became the basis of the definition, which was first printed in 1977 in Public Law 94–142 and continues in the latest 1997 reauthorization of IDEA:

> *a disorder in one or more of the basic psychological processes involved in understanding or in using language, spoken or written, which disorder may manifest itself in an imperfect ability to listen, speak, read, write, spell, or to do mathematical calculations. The term includes such conditions as perceptual difficulties, brain injury, minimal brain dysfunction, dyslexia, and developmental aphasia . . . in the definition, but learning problems that are primarily the result of visual, hearing, or motor impairments; mental retardation; emotional disturbance; or environmental, cultural, or economic disadvantage are excluded.* (Federal Register, *1999*).

Since 1977 there have been several other definitions of learning disabilities. In 1984 the Association for Children and Adults with Learning Disabilities (ACALD) adopted a definition that broadened the scope of the problem beyond academics. Another definition was adopted in 1988 by the National Joint Committee for Learning Disabilities (NJCLD). The definition put forth by this coalition of professional and parent organizations defines learning disabilities as:

> *a generic term that refers to a heterogenous group of disorders manifested by significant difficulties in the acquisition and use of listening, speaking, reading, writing, reasoning, or mathematical abilities. These disorders are intrinsic to the individual and presumed to be due to central nervous system dysfunction, and may appear across the life span. Problems of self-regulatory behaviors, social perception, and social interaction may exist with learning*

disabilities but do not themselves constitute a learning disability. Although learning disabilities may occur concomitantly with other handicapping conditions (for example, sensory impairment, mental retardation, serious emotional disturbance) or with extrinsic influences (such as cultural differences, insufficient or inappropriate instruction), they are not the result of those conditions or influences (National Joint Committee on Learning Disabilities, *1994*).

This definition stresses the general nature of problems grouped under the term *learning disabilities*. It also refers to more specific abilities such as reading and writing, and it allows some overlap with other disabilities. Note that both definitions cited above have one thing in common: They define a learning disability by what it is *not*.

Most states and local districts require that the following criteria be met for a student is to be classified and served as learning disabled:

- ***Discrepancy criterion:*** This criterion states that there must be a discrepancy between the student's potential (as measured by a standardized intelligence test) and actual achievement (as measured by a standardized achievement test). Each state determines how large a discrepancy must be in order for the student to meet the inclusionary criterion. Many states have complicated discrepancy formulas to calculate this difference. The considerable debate over the use of discrepancy scores has focused on (1) the difficulty with reliable calculations, (2) problems related to the fact that test scores are likely to be negatively influenced by attention problems and lack of motivation, and (3) the enormous time and effort required (Gerber, 1993).

- ***Exclusionary criterion:*** The exclusionary criterion states that the learning disability is not the result of other known factors such as mental retardation, sensory impairment, physical disabilities, emotional disturbance, or environmental disadvantage. If other disabilities are suspected, the student is evaluated in that area. If the student has another disability that does not cause the learning disability (e.g., a physical disability), then the student is eligible for learning disabilities services and may also be eligible for other services. If there is no other disability or factor present, the student must still meet the third criterion.

- ***Need criterion:*** The third criterion is a demonstrated need for special education services. There must be a demonstrated need for individualized curriculum and procedures.

While there is no such thing as a "typical" profile of a student with learning disabilities, there is extensive research documenting the characteristics associated with learning disabilities and the difficulties that these students experience, particularly in reading and written language. A summary of the characteristics associated with learning disabilities is presented in Table 3.1.

TABLE 3.1 Summary of characteristics associated with learning disabilities

Characteristic	Description
Reading difficulties	Student makes many word recognition and comprehension errors; has difficulty keeping his place while reading.
Written language difficulties	Student has difficulties with handwriting, spelling, text structure, sentence structure, lexicon, and composition.
Deficits in the area of metacognition	Student uses inefficient or inappropriate learning strategies or is completely lacking in learning strategies.
Disorders of attention	Student is highly distractable, impulsive (responds very quickly without monitoring accuracy), and/or perseverative.
Poor spatial orientation	Student seems to become lost easily and has great difficulty orienting to new surroundings.
Difficulty with polar relationships	Student has particular difficulty with the concepts *big–little, light–heavy,* and *close–far.*
Confusion with directions	Student has difficulty with the concepts *right, left, north, south, east, west, up, down,* etc.
Poor motor coordination	Student is generally clumsy and poorly coordinated and has great difficulty achieving balance.
Poor fine motor ability	Student has difficulty manipulating small objects such as pencils, paintbrushes, and scissors.
Insensitivity to social nuances	Student does not read facial expressions and body language or seem to know when actions are not socially appropriate.
Inability to follow directions	Student has difficulty following oral directions, particularly the first time they are given.
Inability to keep up with group discussions	Student cannot seem to follow the flow of thought and conversation in class discussions.
Inadequate time concepts	Student is frequently late and often does not seem to have a concept of time or responsibilities related to time.
Perceptual problems	Student cannot copy letters (without reversals) or discriminate shape differences; also has difficulty discriminating sound differences.
Memory problems	Student cannot remember simple sequences or find objects that are always in the same location.
Social immaturity	Student seems unable to predict the consequences of his behavior and tends to use less socially acceptable behaviors.
Auditory processing difficulties	Student has difficulties when there is competing noise in the background.

The etiology of the deficits associated with learning disabilities is not fully understood. Both the IDEA and the NJCLD definitions presume an underlying neurological problem, but neurological evidence is inconclusive. What we do know is that (1) children with the characteristics associated with learning disabilities are ill-equipped to function without special assistance in school settings, and (2) problems with language and learning are connecting and overlapping.

The American Speech-Language-Hearing Association's Committee on Prevention of Speech-Language and Hearing Problems (1984) estimated that 71 percent of all preschoolers with disabilities are diagnosed as having a speech or language disorder as their primary disability. It is interesting to speculate as to why this percentage does not continue throughout the school years. Possible explanations are that: (1) early intervention efforts are enormously effective; (2) language problems resolve with age; or (3) these children are reclassified into another disability category when they enter school. It is highly probable that the majority of learning disabilities are really language disabilities. At school-age, the label is changed to fit the school context. This conclusion is supported by a study by Gibbs and Cooper (1989). In their study of 242 eight- to twelve-year-old children with learning disabilities, they found that 96.2 percent of these students exhibited a speech, language, or hearing problem. Slightly over 90 percent demonstrated language problems, 23 percent had articulation disorders, and 12 percent had voice disorders.

The label **language-learning disabled** is often used to refer to the substantial percentage of children in the learning disabilities category whose problems are exclusively in the areas of speech and language. Estimates of the percentage of students with learning disabilities who have difficulty learning and using symbols are as high as 75 percent (Miniutti, 1991). Table 3.2 provides an overview of the language difficulties associated with learning disabilities.

Attention Disorders

Attentional problems include attention deficit disorder (ADD) and related disorders of behavior and learning (e.g., attention deficit-hyperactivity disorder [ADHD]). They are thought to affect as much as 20 percent of the school-age population. Children classified as *ADD* demonstrate inattention and impulsivity. Some also experience hyperactivity. The term used for this disorder by family physicians, pediatricians, psychiatrists, and other mental health clinicians is *ADHD* because this is the diagnostic label in the psychiatric classification scheme (i.e., the *Diagnostic and Statistical Manual of Mental Disorders* [*DSM-IV*], 1994).

The regulations of the reauthorization of IDEA (Federal Register, 1999) add ADD and ADHD to the list of conditions that make a child

TABLE 3.2   Language difficulties associated with learning disabilities

Language Dimension	Difficulties
Phonology	Delayed acquisition of sounds Inferior perception and/or production of complex sound configurations Inefficient use of phonological codes in short-term memory Impaired sensitivity to sounds
Morphology/Syntax	Production of shorter and less elaborated sentences than peers Failure to encode all relevant information in sentences Difficulty with negative and passive constructions, relative clauses, contractions, and adjectival forms Confusion of articles (*a, an, the*) Difficulty with verb tense, plurality, possession, and pronouns Delayed acquisition of morphological rules Difficulty learning the rules for using auxiliaries, modals, prepositions, conjunctions, and other grammatical markers
Semantics	Word-finding and definitional problems Restricted word meanings (too literal and concrete) Difficulty with multiple word meanings Excessive use of nonspecific terms (e.g., *thing, stuff*) and indefinite reference Difficulty comprehending certain conjunctions (e.g., *but, or, if, then, either*) Difficulty with relational terms (comparative, spatial, temporal)
Pragmatics	Difficulty with questions and requests for clarification Difficulty initiating and maintaining conversation

eligible for services under the "other health impaired" category. Children with ADD/ADHD may be eligible under other disability categories if they meet the criteria for those disabilities. If not eligible for special services under IDEA, they may be served under Section 504 of the Rehabilitation Act of 1973 (Section 504) or the Americans with Disabilities Act of 1990 (ADA). (This legislation is described in Chapter 5.)

The diagnosis of ADD is separate from the diagnosis of specific learning disabilities, but there is considerable overlap in the two groups. It has been estimated that 30 to 60 percent of children classified as ADD are learning disabled (Tarnowski and Nay, 1989). The remaining children with a diagnosis of ADD are hyperactive. Early ADHD may predispose children toward reading problems (Ferguson & Horwood, 1992), but it is not possible to determine whether the source of the reading difficulties is the attention problems or language problems.

Research considering the language difficulties associated with ADHD has produced contradictory findings. Some studies have found delay in developing language in children with ADHD (Hartsough & Lambert, 1985; Szatmari, Offord, & Boyle, 1989): The percentage of children with ADHD who are delayed in developing language is estimated to be in the range of 6 to 35 percent, compared to 2 to 5.5 percent for children without the ADHD label. Other studies have found no delays (Barkley, DuPaul, & McMurray, 1990).

The substantial differences in the impulsivity, poor attention, and excessive activity among children with ADHD and across situations calls for a multidimensional approach to assessment. Parent, teacher, and even peer reports, plus observation in the classroom and other school settings, are essential.

Specific Language Impairment

When students demonstrate communication difficulties that do not seem to be the result of or directly associated with a hearing loss or another disability, they are labeled as having a speech or language impairment.

The American Speech-Language-Hearing Association's (ASHA) (April 1980) definition of language disorders is

> *the abnormal acquisition, comprehension or expression of spoken or written language. The disorder may involve all, one, or some of the phonologic, morphologic, semantic, syntactic, or pragmatic components of the linguistic system. Individuals with language disorders frequently have problems in sentence processing or in abstracting information meaningfully for storage and retrieval from short and long term memory (ASHA, 1980, pp. 317–318).*

The label **specific language impairment** (SLI) is used for children with language impairment that "cannot be attributed to deficits in hearing, oral structure and function, or general intelligence" (Leonard, 1987, p. 1). It is important to note that, while the term "specific language impairment" (SLI) is used as if it refers to a clearly defined group of children, in fact there is no generally recognized or accepted definition for SLI (Aram, Morris, and Hall, 1993). Moreover, despite a great deal of research and thought committed to trying to understand why children with no other apparent problems have so much difficulty learning and using language, it is not clear what causes SLI. It does not seem to affect or be affected to anatomical, physical, or intellectual problems.

In contrast to the lack of definitive information regarding the cause or causes of SLI, there are considerable data concerning the educational and social impact of language impairment. There is a strong relationship between early speech-language impairments and reading disabilities (Tallal, Curtiss, and Kaplan, 1989). As noted in the section on learning disabilities, many children identified as having language difficulties in the preschool years (whether they are specifically labeled SLI or not), are later relabeled as language-learning disabled or learning disabled. Retrospective follow-up studies report that, when they enter school, 40 to 60 percent of these children will continue to experience difficulties with spoken language, and they will also have problems with reading and spelling (Aram, Ekelman, & Nation, 1984). Not unexpectedly, problems with social interaction are prevalent because relationships are based on communication (Bashir, 1989). Most students with language impairment have difficulty making friends, as they are not as likely to be selected as partners in social situations (Rice, 1993).

There is some agreement that the following factors should be excluded in defining SLI: peripheral hearing loss, neuromuscular disabilities, emotional disturbance, and mental deficiency. There is also some agreement concerning the requirement that there be a discrepancy between actual language and expected language. However, there is no consensus regarding how this discrepancy should be established.

Despite the fact that they constitute a heterogeneous group, it is possible to delineate a set of language difficulties that are common to the majority of children labeled STI (see Table 3.3). Most do not speak their first words until age 2, do not combine words until age 3, and demonstrate a mild to moderate deficit in a range of language areas (Leonard, 1990).

As there is lack of consensus as to a precise definition of SLI, there are also differences of opinion as the underlying problem. Some have suggested that the mechanisms of language acquisition are impaired by an inability to process the incoming stream of speech (e.g., Tallal & Piercy, 1973). Others suggest that a language impairment represents the low end of the normal continuum of linguistic aptitude, not a different set of skills (e.g., Leonard, 1998). This view considers children with SLI as simply less skillful when it comes to mastering the complexities of language, rather than "disabled."

Motor Disabilities

Two of the IDEA disability categories include children with motor disabilities: orthopedic impairments and multiple disabilities.

Orthopedic Impairments

Many special educators and state and local educational agencies use the term *physical disabilities* for children with orthopedic

TABLE 3.3   Language difficulties associated with specific language impairment

Language Dimension	Difficulties
Phonology	Failure to capitalize on regularities across words Slow development of phonological processes Unusual errors across sound categories
Morphology/Syntax	Co-occurrence of more mature and less mature forms Fewer lexical categories per sentence than peers More grammatical errors than peers Slow development of grammatical morphemes Many pronoun errors
Semantics	Delayed acquisition of first words Slower rate of vocabulary acquisition Less diverse repertoire of verb types
Pragmatics	Intent not signalled through linguistic means Difficulty gaining access to conversations Less effective at negotiating disputes Less use of the naming function Difficulty tailoring the message to the listener Difficulty repairing communication breakdowns

impairments. The IDEA definition for this category is a severe orthopedic impairment

> *that adversely affects a child's educational performance. The term includes impairments caused by congenital anomaly (e.g., clubfoot, absence of some member, etc.), impairments caused by disease (e.g., poliomyelitis, bone tuberculosis), and impairments from other causes (e.g., cerebral palsy, amputations, and fractures or burns that cause contractures)* (Federal Register, *1999*).

There are two common classifications of physical disabilities: neurological and musculoskeletal. Neurological disabilities are caused by or related to the nervous system (e.g., spina bifida, cerebral palsy). Musculoskeletal disabilities are caused by or related to the muscles and skeleton (e.g., muscular atrophy). It is not difficult to understand why virtually all children with motor disabilities caused by damage to the brain or spinal cord experience problems with speech and language. Speech requires motor planning and precise and complex coordination of breathing, sound production, and articulation. Language requires complex and integrated brain function.

Imagine a continuum of motor involvement. The intellectual functioning of many of the children on this continuum will be within or above the normal range. Others, particularly many at the severe motor involvement end of the continuum, will demonstrate severe to profound retardation. Most children with minimal damage to the neuromotor system (at one end of the continuum) and many children with severe involvement (at the other end of the continuum) will learn to produce functional speech. Those who cannot use speech need to learn and use augmentative and alternative communication systems (see Chapter 13).

The condition that accounts for the largest percentage of students with motor disabilities is cerebral palsy. Cerebral palsy is an umbrella term for any disorder of movement or posture that results from a nonprogressive abnormality (either damage or disease) to the immature brain. Some children with cerebral palsy have only very minimal fine motor coordination problems; others are affected to the extent that they cannot move without assistance. Many children with cerebral palsy also have other disabilities such as retardation and sensory impairments. Students with severe and/or multiple disabilities are served in the category multiple disabilities.

A term that is often used in reference to the speech of children with cerebral palsy is **dysarthria.** Dysarthria is a group of related speech disorders that result from disturbed voluntary control over the speech mechanism. It includes impairment in the motor processes of respiration, phonation, articulation, and resonance. At the broadest level, dysarthria is a disturbance of motor function caused by damage to the nervous system. Children with dysarthria cannot speak with normal muscular speed, strength, precision, or timing because they cannot coordinate their resonation, articulation, and respiration mechanisms. In some children with cerebral palsy, dysarthria is relatively mild; in others it is so severe that speech is virtually unintelligible. Dysarthria should not be confused with **apraxia,** a neurological, phonologic disorder resulting from sensorimotor impairment of the capacity to select, program, or execute the positioning of the speech muscles for speech sound production. It affects the ability to *plan* speech movements. In apraxia, the speech mechanisms are functioning, but the child cannot get them to operate properly.

The type and extent of the speech, language, and communication difficulties of children with cerebral palsy depend on the degree of involvement of the neuromuscular system and the child's unique complex of associated disorders (i.e., sensory and perceptual impairments, retardation, seizures). However, there are some speech problems that are associated with specific types of cerebral palsy. Children with a general pattern of spasticity (high muscle tone with tight, stiff, and overactive muscles) typically demonstrate slow, labored speech.

Children with what is called an athetoid pattern (fluctuating muscle tone with uncontrolled writhing movements) tend to have jerky speech. Children with an ataxic pattern (awkward and clumsy, poorly controlled movements) have a tremorous, quavering voice.

Multiple Disabilities

Students with multiple disabilities are those who have

> *concomitant impairments (such as mental retardation-blindness, mental retardation-orthopedic impairment, etc.), the combination of which causes such severe educational problems that they cannot be accommodated in special education programs solely for one of the impairments. The term does not include deaf-blindness* (Federal Register, *1999*).

Another IDEA regulation, related to programs and services, defines children with severe disabilities as

> *children who, because of the intensity of their physical, mental, or emotional problems, need highly specialized education, social, psychological, and medical services in order to maximize their full potential for useful and meaningful participation in society and for self-fulfillment* (Federal Register, *1999*).

Notable characteristics of students with severe and multiple disabilities are (1) they have severe impairments in intellectual functioning, (2) they have two or more disabilities, and (3) they require intensive levels of support across all adaptive skill areas and all environments. Most have both sensory and motor impairments (Chapters 12 and 13 deal extensively with assessment and intervention approaches for students with multiple and severe disabilities).

Sensory Impairments

An impairment or limitation of any of the senses—auditory, visual, tactile, olfactory, or gustatory—deprives the child of critical information about the environment.

Hearing Impairment

Any loss or distortion of auditory input will have some effect on speech and language development but, as would be expected, children who are totally deaf have the greatest problems. The IDEA regulations define deafness as

> *hearing impairment that is so severe that the child is impaired in processing linguistic information through hearing, with or without amplification, and that adversely affects a child's educational performance* (Federal Register, *1999*).

The IDEA regulations define hearing impairment as

> *an impairment in hearing, whether permanent or fluctuating, that adversely affects a child's educational performance but which is not included under the definition of deafness* (Federal Register, *1999*).

Hearing loss may occur before or after birth. When it is present at birth the medical term for the condition is **congenital hearing loss.** When acquired later in life it is called **adventitious hearing loss.** More important from an educational perspective is whether the loss is prelingual or postlingual. If present at birth or before the child has learned language (around age two) the loss is called a **prelingual hearing loss.** A hearing loss that occurs after the child has developed language is called a **postlingual hearing loss.**

The three major categories of hearing loss are **conductive, sensorineural,** and **mixed.** Each has a different prognosis and a somewhat different effect on language and communication. Conductive hearing losses are due to abnormalities or problems associated with the outer or middle ear. The problem is usually a malfunction or blockage that prevents clear transmission of sound waves to the inner ear. Examples are impounded wax, infections in the middle ear, excess fluid in the eustachian tube, or interruptions in the middle ear bones. The primary effect of a conductive problem is loss of hearing sensitivity because the level of sound reaching the inner ear is reduced. Conductive impairments are usually amenable to medical intervention (removal of the blockage) or amplification (a hearing aid).

Sensorineural hearing loss is the result of damage or disease in some portion of the inner ear, auditory nerve, and/or the neural pathways. The signal may not reach the brain at all or may arrive in a highly distorted form. Usually sound impulses remain unclear and distorted even when amplification is provided. Medical and surgical procedures are of limited usefulness with this type of hearing loss.

Sensorineural hearing loss may be genetic in origin, or it may be caused by disease or injury before, during, or after birth. Genetic causes are thought to account for approximately 50 percent of all cases of severe loss (Northern & Downs, 1991). There are more than 50 genetic syndromes in which hearing loss may occur. Nongenetic causes of hearing loss include maternal rubella (commonly called German measles), meningitis, otitis media (middle ear infection), and congenital cytomegalovirus infection (CMV). (CMV is a viral infection in newborns that is transmitted through the placenta or picked up during the birth process.)

A mixed loss is a combination of conductive and sensorineural losses. The two exist simultaneously. There may be some benefits from amplification if the conductive loss is the greater; but, even then, the prognosis for sound discrimination is generally poor. In approximately half the population of students with hearing impairment, the cause or causes of the loss are not known.

Children who cannot hear speech cannot learn to produce it without special training. Relatively few children with *significant* hearing loss develop *normal* oral language comprehension and production abilities. Ultimately, how much hearing impairment affects a child's speech and language development will depend on

- the severity of the hearing loss
- age of onset of the hearing loss
- frequencies at which hearing loss is greatest
- age when loss was identified and intervention was initiated
- amount and type of intervention, and
- the child's communication mode (whether manual, oral, or combined).

The effects of hearing loss are most deleterious when the loss is severe and is present at birth or occurs shortly thereafter.

The interactive nature of cognitive, language, social, and motor development means that speech and language difficulties will invariably affect performance in other domains. Children have to learn to make more out of less information if whatever hearing they have is to be useful. Thus, in addition to a language interventionist and a special education teacher specialized in education for the deaf, the support team for students with hearing impairment will include an audiologist. The fitting of amplification as early as possible is critical.

Teachers are a major source of referrals for audiometric evaluation. Table 3.4 provides a list of physical and behavioral signs suggesting the need for audiometric evaluation. The professional primarily responsible for this evaluation is the audiologist. However, screening may be done by language interventionists and school or public health nurses because audiologists are not available in many school systems and all school systems do not have access to audiological services in the community.

Hearing is measured and reported in **decibels (dB),** which are a measure of the intensity of sound relative to a reference point. Zero decibels (0 dB) does not mean the absence of sound. Rather it is the point at which people with normal hearing can barely detect sound. Each succeeding number of decibels indicates some loss. The point at which an individual responds to sound 50 percent or more of the time is that person's hearing level, or *threshold of hearing.* Thus, the lower the threshold, the more acute or sensitive the child's hearing.

Once the child's hearing has been evaluated and described in decibels, it is possible to *estimate* the potential effect of the loss on speech and language acquisition. Estimates of potential effect are presented in Table 3.5. At this point the audiologist may recommend hearing aids. A **hearing aid** does not correct the loss and there is always

TABLE 3.4 Indicators for referral for audiometric assessment

Physical Indicators
  1. Frequent complaints of earaches and colds
  2. Discharge from the ears
  3. Complaints of buzzing or ringing in the ears
  4. Breathing through the mouth

Behavioral Indicators
  1. Does not seem to understand simple directions
  2. Fails to respond to questions
  3. Requests many word and sentence repetitions
  4. Frequently fails to respond when spoken to
  5. Inattention and daydreaming
  6. Articulation difficulties
  7. Voice problems
  8. Shows a preference for high- or low-pitched sounds
  9. Disorientation and confusion when noise levels are high

Source: "Working with sensorily impaired children" by R. F. DuBose, in S. G. Garwood (Ed.), *Educating young handicapped children: A developmental approach* (2nd ed., pp. 235–276), 1983, Rockville, MD: Aspen Publications.

TABLE 3.5 Relationship of degree of impairment to understanding of speech and language

Decibel (dB)	Effects
25–35 dB	Some difficulty hearing faint or distant speech and discriminating sound combinations.
36–54 dB	Understands conversational speech at 3–5 feet but may miss a significant percentage (as much as 50%) of class discussions. May demonstrate limited vocabulary and speech anomalies.
55–69 dB	Only hears/understands loud conversations and experiences difficulties with phone conversations and class discussions. Limited vocabulary and deficient in language usage and comprehension.
70–89 dB	May hear loud voices (about a foot from the ear) and may be able to identify environmental sounds and discriminate vowels (but not all consonants). Speech and language defective and likely to deteriorate (without therapy).
90 +	May hear some loud sounds but is more aware of vibrations. Relies on vision as the primary avenue for communication. Speech and language are of very poor quality and likely to deteriorate (without therapy).

some sound distortion. What an aid does is make sounds louder. Hearing aids may be worn behind the ear, in the ear canal, or built into eyeglasses. A child may have an aid in one ear or in both ears.

Another consideration after the audiological evaluation is completed is whether a cochlear implant would be helpful. A **cochlear implant** provides sound information by directly stimulating the functional auditory nerve fibers in the cochlea. This device has two parts: an internal part surgically implanted under the skin with electrodes inserted into the cochlea and an external part, which consists of a microphone, speech processor, and transmitting coil. There is come controversy about cochlear implants for children because of the surgical risks, the potential discomfort, and the belief of many individuals that deafness is not a disorder that should be "cured."

A third approach is assistive listening devices. With an **assistive listening device** (sometimes called an FM system) the child's hearing aid will only pick up sounds from a wireless microphone worn by the teacher. An advantage is that the assistive listening device can work better in noisy environments (as school environments tend to be). A disadvantage is that the microphone must be passed around to different speakers in group discussions and other group activities.

There is considerable controversy over how and where students who are deaf or severely hearing impaired should be educated. One side of this continuing debate argues that they should be educated to become as much like their hearing peers as possible; that the goal should be for them to live and participate in "normal" society. There is a fear that if children are taught a manual form of communication they will prefer it and never develop auditory and oral skills. Advocates of this position believe that students with severe hearing impairment should learn to read lips, use their residual hearing, and use speech. The other position is in favor of teaching children to use manual communication, either alone or in combination with speech. They disagree with the argument that children with severe hearing impairment should strive for the goal of "normalcy." Rather, students should be given the communication skills they need (in any form possible), oral, manual, and written. It also has been argued that children who learn American Sign Language are able to establish a language base, which is crucial in the early developing years. The foremost goal is integration into the world of work, and independence so that they can socialize with other persons with hearing impairments, as well as hearing peers.

Arguments concerning inclusion of children who are deaf or severely hearing impaired in general education classes parallel the oral–manual communication debate. One side argues that, while the inclusive classroom may offer maximum opportunity for interactions with peers who are not disabled, it provides few opportunities for communication and socialization with peers and adults who are deaf or hearing impaired. When adolescents who are deaf are asked to reflect on their experiences in public schools and schools for the deaf, they emphasize the importance of a social and cultural education as well as an academic education (Wilson, 1997). Further, they urge their peers to play a major role in their own placement decisions and make an effort to experience different placement options. The other side contends that placing students who are deaf or hearing impaired in carefully chosen general education classes with appropriate support services (e.g., note takers, interpreters, tutors) is academically and socially beneficial. This is borne out by research that reports increased achievement in both reading and mathematics for students in inclusive settings (Holt & Allen, 1989).

Visual Impairment

The IDEA definition for this category is

> *an impairment in vision that, even with correction, adversely affects a child's educational performance. The term includes both partial sight and blindness* (Federal Register, *1999*).

Most educators classify students with visual impairments according to their ability to use their vision versus the need to use tactile input. Students with **low vision** can generally read print, although they may depend on optical aids, such as magnifying lenses or other means to enlarge the size of the print. A few may read both Braille and print. They may or may not be legally blind. Students labeled as **functionally blind** typically use Braille for efficient reading and writing but they supplement their limited vision by using a combination of tactile and auditory learning methods. They may be able to depend on their functional vision for such activities as moving through the environment or sorting clothes by color. Those students who do not receive any meaningful input through the visual sense are **totally blind.** They are totally dependent on tactile and auditory input to learn about their environment and they read only Braille. Only about 1 percent of students receiving special education services are totally blind.

Students in this category are similar to those in the other disability groups in that they are a heterogeneous population. Some are gifted or have special talents while others have severe and multiple disabilities. They also vary with respect to type of visual disorder, degree of visual limitation, and extent to which the reduced visual capacity interferes with daily functioning. The one commonality among these students is that their visual impairment creates a barrier to learning. How much of a barrier depends on age of onset, degree of vision loss, etiology of the visual impairment, and the presence of other disabilities.

Delayed cognitive development and difficulties with social interactions are the major contributors to the language delay observed in infants and very young children who are severely visually impaired. Unless the child has another disability, the delayed cognitive development is a result of restricted mobility, which limits experiences with objects and activities in the physical environment. Because incidental learning is limited, children blind from birth need special help to learn many concepts (including social skills) that are relevant to language acquisition.

There are remarkable similarities in the language of children who are blind and the language of their sighted peers. Like their sighted peers, they use "sighted" words such as *look*. By age 3 most have an MLU comparable to that of same-age peers (Landau & Gleitman, 1985). However, there are also some differences. In a longitudinal study of the language development of children with visual impairment, Orwin (1984) found limited naming or requesting and a heavy reliance on routine phrases and people's names. The children in this study did not refer to objects and events beyond their reach or touch and they rarely used function words (*there, more, no, gone*).

Limitations in the range and variety of experiences, mobility, and interactions with the environment have an impact on how students with visual impairment experience the world. Visual impairment can result in experiential and environmental deprivation, which, in turn, affects language. Because they lack the breadth of experiences of their peers without disabilities, children with visual limitations may learn the names for objects in their environment but not acquire words to describe object characteristics. In addition, they may provide detailed explanations of objects and events with little real understanding. Because communication is based on common experiences, both circumstances have an impact on social interactions. Another commonly observed consequence of severe visual impairment is the development of unusual mannerisms. Because children cannot observe their partner's distance away when communicating, they may speak too loudly, smile too often, and use eyebrow movements that appear inappropriate to what is being said.

Some children with visual impairment produce echolalic utterances. In one study, the percentage of echolalic utterances in the spontaneous speech of a 3-year-old was 20.7 percent with her mother and 35.7 percent with another adult (with whom she was not well-acquainted) (Kitzinger, 1984). Another consequence of visual impairment and not being able to move around in the environment is a sense of anxiety related to not knowing whether someone is watching or to whom someone is directing verbal or physical anger. A child with visual impairment will not know whether the teacher is reprimanding her or another student.

As is the case with children who have hearing impairments, teachers are a major source of referrals for children with mild to moderate visual impairment. Table 3.6 provides a list of physical and behavioral signs suggesting the need for referral for visual assessment.

TABLE 3.6 Indicators for referral for vision assessment

Physical Indicators
  1. Crossed eyes
  2. Watery or inflamed eyes
  3. Recurring sties
  4. Red, swollen, or encrusted eyelids
  5. Dizziness, nausea, and frequent headaches

Behavioral Indicators
  1. Frequent rubbing of the eyes
  2. Tilting the head when looking at printed materials
  3. Holding material close to the face
  4. Squinting and/or frowning
  5. Shutting or covering one eye when looking at printed material
  6. Complaints about being unable to see distant objects

The best estimates suggest that approximately one student in a thousand has a visual disorder that interferes with learning. Visual impairment accounts for less than 0.5 percent of the total special education population (U.S. Department of Education, 1999). Most students with visual impairment attend general education classes with their sighted peers.

Behavior Disorders and Autism

Our inclusion of language difficulties associated with behavior disorders and those associated with autism in the same section does not suggest a relationship between the cause (or causes) or the characteristics of the language difficulties exhibited by children with behavior disorders and those of children with autism. The one commonality between the two groups is that the language difficulties of both are poorly understood.

Emotional Disturbance

The area of serious emotional disturbance, sometimes called *behavior disorders,* tends to be a catch-all category for myriad child behaviors that are disturbing to adults, such as defiance, aggression, self-stimulation, depression, destructive behavior, social withdrawal, and noncompliance. The IDEA definition for emotional disturbance is virtually the same as the definition in the original legislation:

> *a condition exhibiting one or more of the following characteristics over a long period of time and to a marked degree that adversely affects a child's educational performance:*
>
> *(A) An inability to learn that cannot be explained by intellectual, sensory, or health factors.*
>
> *(B) An inability to build or maintain satisfactory interpersonal relationships with peers and teachers.*

(C) Inappropriate types of behavior or feelings under normal circumstances.

(D) A general pervasive mood of unhappiness or depression.

(E) A tendency to develop physical symptoms or fears associated with personal or school problems.

The term includes schizophrenia. The term does not apply to children who are socially maladjusted, unless it is determined that they have an emotional disturbance (Federal Register, *1999*).

This definition specifies three conditions that must be met: chronicity (the behavior must occur over a long period of time); severity (the behavior must occur "to a marked degree"); and difficulty in school (the behavior must adversely affect educational performance). The dissatisfaction with this definition expressed by many professionals is related to the fact that such terms and phrases as "normal," "over a long period of time," "to a marked degree," "adversely affect educational performance," and "satisfactory interpersonal relationships" are not quantifiable (Kauffman, 1993).

It is virtually impossible to determine with any certainty the cause of students' emotional or behavioral disorders. Possible contributors include biological causes, environmental factors, genetics, living conditions (e.g., poverty, single-parent households), and child abuse.

Given the characteristics of this disability, it is not surprising to find that many children (at least 50 to 60 percent) in this group have speech, language, and communication difficulties (e.g., Baltaxe & Simmons, 1990; Ruhl, Hughes, & Camarata, 1992). Children referred for speech/language evaluations have a higher rate of emotional/behavior problems than the noncommunication disordered population and, vice versa, children labeled as behavior disordered or emotionally disturbed have higher rates of communication disorders. One study, which looked at 38 children (8- to 12-year-olds) with mild to moderate behavior disorders, found an incidence of 71 percent of communication problems (Camarata, Hughes, & Ruhl, 1988). Another study, which reviewed the histories of ten children with prepubertal onset of schizophrenia found that all had a language delay, communication disorder, or learning and school problems prior to the appearance of their psychiatric disorder (Baltaxe, Russell, Simmons, & Bott (1987). The same study found language delay, communication disorder, or learning and school problems in three quarters of the children with prepubertal onset of schizotypal personality disorder. Language assessment (morphology, syntax, semantics) of thirty students (ages 9 to 16 years) labeled as having behavior disorders by Ruhl and colleagues (Ruhl et al., 1992) indicated (1) difficulty understanding and producing complex sentences; (2) delayed semantic functioning; and (3) delayed grammatical skills.

Autism

The terms *autism spectrum disorders* (ASDs) and *pervasive develop-ment disorder* (PDD) are used to refer to the wide spectrum of neu-rodevelopmental disorders. These terms are used to describe a cluster of five disorders that have their onset in childhood. The five disorders are (1) autistic disorder (autism), (2) Rett's disorder, (3) childhood dis-integrative disorder, (4) Asperger's syndrome, and (5) pervasive de-velopmental syndrome (not otherwise specified). These students share three major characteristics: They have impairments in social in-teraction, nonverbal and verbal communication, and restricted and repetitive patterns of behavior (American Psychiatric Association, 1994), each of which can occur at different levels of severity.

Autism, the most severe of the five disorders, is also differentiated from the other disorders by the number of domains affected. In 1991, Congress made autism a separate disability category. The IDEA defin-ition of autism considers a broad range of characteristics: (1) language development, (2) social interaction, (3) repetitive behavior, (4) im-peding behavior, (5) the need for environmental predictability, (6) sensory and movement disorders, and (7) intellectual functioning. Autism is defined as:

> *a developmental disability significantly affecting verbal and nonver-bal communication and social interaction, generally evident before age 3, that adversely affects a child's educational performance. Other characteristics often associated with autism are engagement in repet-itive activities and stereotyped movements, resistance to environmen-tal change or change in daily routines, and unusual responses to sensory experiences. The term does not apply if a child's educational performance is adversely affected primarily because the child has an emotional disturbance* (Federal Register, *1999*).

After many years of searching for causal factors, there is now con-sensus that autism is a neurological disorder that is probably caused by a number of biological defects (Akshoomoff, 2000). Approximately 65 percent of persons with autism have abnormal brain patterns and most have unusually high levels of serotonin, a neurotransmitter and natural opiate (Schreibman, 1988). Autopsies of persons with autism show abnormalities in the cerebellum, the section of the brain that regulates incoming messages, and in the cerebral cortex (Courchesne, 1987). Although there have been great advances in identifying neuro-logical abnormalities that are fairly consistent across individuals with autism, the disorder remains one that is heterogeneous in terms of etiology, neurobiology, and behavioral abnormalities.

Current research indicates that children with autism can be iden-tified as early as 18 months of age. Some of the behaviors to look for include (1) the lack of or a delay in pointing behavior; (2) hand lead-ing rather than pointing; (3) lack of joint attention and symbolic play;

(4) not showing objects to others; (5) lack of eye gaze with others; (6) fewer than five words at 24 months of age; (7) unusual hand or finger movements; (8) not attending to the source of sound; and (9) not wanting to touch others (Prelock, 2001).

While autism occurs in children at all levels of intellectual functioning (from gifted to profoundly mentally retarded), approximately two thirds of individuals with autism have been described as having intellectual impairments on the basis of their performance on standard IQ tests (DeMyer, 1975). The majority of these are categorized as having mental retardation (Gillberg, 1991).

At least 50 percent of children with autism have some functional speech and language abilities (Lord & Paul, 1997) but still they are likely to use challenging behaviors (e.g., self-injurious behavior, aggression, tantrums, stereotypical behaviors) rather than speech or language to get attention, escape a task or activity, protest changes, or regulate social interactions. They seem to use such repetitive, rhythmic actions as rocking, twirling objects, and waving fingers in front of the face to communicate boredom and agitation or, perhaps, to achieve some type of self regulation (Helmstetter & Durand, 1991; LaVigna & Donnellon, 1986). Self-injurious behaviors exhibited by children with autism include head banging, biting, and scratching. Students who demonstrate severe forms of these behaviors may permanently injure themselves. Aggressive behaviors are similar to self-injurious behaviors except that they are directed toward others. It is important to note that students with autism are much less likely to engage in any of these challenging behaviors when they are involved in preferred and meaningful activities.

The language abilities of children with autism range from total absence of speech to language and communication that is generally adequate in terms of phonological and grammatical form but disordered from the perspective of semantic and pragmatic skills (e.g., poor eye contact, poor observance of the rules for referencing old and new information) (Prizant, Wetherby, & Rydell, 2000). Much of the language research with these children has focused on communicative and symbolic abilities. Greenspan and Wieder (1997) reviewed the records of 200 children who received treatment and were followed for at least two years. The children were diagnosed between 22 months and 4 years of age. Ninety-six percent showed significant receptive language deficits (difficulties understanding single words and simple directions). Sixty-eight percent of the children had not used complex gestures involving chains of reciprocal interactions (e.g., taking a caregiver to the door and motioning to go outside) prior to age 2. Table 3.7 provides an overview of the language difficulties associated with autism.

Wetherby, Prizant, and Hutchinson (1998) compared the developmental profiles of children with ASD with children with delayed

TABLE 3.7   Language difficulties associated with autism

Language Dimension	Difficulties
Phonology	Difficulty with expressive prosody (e.g., fluctuations in vocal intensity, monotonous pitch, tonal contrasts inconsistent with the meanings expressed)
Morphology/Syntax	Confusions of pronominal forms (e.g., gender confusion [*he* for *she* or *it*], case substitution [*him* for *he*], first- and second-person singular forms [*you* for *I* or *me*]) Use of less complex sentences than peers
Semantics	Word-finding problems Inappropriate answers to questions
Pragmatics	Limited range of communicative functions Difficulty initiating and maintaining a conversation Few gestures Failure to make eye contact prior to or during communicative interactions Preference to follow rather than lead in a conversation Engaging of potential communication partners at a level that requires little actual sharing

language (DL) who were at the same language stage. The ages of the children ranged from 17 to 60 months. The two groups had distinctly different profiles of relative strengths and weaknesses. The children with DL had relative strengths in communicative functions, reciprocity, social-affective signaling, and symbolic behavior and relative weaknesses in vocal and verbal means. While similar to the DL children in vocal and verbal communication means, the children with ASD demonstrated substantially poorer scores in communicative functions, gestural communicative means, reciprocity, social-affective signaling, and symbolic behavior. Their strengths were in behavior regulation and constructive play. Correlational findings from this study pointed to three clusters of impairments that characterized these young children: (1) joint attention, (2) symbolic play, and (3) social-affective signaling.

Some students with autism never develop sufficient speech for oral communication to be a functional communication mode. The majority of these children will use an augmentative and alternative system (e.g., manual language, technology-assisted communication, communication boards) as described in Chapter 13.

Echolalia is a form of communication often observed in children with autism. Echolalia (repeating a portion of the speaker's utterance) may be immediate (an exact repetition produced within seconds) or delayed (an approximation produced some time after the original utterance). Adopting a developmental perspective helps us get a better understanding of ecolalia and other forms of unconventional verbal behavior observed in children with autism (Prizant & Rydell, 1993). (*Unconventional verbal behavior* in this context refers to signals that are not shared or understood by the social community.) Their early speech may be predominately echolalic and serve only limited communicative functions (Prizant & Rydell, 1984). For example, a child might use echolalia to gain an adult's attention, to indicate a lack of understanding, or to fill a conversational turn.

With development in social-cognitive and linguistic areas, echolalic speech comes to be used for a greater variety of communicative functions and more creative language patterns also emerge. As the children learn a more rule-governed and generative linguistic system, echolalic speech decreases and speech repetition becomes more flexible and less rigid. Many children progress to creative and spontaneous language. Echolalia does not completely disappear in these children. However, it is only observed during states of confusion and fatigue or during highly stressful adult-directed interactions when it seems to serve the function of conversational turn-taking. For other children, patterns of echolalia and other forms of unconventional verbal behavior may not change.

Children with autism also appear to lack intersubjectivity—the recognition that another person has a point of view—and they rarely show an interest in objects or activities that can be mutually shared (Kasari, Sigman, Yirmiya, & Mundy, 1993). Their lack of responsiveness to other people is pervasive. Most avoid eye contact or other forms of interaction with others, even when they are hurt or upset (Schreibman, Koegel, Charlop, & Egel, 1990). They voluntarily spend a disproportionate amount of time alone, developing a strong attachment to particular objects (Mundy, Sigman, & Kasari, 1990). Children with autism appear to be impaired in their ability to understand and interpret social cues accurately: They seem totally lacking in the ability to identify what others think and feel (Wing, 1988). The gestures and expressions that are an integral part of human communication are confusing and lack meaning. Additionally, they have deficits in joint attention, shared affect, and symbolic play, all of which are strongly associated with development of language and communication abilities.

Stimulus overselectivity, the tendency to attend to and focus on a small, often irrelevant subset of stimuli, is another contributor to the language difficulties of children with autism (Kauffman, 1993). Deriving meaning and sense from an array (whether features of a single object or the multiple aspects of an array) requires the child to perceive and organize the parts into a cohesive whole. This is virtually impossible for the child with stimulus overselectivity. When presented with a complex array of objects or object features, he focuses on and responds to only one aspect of that array or a particular set of cues to the exclusion of all others. To acquire meaningful language, a child needs to hear the word representing a concept while simultaneously experiencing the labeled object, relation, or event. Because the tendency for stimulus overselectivity is evident with both auditory and visual stimuli, it hinders these visual-auditory associations. Stimulus overselectivity also affects social learning. The child can easily miss nonverbal social cues because of preoccupation with what is being said, or may miss what is being said because of attending exclusively to the speaker's facial expressions. Thus, overselectivity interferes with both concept development, the association of labels with objects and events, and social learning, all of which are necessary for language learning.

Asperger Syndrome

Increasingly, preschool and school-age children are being diagnosed with Asperger Syndrome (AS). Characteristics of AS include impairment in social interaction skills, repetitive behavior patterns, yet no cognitive or language delays in areas other than pragmatics. The pragmatic profiles of children with AS include significant problems with social interactions, in particular with peers. Eye contact is variable and unique repetitive patterns such as spinning or hand-flapping may be present in the preschool years. Children with AS have difficulty taking the perspective of the listener in their interactions and frequently misread social cues. They have tremendous difficulty forming bonds and friendships with other children. These children can be found at the extremes of interaction with some being very shy and undemanding and others being verbally aggressive and belligerent. Prosody also has been reported to be problematic, characterized by flat intonation.

Church, Alisanski, and Amanullah (2000) followed forty children with AS from 3 to 15 years of age. They found that many children with AS were not identified as needing special services as preschoolers; however, most parents reported that they were very concerned with their child's social skills. By elementary school, 96 percent of the children were receiving speech and language services for their pragmatic problems. In addition to their severe problems with social skills and pragmatic skills, many children with AS show delays in motor development and may have been referred to as clumsy or awkward. AS appears to be more prevalent in males and there appears to be a familial pattern present.

The Committee on Educational Interventions for Children with Autism proposes that services for children with autism should be intensive (at least twenty-five hours per week) and year-round. Prelock (2001) presents guidelines for best practices when working with children with ASD based on the work of Prizant and Rubin (1999) and Freeman (1997). Some of these include: (1) work at the child's developmental level and take into consideration each child's individual needs; (2) understand the theory behind interventions as well as any data-based reports that speak to the efficacy of a given intervention; (3) take into consideration the cultural values and the priorities of the family; and (4) use a functional approach to intervention.

Cognitive Difficulties

The fundamental role of social and cognitive functioning in the development of language and communication is most evident when these areas fail to develop at a normal rate. This section considers characteristics of children with mental retardation and characteristics associated with traumatic brain injury.

Mental Retardation

The IDEA defines mental retardation in terms of educational performance. Mental retardation is

> *significant subaverage general intellectual functioning existing concurrently with deficits in adaptive behavior and manifested during the developmental period that adversely affects a child's education performance* (Federal Register, *1999*).

The American Association on Mental Retardation's (AAMR) definition, published in 1992, places more emphasis on the interaction of a person's intellectual and adaptive behavior impairments with the environment.

> *Mental retardation refers to substantial limitations in present functioning. It is characterized by significantly subaverage intellectual functioning, existing concurrently with related limitations in two or more of the following applicable adaptive skill areas: communication, self-care, home living, social skills, community use, self-direction, health and safety, functional academics, leisure, and work. Mental retardation manifests before age 18* (Luckasson et al., 1992, p. 5).

In its most recent manual, the AAMR (Luckasson et al., 1992) goes beyond recognition of intellectual and adaptive behavior limitations and their effects to the importance of the person's environments and the impact of the environments on functioning. The importance of coordinated services and accommodations (*systems of support*) matched to the person's needs is emphasized. The manual sets forth these assumptions as essential to the application of the AAMR definition:

- There must be valid assessment that considers cultural and linguistic diversity as well as differences in communication and behavioral factors.

- Limitations in adaptive skills must occur in the context of age-appropriate community environments and be indexed to the person's individualized needs for supports.
- Recognize that specific adaptive limitations often coexist with strengths in other adaptive skills or other personal capabilities.
- Life functioning will generally improve if the person is provided with appropriate supports over a sustained period of time.

Under the 1992 AAMR diagnostic and classification system we no longer make distinctions between mild, moderate, severe, or profound retardation. Instead, the individual is described using a multidimensional assessment approach. After assessing the student's intellectual and adaptive skills, and considering psychological/emotional, physical/health, and environmental factors, the team then considers what types of support the student needs. The AAMR describes four levels of support: intermittent, limited, extensive, and pervasive. *Intermittent support* is support that is provided on an "as needed basis." It may be high or low intensity and provided on an episodic or short-term basis. *Limited support* is characterized by consistency over time, and is time-limited but not of an intermittent nature. It generally requires fewer staff members and involves less cost than more intense levels of support. *Extensive support* is characterized by regular (usually daily) involvement in at least some environments. It is not, however, long-term living support. *Pervasive support* is constant, high intensity support that is provided across environment of a potentially life-sustaining nature. Pervasive support involves more staff and greater intrusiveness than the other levels of support. How intense an individual's systems of support should be depends on the person's needs in one or more situations. Types of support will vary across students and across skill areas for a specific student.

The cause of mental retardation is known only about 50 percent of the time. When it is known, it is usually rooted in biological processes (Coulter, 1992). The AAMR groups the biological causes of mental retardation into seven categories:

1. infection and intoxification (e.g., rubella, syphilis, maternal use of drugs or alcohol)
2. chromosomal abnormalities (e.g., fragile-X syndrome, Down syndrome)
3. gestation disorders (e.g., prematurity and low birthweight)
4. unknown prenatal influences (e.g., hydrocephalus, microcephalus)
5. traumas or physical agents occurring prior to birth, during delivery, or after birth (e.g., anoxia)
6. metabolic or nutritional problems (e.g., phenylketonuria [PKU], Tay-Sachs disease)
7. gross postnatal brain disease (e.g., neurofibromatosis)

The less severe the retardation, the less likely it is that a single cause can be specified. The majority of cases of mental retardation are the result of adverse psychosocial influences. Psychosocial causes can be categorized broadly into three subcategories: social, behavioral, and educational. Because the boundaries of these categories overlap, it is often difficult to isolate their effects. Mental retardation is frequently the result of complex interactions of multiple factors in all three subcategories. For example, teenage births are behavioral factors, but social factors (economic disadvantage) and educational factors (dropping out of school) complicate the picture.

While the label *mental retardation* does not describe a unique language pathology, it is safe to say that virtually all children with mental retardation experience some difficulties learning and using development language. Table 3.8 provides an overview of the language difficulties associated with mental retardation.

What is most helpful when working with children with mental retardation (as in working with other children with disabilities) is information concerning learning characteristics. Many of their learning problems are a consequence of learning strategy deficiencies or poor auditory processing.

- *Learning strategy deficiencies:* They lack the learning strategies necessary to benefit from their experiences, frequently overlooking cues that could help them solve problems and they generally fail to take outcomes of previous trials into account.
- *Poor auditory processing:* They typically perform poorly on tasks requiring auditory memory and problem solving and they fail to examine and evaluate their understanding of incoming messages.

TABLE 3.8   Language difficulties associated with mental retardation

Language Dimension	Difficulties
Phonology	Delayed development of phonological rules Problems with speech production
Morphology/Syntax	Production of shorter, less complex sentences with fewer subject elaborations or relative clauses Delayed morpheme development Delayed development of syntax
Semantics	Use of more concrete word meanings Slower rate of vocabulary acquisition
Pragmatics	Difficulty with speech–act developmemt Difficulty with referential communication Difficulty initiating and maintaining a conversation Difficulty repairing communication breakdowns

Cognitive impairments place strong constraints on many aspect of linguistic communication. However, the severity and pervasiveness of the language difficulties that a particular child with mental retardation experiences will be related to a host of factors other than cognitive limitations alone. These include sensory acuity, motivation, lack of social competence, and past instruction.

Traumatic Brain Injury

More than one million children and adolescents incur traumatic brain injury every year as a result of external physical force, such as a blow to the head received in an auto accident (Russell, 1993). A child who has suffered brain injury is likely to demonstrate:

- slowed processing and poor memory for new information and personal experiences;
- disorientation, confusion, and disorganization;
- problems with behavioral self-regulation and effective social interaction; and
- inconsistent performance (due to physical and mental fatigue) (Szekeres & Meserve, 1994).

The IDEA regulations define traumatic brain injury as:

an acquired injury to the brain caused by an external physical force, resulting in total or partial functional disability or psychosocial impairment, or both, that adversely affects a child's education performance. The term applies to open or closed head injuries resulting in impairments in one or more areas, such as cognition; language; memory; attention; reasoning; abstract thinking; judgment; problemsolving; sensory, perceptual and motor abilities; psychosocial behavior; physical functions; information processing; and speech. The term does not apply to brain injuries that are congenital or degenerative, or brain injuries induced by birth trauma (Federal Register, *1999*).

There are two types of brain injury that are not served under the IDEA's traumatic brain injury category. One is **anoxia.** Anoxia is brain injury from loss of oxygen to the brain. It may be an outcome of illness or an accident such as stroke, choking, or drowning. The other is brain damage from diseases such as meningitis or tumors. When students have brain damage resulting from these causes they are served in the Other Health Impairments category. The injury may be localized, confined to specific areas, or diffuse (spread over many brain regions).

In general, the smaller the damaged area, the better the prognosis for recovery. The damage is a result of nerve cell death. It may come about directly (a result of the cells being removed or lack of oxygen) or indirectly (a result of degeneration of nerve cell connections). Functioning after brain trauma depends on a variety of factors, including preinjury characteristics (e.g., age, intellectual functioning, educational and vocational levels, personality); location and severity of the injury; and postinjury treatment, support systems, and emotional and behavioral reactions.

Many students with brain injuries regain some of their speech and language abilities (DePompei, 1999). Expressive language seems to recover the most with receptive and written language difficulties continuing to be challenges. Acquisition of new concepts and vocabulary may be particularly troublesome (Lash, 2000). Some students experience acquired childhood **aphasia** for a period of time after the injury (Tyler & Mira, 1999). This disorder, which is associated with loss or disturbance of speech, language, and communication skills occurring after a period of time of normal language development, has the following characteristics: initial mutism followed by a period of reduced speech initiative; nonfluent speech output; simplified syntax; impaired auditory comprehension abilities; problems understanding language and following directions (Appleton & Baldwin, 1998). The language difficulties associated with traumatic brain injury are summarized in Table 3.9.

Because traumatic brain injury may affect children in any number of ways, they share characteristics with students with physical disabilities: health impairments, learning disabilities, mental retardation, emotional or behavioral disorders of speech, and language disorders. On the positive side, many children with traumatic brain injury show significant improvement in skills as the injury heals or the brain learns to bypass the damaged area. Improvement is typically most dramatic during the early stages following the injury.

Children with TBI are certain to demonstrate a range and variety of social, cognitive, academic, and language problems. Traditional

TABLE 3.9 Language difficulties associated with traumatic brain injury

Language Dimension	Difficulties
Phonology	Sound substitutions and omissions Slurred speech Difficulties with speech prosody (pitch, loudness, rate, and rhythm)
Morphology/Syntax	Deficits in syntactic comprehension Fragmented, irrelevant, and lengthy utterances Mutism immediately after the injury, followed by telegraphic production
Semantics	Small, restricted vocabulary Word-finding problems
Pragmatics	Difficulty with organization and expression of complex ideas Socially inappropriate and off-topic comments Less use of the naming function

wisdom suggested that the younger the child when the injury occurred, the better the prognosis. However, the picture may be more complicated than this. Although spontaneous and complete recovery following brain injury often occurs, a substantial number of children will continue to exhibit persistent cognitive and language deficits (Blosser & DePompei, 1992; Ewing-Cobbs, Fletcher, & Levin, 1985). Counter to conventional wisdom, some younger children experience more severe and persistent cognitive and language deficits following brain injury than either older adolescents or adults.

SUMMARY

After reading this chapter, three points related to the characteristics of students with language and communication difficulties should be patent: (1) the pervasiveness of language and communication disorders among children with disabilities (in all disability categories); (2) the challenges that acquisition of language and communication skills poses for children with disabilities; and (3) the heterogeneity of language abilities and disabilities demonstrated by children both within and across categories. We reiterate our cautionary note about labels: Labels provide little information about children's language intervention needs. They should be avoided to the extent possible in favor of explicit and comprehensive descriptions of the child's speech, language, and communication abilities and learning and behavioral characteristics. It is difficult to avoid labeling altogether, but recognizing the pitfalls in the use of disability categories can help us deal with the practice more intelligently.

Because the numbers of children with disabilities being included in regular education classes and other integrated environments continue to increase, language interventionists and teachers are realizing that they need more knowledge and expertise about all aspects of language and communication intervention, including augmentative and alternative communication. New responsibilities means new skills. As special and general education become more and more enmeshed, professionals see the need for skills related to team collaboration and problem solving, consultation, and peer mentoring.

The least restrictive environment (LRE) mandate of the IDEA states that school systems must educate students with disabilities, to the maximum extent appropriate for the individual student, with students who do not have disabilities. This is called the "presumption of inclusion." It cannot be set aside unless there is evidence that the student cannot be educated appropriately with students who do not have disabilities.

Schools may not remove a student from general education unless the student cannot be educated successfully there even when supplementary aids and support services are provided. The premise underlying the LRE principle is explained in this statement by Turnbull, Turnbull, Shank, and Leal (1995):

> *No matter what name you attach to the principle, its premise remains basically the same. When a state has a legitimate reason to intervene in a person's life (and educating its citizens certainly is such an interest), it must use the means that restrict the person's freedom to the least degree necessary to accomplish the state's purposes* (p. 106).

In the minds of many, the LRE translates to inclusion (e.g., Stainback & Stainback, 1990). Successful inclusion depends on the commitment of the entire school community from superintendents and supervisors to principals, teachers, ancillary staff, coaches, aides, students, parents, and families.

There is no intent to suggest that placement in general education classrooms means that the student never leaves the class. Inclusion advocates note that there is a significant difference between being "based-in" and "confined to" general education classrooms (Brown, Schwarz, Udvari-Solner, Kampschroer, Johnson, Jorgansen, & Gruenewald, 1991). "Based-in" means belonging, "being a member of." While a student may not spend all his time there, it is still *his* class and *his* classroom and "everyone knows it." "Confined to," on the other hand, is not flexible: It means "spending 100 percent of each day" in the regular classroom and not leaving unless one's classmates without disabilities leave. Such a lack of flexibility and responsiveness to individual needs would be inimical. How much time a student with disabilities should spend in the general education classroom depends on how much time it takes for the student to be considered a member of the class rather than a visitor. Only students who are engaged in meaningful, productive, and functional activities should spend most, if not all, of the school day there.

This textbook takes the position that the vast majority of students with disabilities can and should be educated in, and be members of, general education classes. We acknowledge, however, that inclusion will be successful only to the extent that students are provided with the supplementary services and supports they need (as specified in the IDEA). Our responsibility where inclusion is concerned is to prepare ourselves to provide appropriate curricula, instruction, supplementary services, and related services in the settings where they will most benefit the students.

DISCUSSION QUESTIONS

1. Discuss possible uses for Miller's list of the factors necessary for normal development of speech, language, and communication.

2. Discuss differences between descriptive classification systems and disability classification systems for language and communication difficulties. What are the advantages and disadvantages of the two types of systems?

3. Discuss commonalities and differences among children labeled as having learning disabilities, attention disorders, and specific language impairment. What are the effects (if any) of the differences on intervention?

4. Discuss differences between the five disorders clustered under the heading of autism spectrum disorders and the implications of the differences for intervention.

5. Assemble students into 4- or 5-member groups. Ask them to imagine that they are members of an interdisciplinary team that has just learned that the inclusive second-grade classroom in their school will have six new children on Monday of next week. The six children have the following labels, respectively: learning disabilities, severe motor disabilities, visual and hearing impairments, autism, and mental retardation. All have language and communication difficulties. The groups should describe the *specific* information they will need in order to plan for these children.

REFERENCES

Akshoomoff, N. (2000). Neurological underpinnings of autism. In A. M. Wetherby & B. M. Prizant (Eds.), *Autism spectrum disorders* (pp. 167–191). Baltimore: Brookes.

American Psychiatric Association. (1994). *Diagnostic and statistical manual of mental disorders* (4th ed.). Washington, DC: Author.

Appleton, R., & Baldwin, T. (1998). *Management of brain-injured children*. New York: Oxford University Press.

Aram, D. M., Ekelman, B. L., & Nation, J. E. (1984). Preschoolers with language disorders: 10 years later. *Journal of Speech and Hearing Research, 27,* 232–244.

Aram, D., Morris, R., & Hall, N. (1993). Clinical and research congruence in identifying children with specific language impairment. *Journal of Speech and Hearing Research, 36,* 580–591.

ASHA Committee on Language-Speech and Hearing Services in the schools. (1980, April). Definitions for communicative disorders and differences. *ASHA, 22,* 317–318.

ASHA Committee on Prevention of Speech-Language and Hearing Problems (1984). Prevention: A challenge for the profession. *ASHA, 26,* 35–37.

Baltaxe, C., Russell, A., Simmons, J. Q., & Bott, L. (1987, October). *Thought, language and communication disorder in prepubertal onset of schizophrenia and schizotypal personality disorders.* Paper presented at the Academy of Child and Adolescent Psychiatry, Washington, DC.

Baltaxe, C., & Simmons, J. Q. (1990). The differential diagnosis of communication disorders in child and adolescent psychopathology. *Topics in Language Disorders, 10*(4), 17–31.

Barkley, R. A., DuPaul, G., & McMurray, M. (1990). A comprehensive evaluation of attention deficit-disorder with and without hyperactivity as defined by research criteria. *Journal of Consulting and Clinical Psychology, 29,* 546–559.

Bashir, A. S. (1989). Language intervention and the curriculum. *Seminars in Speech and Language, 10*(3), 181–190.

Blosser, J. L., & DePompei, R. (1992). A proactive model for treating communication disorders in children and adolescents with traumatic brain injury. *Clinics in Communication Disorders, 2*(2), 52–65.

Brown, L., Schwartz, P., Udvari-Solner, A., Kampschroer, E. F., Johnson, F., Jorgansen, J., & Gruenewald, L. (1991). How much time should students with severe intellectual disabilities spend in regular education classrooms and elsewhere? *Journal of the Association for Persons with Severe Handicaps, 16,* 39–47.

Camarata, S. M., Hughes, C. A., & Ruhl, K. L. (1988). Mild/moderately behaviorally disordered students: A population at risk for language disorders. *Language, Speech, and Hearing Services in Schools, 19,* 191–200.

Church, C., Alisanski, S., & Amanullah, S. (2000). The social, behavioral, and academic experiences of children with Asperger Syndrome. *Focus on Autism and Other Developmental Disabilities, 15*(1), 12–20.

Cole, K. N., Coggins, T. E., & Vanderstoep, C. (1999). The influence of language/cognitive profile on discourse intervention outcome. *Language, Speech and Hearing Services in the Schools, 30,* 61–67.

Coulter, D. L. (1992). Reaction paper: An ecology of prevention for the future. *Mental Retardation, 30,* 363–369.

Courchesne, E. (1987). A neurophysiological view of autism. In E. Schopler & G. B. Mesibov (Eds.), *Neurobiological issues in autism* (pp. 285–324). New York: Plenum.

DeMyer, M. K. (1975). Research in infantile autism: A strategy and its results. *Biological Psychiatry, 10,* 433–540.

DePompei, R. (1999). Run a reverse left; Communication disorders after brain injury. *Brain Injury Source, 3*(3) 22–25.

Ewing-Cobbs, L., Fletcher, J. M., & Levin, H. S. (1985). In M. Ylvisaker (Ed.), *Head injury rehabilitation: Children and adolescents* (pp. 71–89). Austin, TX: PRO-ED.

Federal Register. (1992). Washington, DC: U.S. Government Printing Office, September 29.

Federal Register. (1999) Washington, DC: U.S. Government Printing Office, March 12.

Ferguson, D. M., & Horwood, L. J. (1992). Attention deficit and reading achievement. *Journal of Child Psychology and Psychiatry, 33,* 375–385.

Freeman, B. J. (1997). Guidelines for evaluating intervention programs for children with autism. *Journal of Autism and Developmental Disorder, 27,* 641–650.

Gerber, A. (1993). *Language-related learning disabilities.* Baltimore: Brookes.

Gibbs, D. P., & Cooper, E. B. (1989). Prevalence of communication disorders in students with learning disabilities. *Journal of Learning Disabilities, 29,* 60–63.

Gillberg, C. (1991). Outcome in autism and autistic-like conditions. *Journal of the American Academy of Child and Adolescent Psychiatry,* 30, 375–382.

Greenspan, S. I., & Wieder, S. (1997). Developmental patterns and outcomes in infants and children with disorders in relating and communicating: A chart review of 200 cases of children with autistic spectrum diagnoses. *Journal of Developmental and Learning Disorders, 1,* 87–141.

Hartsough, C. S., & Lambert, N. M. (1985). Medical factors in hyperactive and normal children: Prenatal, developmental, and health history findings. *American Journal of Orthopsychiatry, 55,* 190–201.

Helmstetter, E., & Durand, V. M. (1991). Non-aversive intervention for severe behavior problems. In L. Meyer, C. Peck, & L. Brown (Eds.), *Critical issues in the lives of people with severe disabilities* (pp. 559–600). Baltimore: Brookes.

Holt, J. A., & Allen, T. E. (1989). The effects of schools and their curricula on the reading and mathematics achievement of hearing impaired students. *International Journal of Education Research, 13,* 547–562.

Kanner, L. (1943). Autistic disturbances of affective contact. *Nervous Child, 2,* 217–250.

Kasari, C., Sigman, M., Yirmiya, N., & Mundy, P. (1993). Affective development and communication in young children with autism. In A. P. Kaiser & D. B. Gray (Eds.), *Enhancing children's communication* (pp. 201–222). Baltimore: Brookes.

Kauffman, J. M. (1993). *Characteristics of emotional or behavioral disorders of children and youth* (5th ed.). New York: Macmillan.

Kitzinger, M. (1984). The role of repeated and echoed utterances in communication with a blind child. *British Journal of Disorders of Communication, 19,* 135–146.

Landau, B., & Gleitman, L. (1985). *Language and experience: Evidence from the blind child.* Cambridge, MA: Harvard University Press.

Lash, M. H. (2000). *Resource guide: Children, adolescents, and young adults with brain injuries.* Wake Forest, NC: L & A Publishing Training.

LaVigna, G. W., & Donnellon, A. M. (1986). *Alternatives to punishment: Solving behavior problems with non-aversive strategies.* New York: Irvington.

Leonard, L. (1987). Is specific language impairment a useful construct? In S. Rosenberg (Ed.), *Applied psycholinguistics* (pp. 1–39). New York: Cambridge University Press.

Leonard, L. (1987). Language learnability and specific language impairment. *Applied Psycholinguistics, 10,* 179–202.

Leonard, L. (1990). Language disorders in preschool children. In G. H. Shames & E. H. Wiig (Eds.), *Human communication disorders* (3rd ed., pp. 159–192). Columbus, OH: Merrill.

Leonard, L. B. (1998). *Children with specific language impairment.* Cambridge, MA: MIT Press.

Lord, C., & Paul, R. (1997). Language and communication in autism. In D. Cohen & F. Volkmar (Eds.), *Handbook of autism and pervasive developmental disorders* (2nd ed., pp. 195–225). New York: Wiley.

Luckasson, R., Coulter, D. L., Polloway, E. A., Reiss, S., Schalock, R. L., Snell, M. E., Spitalnik, D. M., & Stark, J. A. (1992). *Mental retardation: Definition, classification, and systems.* Washington, DC: American Association on Mental Retardation.

Miniutti, A. (1991). Language deficiencies in inner-city children with language and behavioral problems. *Language, Speech, and Hearing Disorders, 55,* 665–678.

Miller, J. F. (1983). Identifying children with language disorders and describing their language performance. In J. F. Miller, D. E. Yoder & R. Schiefelbusch (Eds.), *Contemporary issues in language intervention* (pp. 67–74). Rockville, MD: American Speech-Language-Hearing Association.

Mundy, P., Sigman, M., & Kasari, C. (1990). A longitudinal study of joint attention and language development in autistic children. *Journal of Autism and Developmental Disorders, 20,* 115–128.

National Joint Committee on Learning Disabilities. (1994). Learning Disabilities: Issues on definition, a position paper of the National Joint Committee on Learning Disabilities. In *Collective perspectives on issues affecting learning disabilities: Position papers and statements.* Austin, TX: PRO-ED.

Nippold, M. A. (1992). The nature of normal and disordered word finding in children and adolescents. *Topics in Language Disorder, 13,* 1–14.

Northern, J., & Downs, M. (1991). *Hearing in children* (4th ed.). Baltimore: Williams and Wilkins.

Orwin, L. (1984). Language for absent things: Learning from visually handicapped children. *Topics in Language Disorders, 4*(4), 24–37.

Prelock, P. (2001). Understanding autism spectrum disorder: The role of speech-language pathologists and audiologists in service delivery. *The ASHA Leader, 6*(17), 4–7.

Prizant, B. M., & Rubin, E. (1999). Contemporary issues in interventions for autism spectrum disorders: A commentary. *Journal of the Association for Persons with Severe Handicaps, 24,* 199–208.

Prizant, B. M., & Rydell, P. J. (1984). Analysis of functions of delayed echolalia in autistic children. *Journal of Speech and Hearing Research, 27,* 183–192.

Prizant, B. M., & Rydell, P. J. (1993). Assessment and intervention strategies for unconventional verbal behavior. In S. F. Warrren & J. Reichle (Series Eds.) & J. Reichle & D. P. Wacker (Vol. Eds.), *Communication and language intervention series: Vol. 3. Communicative approaches to challenging behavior* (pp. 263–297). Baltimore: Brookes.

Prizant, B. M., Wetherby, A. M., & Rydell, P. J. (2000). Communication intervention issues for young children with autism spectrum disorders. In A. M. Wetherby & B. M. Prizant (Eds.), *Autism spectrum disorders* (pp.193–224). Baltimore: Paul H. Brookes.

Rice, M. (1993). "Don't talk to him; He's weird" A social consequences account of language and social interactions. In A. Kaiser & D. Gray

(Eds.), *Enhancing children's communication: Research foundations for intervention.* Baltimore: Brookes Publishing.

Ruhl, K. L., Hughes, C. A., & Camarata, S. M. (1992). Analysis of the expressive and receptive language characteristics of emotionally handicapped students served in public school settings. *Journal of Childhood Communication Disorders,* 14, 165–176.

Russell, N. K. (1993). Educational considerations in traumatic brain injury: The role of the speech-language pathologist. *Language, Speech, and Hearing Services in Schools,* 24, 67–75.

Rutter, M. (1978). Diagnosis and definition of childhood autism. *Journal of Autism and Childhood Schizophrenia,* 8, 139–161.

Schreibman, L. (1988). *Autism.* Newbury Park, CA: Sage.

Schreibman, L., Koegel, R. L., Charlop, M. H., & Egel, A. L. (1990). Infantile autism. In A. S. Bellack, M. Hersen, & A. E. Kazdin (Eds.), *International handbook of behavior modification and therapy* (2nd ed.) (pp. 763–789). New York: Plenum.

Siegal, L. S., & Ryan, E. B. (1984). Reading disability as a language disorder. *Remedial and Special Education* (RASE), 5, 28–33.

Snyder, L. S., & Downy, D. M. (1991). The language-reading relationship in normal and reading-disabled children. *Journal of Speech and Hearing Research,* 34, 129–140.

Stainback, W., & Stainback, S. (1990). *Support networks for inclusive schooling.* Baltimore: Paul H. Brookes.

Szatmari, P., Offord, D. R., & Boyle, M H. (1989). Ontario child health study: Prevalence of Attention deficit disorder with hyperactivity. *Journal of Child Psychology and Psychiatry,* 30, 219–230.

Szekeres, S. F., & Meserve, N. F. (1994). Collaborative intervention in schools after traumatic brain injury. *Topics in Language Disorders,* 15, 21–36.

Tallal, P., Curtiss, S., & Kaplan, R. (1989). *The San Diego longitudinal study: Evaluating the outcomes of preschool impairment in language development.* Final Report, National Institute of Neurological Communication Disorders.

Tallal, P., & Piercy, M. (1973). Defects of nonverbal auditory perception in children with developmental aphasia. *Nature,* 241, 468–469.

Tarnowski, K. J., & Nay, S. M. (1989). Locus of control in children with learning disabilities and hyperactivity: A subgroup analysis. *Journal of Learning Disabilities,* 22, 381–399.

Tomblin, J. B., & Records, N. L., Buckwalter, P., Zhang, X., Smith, E., & O'Brien, M. (1997). Prevalence of specific language impairment in kindergarten children. *Journal of Speech, Language, and Hearing Research,* 40, 1245–1260.

Turnbull, A. P., Turnbull, H. R., Shank, M., & Leal, D. (1995). *Exceptional lives.* Columbus, OH: Merrill.

Tyler, J. S., & Mira, M. P. (1999). *Traumatic brain injury in children and adolescents: A sourcebook for teachers and other school personnel.* Austin, TX: PRO-ED.

U.S. Department of Education. (1999). *Twenty-first annual report to Congress on the implementation of the Individuals with Disabilities Education Act.* Washington, DC: Author.

Vogel, S. A. (1977). Morphological ability in normal and dyslexic children. *Journal of Leaning Disabilities,* 10, 35–43.

Wetherby, A. M., Prizant, B. M., & Hutchinson, T. (1998). Communicative, social-affective, and symbolic profiles of young children with autism and pervasive developmental disorder. *American Journal of Speech-Language Pathology,* 7, 79–91.

Wiig, E. H. (1990). Language disabilities in school-age children and youth. In G. H. Shames & E. H. Wiig (Eds.), *Human communication disorders* (3rd ed.), (pp. 193–220). Columbus, OH: Merrill.

Wilson, C. (1997). Mainstream or "deaf school"? Both! Say deaf students. *Perspectives in Education and Deafness, 16*(2), 10–13.

Wing, L. (1988). The continuum of autistic characteristics. In E. Schoper & G. Mesibov (Eds.), *Diagnosis and assessment.* New York: Plenum.

CHAPTER 4

Families: The First Communication Partners

Nancy B. Robinson

In the previous edition of this book, this chapter stressed the importance of preparing professionals to work effectively with families in communication and language intervention programs with children. The importance of building partnerships with families of children with communication needs is even more critical now. In the United States and other countries, globalization of the population means that cultural and language diversity are increasing at unprecedented rates. As the population of the United States becomes increasingly diverse, professionals in education, special education, speech-language pathology, early childhood education and related fields are challenged to accommodate their services to meet the needs of families and children with diverse languages and perspectives on child-rearing and parent–child interaction. The importance of early language intervention was established based on the assumption that families interact with their children in a North American model with values placed on achievement of the individual child in a middle-class socioeconomic context. Assumptions that all families in the United States fit the above profile, practice similar child-rearing, and emphasize similar values were always in question. However, the rapid changes in population demographics that include families from many different Hispanic countries including Mexico and South America; Southeast Asia; China; the Pacific Islands; the Middle East; Africa; Eastern Europe; the former Soviet Union; and other locations throws assumptions of homogeneity out the window. Professionals in the area of language intervention with children are required to rethink established practices, reach out, and build effective partnerships with families of widely diverse cultural values, languages, and traditions.

The focus of this chapter is to prepare professionals to involve families in meaningful ways in the assessment and intervention process for their children with communication and language delays and disorders. Family members, in this instance, are defined as the people with primary responsibility for the full-time care of the child. The pervasive nature of communication, occurring throughout the child's day and in all environments, leads to the conclusion that communication and language intervention is most effective when strategies to support children to improve communication skills are generalized to the settings where they are most likely to interact with others. For young children, family members and primary caregivers are the first and most constant communication partners. As children grow and develop through the preschool, elementary, and adolescent stages, communication partners expand and increase to include peers, teachers, and community members. While children do eventually gain independence and family members play a less direct role in influencing the child's development, studies of long-term impacts on child development repeatedly document the lasting impact of early adult–child communicative interactions (Hart & Risely, 1995; Ramey, Campbell, & Ramey, 1999). For this reason, this chapter emphasizes working with families of young children with communication delays and disorders. While many of the principles and practices discussed have applications with family members of elementary age children, the primary emphasis is placed on working with families of infants, toddlers, and preschool children.

The reader will also note that the phrase "communication and language assessment and intervention" is used throughout the chapter to define the parameters of professional and family partnerships in this context. The choice of terms is limited to communication and language, omitting the term *speech*. The rationale for this decision is based on the literature, which describes effective approaches for families to facilitate more general communication and language skills in young children rather than specific speech or articulation skills. A further clarification is provided regarding the term *professional,* which is used to include any professional who works with children in the areas of communication and language intervention such as speech-language pathologists, special education teachers, preschool teachers, early childhood special educators, early intervention specialists, and so on.

This chapter is arranged in six sections. The first four sections provide guidelines for building partnerships with family members based on the following themes: (1) policy and practice; (2) family and cultural diversity; (3) effective language intervention strategies; and (4) emerging literacy research. In the final two sections of the chapter, strategies for applying guidelines for family partnerships are provided in the areas of communication and language assessment and intervention. Strategies are aimed to support professionals in working effectively with family members, who are the key agents to generalized changes in children's communication and language expression.

Paul and Simeonson (1993) have provided six principles to guide professionals in their work with families, and these are adopted for this chapter. Professionals in communication and language intervention with children are encouraged to develop:

1. an appreciation for the developmental course of the life of the family;
2. a central interest in the experiences of individual families;
3. respect for the cultural and linguistic background as an organizing framework for understanding families;
4. a focus on the ethical implications of all aspects of professional decisions that affect families;
5. a particular emphasis on the social and cultural complexity of providing care for and with families who have children with disabilities; and
6. a commitment to both sharing the vision of diversity and sensitivity to the spiritual and social lives of families.

Throughout this chapter, the above guidelines will provide the parameters and quality indicators for family and professional partnerships in communication and language assessment and intervention services with children.

POLICY PERSPECTIVES OF FAMILY INVOLVEMENT

The role of family members as key decision makers in services for their children is strengthened by policy and practice guidelines developed over the last decade. Professionals involved in the identification, assessment, program planning, and remediation of communication disorders are challenged to consider the broader context of family and community environments, with family members at the center of services and supports provided to their children with disabilities. The professional roles and skills that are emphasized in clinical training programs with children are not adequate to accommodate family involvement and support in all phases of services for children with special needs in communication and language development. Attributable largely to the influence of early intervention legislation (Part C of IDEA, 1997), a focus on family roles in the intervention process with children with special needs has emerged. A central focus on family roles is particularly appropriate when applied to children with communication and/or language disorders.

Roles of Family Members in Disability Programs: Changing Perspectives

Parents have always played a critical role in services provided for children with disabilities. Professional perceptions and understanding of parents' roles evolved in an ever-widening circle of awareness, with families at the center of the circle. The roles that family members played in historical developments related to services for their children were always a major force in the development of social policy and legislation for individuals with disabilities. Turnbull and Turnbull (1990) identified eight stages of development over the past seventy years in which professional concepts of parents and family members changed. Professional perceptions of parents and families moved from casting parents in the role of being in some way to "blame" for disability in the child to understanding parents as part of family systems with multiple roles and responsibilities. The historical views of professionals toward parents and families and changing perspectives to the present views are highlighted in Table 4.1. Professional awareness and knowledge of parent and family roles progressed in the past century from one of judging parents by professionals' standards to one of seeing parents and families as diverse systems that require different levels of support and resources to become full partners in the assessment and intervention process.

While current policies and practices with families are more supportive in involving families in flexible ways than in the past, stereotyped attitudes about parents are perpetuated and remain with many professionals today. Social change is uneven, particularly in established institutional practices. Models of service delivery that were created in the 1960s and 1970s, following significant increases in federal and state funds for services to people with disabilities, were largely based on medical intervention and rehabilitation approaches. For example, following World War II, the return of veterans with a range of severe physical, emotional, and intellectual disabilities prompted rapid increases in legislation, funding, and services for veterans. The rehabilitative approach to disabilities carried over to services for children and elderly people who also benefited from increased medical, educational, and social services in the 1960s (Paul, Porter, & Falk, 1993). Educational models, influenced by learning theory and principles, were strengthened through legislation passed in 1975, the Education for Handicapped Act, now known as the Individuals with Disabilities Education Act (IDEA). However, the schism between medical and educational approaches continues today.

Family-Centered Care: Policy and Principles

Recent changes in approaches to parent involvement for children with disabilities occurred through the notion of *family-centered care,*

TABLE 4.1   Historical roles assigned to parents of children with disabilities

Parents as the Problem Source	Prior to the 1930s, the *eugenics movement* was established through documented cases of familial patterns of mental retardation and delinquency over several generations. While the conclusions that parents caused "defective traits" in their children were faulty, laws were made that prevented people with mental retardation from marrying and having children.
Parents as Organization Members	From the 1930s until the 1950s, parent organizations were the primary advocates. Today's organizations have their roots in parent organizations of this period in history, including the Association of Retarded Citizens, United Cerebral Palsy, the National Society for Autistic Children, the National Association for Down Syndrome, and the Association for Children with Learning Disabilities.
Parents as Service Developers	In the 1950s and 1960s, parent organizations took on the development of direct services, because their children were unserved. The focus of early programs was primarily on educational services for children with disabilities who were excluded from public school and recreation, residential, and vocational programs for family members with disabilities.
Parents as Recipients of Decisions	During the 1950s through the 1970s, increased educational services were opened up to children with disabilities. With more professional training available to serve these children, parents began to take a more passive role in the education process. As more children entered specialized services, professionals were expected to make decisions and parents were expected to agree and appreciate the services provided.
Parents as Learners and Teachers	From the late 1960s until the 1980s, intervention programs with children were considered to be most effective when parents also helped in teaching. The success of Head Start to involve parents in "Parent Training" and follow-through with young children was generalized to mean that *all* intervention programs required parent training and parent-as-teacher components.
Parents as Political Advocates	From the late 1960s until the present, parents are recognized as effective legislative advocates for their children with disabilities. Parent advocacy led to increased state services prior to 1975. While parent advocacy was effective in the legal system in landmark court decisions regarding *appropriate education;* the role of advocate also takes a toll on parents and families.
Parents as Educational Decision Makers	In 1975, the passage of the Education of the Handicapped Act (PL 94-142) established the role of parents as decision makers regarding educational programs for their children with disabilities. The role and responsibility to act as decision maker meant that parents were required to participate in educational planning through the IEP. While the intent of the law was to provide for *active decision making,* this expectation is not realistic for every parent.
Parents as Family Members	From the 1980s until the present, awareness of the family as a *system* of interrelated relationships and responsibilities has influenced professional expectations of parents. The needs of every member of the family must be considered for meaningful partnerships to develop.

Adapted from Turnbull and Turnbull (1990).

a concept that shifts the focus of decision making from professionals to family members. The principles, policy, and practice of family-centered care are central to laws and regulations for early intervention services for children with disabilities from birth to three years of age (Part C of IDEA). For a more thorough discussion of family-centered care, the reader is referred to Shelton, Jeppson, and Johnson (1987), who outlined and defined eight guidelines for family-centered care in the design and implementation of early intervention services with infants and toddlers and family members:

1. recognition that the family is the constant in the child's life while the service systems and personnel within those systems fluctuate;
2. facilitation of parent/professional collaboration at all levels of health care including the care of the individual child; program development, implementation, and evaluation; and policy formulation;
3. sharing of unbiased and complete information with parents about their child's care on an ongoing basis in an appropriate and supportive manner;
4. implementation of appropriate policies and programs that are comprehensive to meet family needs, including financial and emotional supports;
5. recognition of family strengths and individuality and respect for different methods of coping;
6. understanding and incorporating the developmental needs of infants, children, and adolescents and their families into health-care delivery systems;
7. encouragement and facilitation of parent-to-parent support;
8. assurance that the design of health-care delivery systems is flexible, accessible, and responsive to family needs (p. 71).

The importance of family-centered care as a philosophy and approach to developing effective partnerships with families, in either medical or educational settings, has far-reaching effects on professionals' interactions with family members.

The most critical elements of family-centered care for communication and language interventions are understanding that: (1) children are part of family systems, and (2) effective interventions are built on positive relationships with individual families. Turnbull and Summers (1985) compared family-centered care to the "Copernican Revolution." Copernicus changed our conceptualization of the universe by placing the Sun, rather than the earth, at the center of the universe. The parents, professionals, and policymakers who advocated for family-centered care principles and practices changed our conceptualization of intervention programs. Rather than professionals at the center of the services system, making decisions about children and families,

families were placed at the center, with programs and services re-volving around them. Nearly fifteen years have passed since the first passage of legislation (PL 99-457) in 1986 to require family-centered practices in early intervention, subsequently reauthorized in 1997 as Part C of IDEA, and challenges for full implementation remain. One of the major barriers to the widespread practice of family-centered care is the need for professionals to become flexible and willing to forego prior agendas.

Family-Centered Care Practices in Communication and Language Intervention

The practice of family-centered care is based on knowledge of *family systems* theory, described by Turnbull and Turnbull (1990) as "viewing the family as a unique social system with unique characteristics and needs." When families are understood as interacting systems, one can appreciate the impact of roles and responsibilities of parents, siblings, and other family members on all parts of the system. For example, if the language interventionist recommends that a mother spend time each day to review vocabulary words with her child, this may mean additional time that is not available in the daily schedule. In order to follow through, the mother will have to give up something else, such as reading the paper or exercise. In subtle but significant ways, the practice of family-centered care requires that professionals work to-gether with family members to determine intervention activities that fit into the context of individual family life, needs, and preferences.

Family-centered approaches provide opportunities to establish positive relationships with families and to create interventions for their children that fit into natural settings where families and children live. Crais (1991) recommends that family-centered care begin when professionals can assume a supportive role to the primary caregivers in the family. Family members are encouraged to state their concerns and needs preferences about the child's communication delay or dis-order. Working together, family members and professionals then reach consensus regarding intervention approaches and goals. In order to build effective partnerships with families, Crais stresses the importance of professionals taking the first step to understand and accept family members' current perception of the child's communica-tion difficulties.

The approach suggested by Crais (1991) is based on a process of self-awareness. Several informal tools are available for this purpose and these include checklists developed by Shelton, Jeppson, and Johnson (1987) and others (Johnson, Jeppson, & Redburn, 1992; Ma-honey, O'Sullivan, & Dennebaum, 1990). Evaluation of personal views and program practices is useful for individuals in preservice training, professions, and program administration. An example of such tools for individual or group discussion is included in Figure 4.1. Challenges remain in putting family-centered care principles into practice, particularly in training professionals in clinical intervention and education settings to move from client- to family-centered practice, and from professional to family-driven services. Practicing professionals are faced with the opportunity to continually examine their personal and professional values regarding partnerships with family members and sharing decision making at all levels of services for children with communication delays and disorders.

FAMILY AND CULTURAL DIVERSITY

Like the changing roles of parents in services for children with disabilities, expectations of parents in language assessment and intervention are also changing. As discussed in the preceding section, a greater understanding exists about the multiple roles that parents play as caregivers, partners to a spouse, family members, and community members. In addition to a more sensitive approach to individual differences among families, better understanding exists among professionals of the role of the caregiving environment on early childhood developmental outcomes. Early intervention and education for young children with disabilities have demonstrated positive effects on developmental skills in both short- and long-term studies. Given the importance of the caregiving environment, the need to support parents to become optimal caregivers is compelling. However, if we are also to integrate sensitivity to differences among families, flexibility in professionals' expectations of family involvement is required. Rather than seeking consistently high levels of family involvement across families, other measures of effectiveness are needed. For example, critical outcomes are to provide services for the child that are perceived by family members as helpful and positive for the child and family. In order to enter into partnerships and to build positive relationships with families, professionals must accommodate changing social, economic, and cultural patterns of families in the United States and its territories and jurisdictions.

Children and Families at Risk

In a recent review of the status of children and families in the United States, the National Commission on Children (1991) identified increased environmental risks for children including poverty, homelessness, AIDS, random violence in urban centers, inadequate child care, and excessive work schedules for single parents. However, these trends are not new and not all are considered to have negative effects on children. The increasing numbers of divorced parents as

FIGURE 4.1 Building family and professional teams: How are we doing?

		Never	Some-times	Always		Change Needed?	
1.	Do we ensure that parents have ready, direct access to all members of the team?	1	2	3	4 5	yes	no
2.	Do we provide parents with frequent opportunities to review the appropriate-ness and effectiveness of the IFSP/IEP?	1	2	3	4 5	yes	no
3.	Do we encourage parents to request a meeting of the team whenever they feel it is necessary? Are such requests honored?	1	2	3	4 5	yes	no
4.	Do we offer parents the option of being present at all team meetings concerning their children or family?	1	2	3	4 5	yes	no
5.	Does the team provide a supportive, comfortable atmosphere in which parents are free to ask questions and discuss their concerns?	1	2	3	4 5	yes	no
6.	Do team members provide parents with information that is understandable, meaningful, and responsive to their needs?	1	2	3	4 5	yes	no
7.	Do we issue a standing invitation for parents to share information with other members of the team and with other parents? Is the information parents provide acknowledged and used?	1	2	3	4 5	yes	no
8.	Are team reports written in clear, understandable language (free of technical "jargon") that is meaningful to parents?	1	2	3	4 5	yes	no
9.	Does the administration provide support to include family members as active participants on the team (e.g., variable scheduling, baby-sitting, access to records)?	1	2	3	4 5	yes	no
10.	Is there administrative support for staff to learn new skills to support each other in building effective teams (e.g., continuing ed.)?	1	2	3	4 5	yes	no

Ratokalu & Tada, 1993. Adapted from Johnson, B. H., Jeppson, E. S., & Redburn, L. (1992). *Caring for Children and Families: Guidelines for Hospitals.* Bethesda, MD: Association for the Care of Children's Health.

well as the resulting increases in the numbers of children who live with a single parent at some time in their developmental years, are considered to have both negative and positive outcomes for children. Some of the impacts include less time for parents to spend with children, yet some children in families of divorce are found to be more independent and self-reliant when compared to matched groups of children in two-parent families.

The reported increases of violence and drugs in school settings leads to increased anxiety for parents about child survival through adolescence. Increases in the numbers of children living in poverty as a result of being homeless or having divorced parents, and the number of single mothers who live below the poverty line all contribute to complex and interacting environmental risk variables for child growth and development. Increased risk factors also add to the needs of these families for external supports through informal means such as churches, family, friends, and formal community organizations. For language interventionists who work with families of children with communication delays who also face numerous environmental risks, including poverty, awareness of family concerns and priorities for their children are ever more important. The challenges facing professionals include the design of appropriate communication and language intervention goals and strategies that fit the lifestyles of individual families. This may result in language intervention strategies implemented in homes, parks, shelters, or day-care centers, wherever families and caregiving adults most frequently interact with their children.

Family Life-Cycle Stages

Another critical factor that influences families and the resources available to them is the life-cycle stage. Given points in the life cycle affect family participation in the system of care or services for the child with disabilities. Turnbull and Turnbull (1990) described four life-cycle stages that influence family development and functioning: (1) early childhood; (2) elementary school years; (3) adolescence; and (4) adult living. Changes within the family during each of these stages influence the level of family involvement in the educational and service system for children with disabilities.

For example, families of very young children often have competing tasks to accomplish, including the establishment of the marital subsystem within the family as well as the parent–child subsystem. The major concerns for families during the early childhood stage involve negotiating roles as couples, as individuals, and as parents. The birth of a child with a communication disorder during this time adds additional stress to the family subsystem that is just becoming established. Parents are typically the ones to first report concerns if a child is not developing speech as expected. Parents are also the first to then take on additional roles and responsibilities to seek appropriate services for the child. Professionals can more effectively build relationships with young families if they are sensitive to possible impacts of the early childhood life cycle for individual families.

Subsequent life-cycle stages, including elementary school, adolescence, and adult living, pose unique challenges for families and individual members within families. Elementary school years are characterized by less intensive parent–child interaction and involvement as the child enters school and develops relationships outside of the family with peers and teachers. Adolescence continues the development of individual values and socialization, with peer networks and sexual development central in this process. Adult living is initiated as children leave their family home to take up independent lives in school or careers. Professional sensitivity to the life-cycle stages of individual families will enhance positive relationships with parents and family members around intervention with individual children.

Family Cultural and Linguistic Diversity

The increasing cultural diversity in the United States in the past decade, when people of Asian, Hispanic, African, Pacific Islander, and other non-White ethnic and cultural backgrounds have immigrated, affects professionals and service systems for families of young children. Current trends for increasing diversity in the United States are projected to continue with the eventual reversal of our concepts of "minority" and "majority" cultural and language groups. For example, over half of the population in the state of California was officially identified as Hispanic in the year 2000. Adler (1990) outlined challenges for educators, stating that professionals who provide communication and language intervention must meet the needs of non-native English speakers more than ever before. Adler further emphasized the need to address bilingualism and biculturalism directly, meaning that professionals recognize and value the primary cultural and language identity for families and children who seek special education and communication intervention supports and services. Policy guidelines throughout special education and related fields refer to the need for specific training at the preservice and inservice levels to provide professions with the appropriate skills for accommodating families and children of **culturally and linguistically diverse** backgrounds, referred to in current literature as CLD. The necessary attitudes, knowledge bases, and skills required to meet the needs of CLD populations is most commonly referred to as **cultural competence** (Cross, Bazron, Dennis, & Issacs, 1989). Cultural competence was initially described and developed as a conceptual and applied model for mental health services with multicultural clients by Cross et al. and subsequently adopted widely in policy, program, and practice guidelines for people with disabilities and family members. Cultural competence is defined by Cross et al. as "a set of congruent behaviors, attitudes, structures, and policies that come together in a system or agency, or amongst those individuals to work effectively in cross-cultural situations" (p. 18). The 1994 Amendments to PL 103-230, the Developmental Disabilities Assistance and Bill of Rights Act, defines cultural competence as follows:

> *The term* cultural competence *means services, supports, or other assistance that are conducted or provided in a manner that is responsive to the beliefs, interpersonal styles, attitudes, language and behaviors of individuals who are receiving services, and in a manner that has the greatest likelihood of ensuring their maximum participation in the program.*

In their model of cultural competence, Cross et al. identify five essential elements that contribute to the ability of an individual professional, agency, or system of services to become culturally competent:

1. accept and value diversity;
2. understand the role of culture in one's own life and show the capacity for cultural self-assessment;
3. understand and identify the dynamics of difference when cultures interact;
4. achieve a knowledge base about diverse cultures including understanding of the attitudes, values, history and communication patterns of diverse cultures among families and children served;
5. develop adaptations to service delivery that reflect an understanding of cultural diversity.

The authors of this model propose that the above elements are required to be present at each level of an organization, including policymaking, administration, and professional practice in order for families and children of CLD backgrounds to be served appropriately. Further, an individual professional's or agency's development of cultural competence is a process that requires progressive development across a six-point continuum of attitudes that range from cultural destructiveness (oppression of one culture by another), cultural incapacity (discriminatory practices), cultural blindness (one size fits all), precompetence (learning about diversity), cultural competence (adaptations for diversity), and cultural proficiency (includes diversity in services). The application of the cultural competence model to professional training and practice is perhaps best understood as a commitment to a long-term process of personal, professional, program, and policy change. Goode (2001) notes that:

> *There is no one method for getting started on the journey toward cultural competence—at either the individual or program/organizational*

level. Individuals and programs/organizations may embark on this journey at different points of departure with different estimated times of arrival for achieving specific goals and outcomes.

Students and professionals who work with families and children of CLD backgrounds may constantly ask themselves, "Am I being culturally competent?" Guidelines for professional training and the practice of cultural competence are plentiful in special education and related services, yet there is no standard set of competencies or skills to become culturally competent. There are several national organizations established to provide clearinghouse functions for cultural competence information, training, research, and services. The National Center for Cultural Competence (NCCC), located at the Georgetown University Child Development Center can be accessed through the Internet URL (gucdc.georgetown.edu/nccc). As with any Internet resource, the reader is cautioned to check for outdated information and to update resources routinely.

The scope of attitudes, knowledge, and practices needed to accommodate families and children of CLD backgrounds are just beginning to be defined. Jamison and Robinson (2000) reviewed cultural competence recommendations for professionals across several disciplines involved in disability programs and services, including psychology, nursing, special education, speech-language pathology, and social work. Through qualitative analysis, they identified nine thematic areas considered essential for professionals to effectively work with families and children from CLD backgrounds: (1) difference versus disorder; (2) cultural awareness; (3) assessment skills; (4) impact of ESL on language learning; (5) impact of culture on service delivery; (6) child-rearing practices; (7) family-centered care principles; (8) policy; and (9) advocacy. A synthesis of recommendations across disciplines was developed with a focus on speech-language pathology graduates. These findings are adapted in Table 4.2 to apply to all professions involved in communication and language intervention with young children.

Several authors (Anderson, 1991; Damico & Damico, 1993; Hanson, Lynch, & Wayman, 1990; Terrell & Hale, 1992) have stressed the importance of professional training and education to increase sensitivity to diverse cultures and traditions among newly immigrated groups for the purpose of improving multicultural services for children with disabilities. Anderson, in particular, emphasized the impact of culture on family roles and expectations for language development among young children, and advised professionals to recognize the limitations of personal beliefs and to learn about specific cultures that are most divergent from one's own frame of reference. Hanson, Lynch, and Wayman provided guidelines summarized

TABLE 4.2   Cultural competence knowledge and skill areas recommended in professions serving CLD families and children with communication delays and disorders

Cultural Competence Knowledge Area	Cultural competence skills the graduate will demonstrate (examples):
Difference/ Disorder	• The ability to differentiate between a communication difference and a communication disorder • The ability to identify features of the major dialects used within the state or region of employment
Cultural Awareness	• The ability to demonstrate respect and value for cultural differences • The ability to evaluate one's own personal cultural heritage and values
Assessment Skills	• The ability to implement nonbiased assessment procedures with English-as-a-Second Language (ESL) clients • The ability to work with interpreters, who have a variety of training and linguistic backgrounds, during the assessment process (e.g., professional interpreter, bilingual professional, family member)
Impact of ESL	• The ability to evaluate linguistic behaviors that might emerge with second-language acquisition • The ability to recognize bilingual code-switching in children learning more than one language or dialect
Impact of Culture on Service-Delivery	• The ability to understand the history of racial discrimination in the United States and its impact on the delivery of medical and educational services • The ability to account for cultural variables such as gender, age, educational status, diverse cultural backgrounds, and language that affect clinician–client interaction
Child-Rearing Practices	• The ability to understand diverse styles of family interaction and communication with children • The ability to understand child-rearing practices cross-culturally
Family-Centered Care	• The ability to understand how various cultures perceive a disability • The ability to gather family input regarding its definition and perceptions of the client's communication disorder
Policy	• The ability to understand federal and state laws and policies governing special education and related services for clients of CLD backgrounds • The ability to understand professional standards and policies governing individual discipline practices for services with clients of CLD backgrounds
Advocacy	• The ability to understand local, state, and national advocacy services individuals with communication disorders of CLD backgrounds • The ability to understand state and local procedures to obtain interpreter services for language assessment for individuals of CLD backgrounds

Adapted from Jamison & Robinson (2000).

below, to increase cultural competence in supporting families of young children with disabilities.

1. Determine the particular cultural and ethnic group with which the family identifies; for example, know the family's country of origin, its language, and the size of the cultural and ethnic community in the local area.
2. Identify the social organization of the cultural/ethnic community, including those organizations with leadership roles and related resources.
3. Describe the current belief system including its values, ceremonies, symbols.
4. Learn about the history of the ethnic group and current events that directly affect family life.
5. Determine how members of the community gain access to and utilize social services.
6. Identify the attitudes of the ethnic community toward seeking help.

The above steps can be applied in the assessment and intervention-planning process with families and children with language delays. As many authors have observed, assessment instruments are often biased in favor of native English speakers. In order to minimize test bias and to obtain valid information about the child's communication and language development status, building a relationship with families prior to assessment can increase the professional's knowledge of family expectations for the child's language development and other potential cultural and linguistic considerations to include in the assessment. Further, the need for an interpreter can be determined through contact with the family prior to beginning the assessment process. Pre-assessment contact with the family will provide a basis for building partnership and increase the professional's understanding of individual family concerns, values, and the degree to which the primary language or English is used at home. Specific areas to include in early contacts with family members who are responsible for the child's daily care are as follows:

1. the issue of deficit or difference, as the child may not be considered to have a language delay or disorder in the primary language;
2. information regarding resources available in the home to follow through on language development in English, i.e., asking about other English speakers in the home;
3. family resources and expectations of the child (including identifying the primary caregivers);
4. paralinguistic information about how the child communicates (including nonverbal communication).

Following the completion of assessment, the determination of appropriate intervention services requires team consensus with key family members as well as professionals in education, special education, and speech/language pathology.

Damico and Damico (1993) focus on the role of language in the socialization of children in a given culture. They suggest that differences in social practices across cultures also result in language development differences. In mainstream culture, children with cultural and linguistic differences may take passive roles as a result of differences in spoken language codes due to stigmatization, thus reducing social learning opportunities. Through involvement and discussion with family members, either through interpreter services or through direct communication with parents, professionals can learn individual families perspectives and expectations regarding young children's use of language and their ability to communicate.

Effectiveness of Early Language Intervention Strategies

For young children, communicative interactions occur most often within the context of the family. Research conducted over the past two decades (Snow, 1979; Snow, 1984; Snow & Ratner, 1984) established the importance of caregivers' communication with young children to influence social, emotional, and language development outcomes. Further, the effectiveness of early intervention is supported in studies of the relationships between positive parent–child interactions and later language development outcomes (Erickson & Kurz-Riemer, 1999; Girolametto, Pearce, Stieg, & Weitzman, 1996; Iacono, Chan, & Waring, 1998; Ramey, Campbell, & Ramey, 1999). Specific linguistic modifications found when adults talk to young children are raised pitch, slowed rate of speech, shortened phrase length, repetition, parallel talking, and simplified vocabulary (Snow & Ratner, 1984). Grieser and Kuhl (1988) reported findings that showed universal characteristics of adult modifications across languages, including Chinese, English, and German. These findings show that adults are keenly aware of the need to structure language input to young children as these modifications are made in a natural and consistent manner. The effect of motherese (the term is used broadly to include other family members and key caregivers) was reported to have variable effects in several studies in the 1980s. Positive findings of the effects of motherese included increased vocabulary and phrase length in the language of normally developing children (Kemler-Nelson, 1989; Weber-Olsen, 1984). More recently, investigators found limited results of motherese on the language development of young children with language delays (Hampson & Nelson, 1990; Kennedy, Sheridan, Radlinshi, & Beeghly, 1991). Individual differences among children with language delays and those who are typically developing were found to have a more significant effect on later language development than the language environment provided by adults.

Researchers who study *parent–child interaction* examined more comprehensive characteristics of adult responsiveness to young children that included the *rate* and *degree of directiveness* that parents use in the context of play and communication with their child. Many studies conducted in past decades led to the conclusion that parents of children with language delays may "work harder" and tend to use a faster rate and more directive communication styles with children who tend to be less responsive to adults (Field, 1983). However, in recent years researchers have reported that parents showed different styles of communication with young children with and without disabilities and that different adult styles were related to a range of variables that included the child's age, developmental level, and characteristics of the parents themselves that were independent of the child's ability to respond (Carson, Perry, Diefenderfer, & Klee, 1999; Girolametto & Tannock, 1994). For example, fathers were found to be more directive in their interactions with children, changing topics and taking more turns in conversation when compared to mothers. Further, the differences in parents' interaction styles continued throughout the early childhood years in one study of parents who reported that they were less "nurturant" to their children with language delays at age 5 to 6 years.

In spite of differences in parent interactions with children, the degree of *responsiveness,* or the adult's ability to recognize the child's behavioral cues and to provide contingent, appropriate, and consistent responses to those cues, is reported to make a difference for language development in young children (Wilcox, Kouri, & Caswell, 1990). The importance of research findings in parent–child interaction for language intervention professionals is the understanding that different adult styles are equally effective to support language development, but that consistent responsiveness by adults is key to expanding the child's understanding and use of language forms and functions.

Reported findings in studies of parent–child interaction yielded guidelines for professional intervention with family members and their young children with communication delays. Key findings that provide a framework for working with family members and other primary caregivers to provide optimal input for language development with young children include the following:

- Adults' positive interactions with young children convey positive affect and security to the child, thus building an environment that invites further interaction.
- Adults' interactions with young children provide "scaffolding" and encourage children to develop progressively advanced communication and language forms.

- Adults' interactions with young children are related to the child's subsequent development of social skills to interact with siblings and peers in multiple settings, such as home, day care, and preschool.
- Responsive interactions between adults and very young children are related to later communication and language development throughout the preschool and early elementary school years.

Parent–Child Interaction: Applications to Language Intervention

Recent methods of early language intervention are based on the finding that adult responsiveness is key to enhancing language development in young children (Johnson, Miller, Curtiss, & Tallal, 1993; Kaiser, Hemmeter, Ostrosky, & Fischer, 1996; Lee & Kahn, 2000; Warren, Yoder, Gazdag, Kim, & Jones, 1993; Yoder, Warren, Kyoungram, & Gazdag, 1994). Further, interventions with parent-implemented language intervention using naturalistic approaches have shown equal effects when implemented by parents in home environments compared to clinical interventions implemented by professional language interventionists (Eiserman, Weber, & McCoun, 1995; Elder, 1995; Kaiser, Hester, Alpert, & Whiteman, 1995). **Milieu approaches** to increase early communication and language skills include specific strategies for family members: **contingent imitation, responsivity, following the child's lead, linguistic mapping,** and **social routines.** The application of milieu approaches requires adults to focus on (1) elicitation of child communication using the above techniques; (2) provide language models in direct response to the child's focus of attention; and (3) embed the above techniques in naturally occurring routines throughout the child's day. Studies using milieu approaches with young children with language delays showed positive effects and increases in *intentional communication skills* through the child's consistent use of gesture, vocal, and gaze behaviors to request and/or comment about items in the immediate environment (Warren et al., 1993; Yoder et al., 1994).

Applications of milieu approaches are also reported in the preschool population, referred to as **enhanced milieu teaching** (EMT). Kaiser and Hester (1994) employed EMT approaches to include environmental arrangement of toys, responsive adult communication, and incidental language teaching techniques, and reported that children increased communicative utterances and vocabulary directed toward adults and peers. Language interventionists have tools to provide support to family members to observe and understand individual communication patterns of their children and to increase opportunities for successful communication interactions throughout the day. Positive effects were found with children with a range of mild to severe language delays, including autism (Kaiser, Hancock, & Nietfeld, 2000). Communication behaviors that increased were not only words, but also included gestures, sounds, words, sign language, and a combination of all of these skills. The primary focus of these interventions is to assist children who have communication and language delays in: (1) enhancing multiple communication skills with gestural, sign, vocal, and verbal forms; (2) expressing functions of communication including pragmatic skills, beginning with early requesting and commenting; and (3) later developing skills including greeting, questioning, turn-taking, sharing affection, and beginning and ending conversations.

Researchers in early language development recently reexamined the role of *adult directives* in interactions with young children, finding positive effects on language development (McCathren, Yoder, & Warren, 1995). Previous researchers had concluded that extensive use of adult directives were not encouraged in naturalistic language intervention because it had been assumed that the child's spontaneous communication was inhibited with a resulting negative effect on language development. (Directives are described as adults' verbal behaviors that communicate to the child the expectation that they do, say, or attend to something.) McCathren and colleagues identified three types of directives employed by adults: (1) *follow-in directives* that follow the child's lead; (2) *redirectives* that initiate a new topic; and (3) *introductions* or directives given to an unengaged child. The importance of the work by McCathren et al. is their specific identification of the facilitative effect of follow-in directives on language development in young children. Follow-in directives are more specifically defined as those adult communications to children that "refer to an event, object, or person to which the child is already attending." (p. 92).

These authors found that follow-in directives had two facilitative effects: (1) joint attention between the child and adult was extended; and (2) the child was more attentive during episodes of joint attention. Follow-in directives were typically parent and adult verbal behaviors that related specifically to the child's focus of attention and "set the stage" for the child to learn salient vocabulary and language concepts. The contribution of the work by McCathren et al. (1995) expands what Bruner (1983) identified as the importance of the facilitative effect of joint attention on early language development. Language interventionists can learn from recent research that a variety of directives can be effective when the context is natural for the individual child and the timing is contingent to the child's focus of attention.

Language interventionists can learn from recent research that a variety of directives used by adults, such as questions, modeling, expansions, and direct requests for child responses, can be effective when the context is natural for the individual child and the timing is contingent on the child's focus of attention. The importance of the contribution of research to practice is that language interventionists can determine interventions that meet family needs and individual interaction styles more easily. That is, adult directives that occur within joint attention episodes and that follow the child's attention focus have the most power to increase the child's word learning and expression. The approach of using follow-in directives described by McCathren et al. is child-centered. For example, adult statements, requests, and models follow the topic and focus of attention of the child rather than an adult-determined focus. However, McCathren et al. recommend judicious use of redirectives and introductions to create opportunities for the child to focus and then benefit from follow-in directives. Further, the role of redirectives is not ignored, as they may be necessary to the behavior and socialization of young children. This review of the effects of parent interaction on early language development identifies six aspects of language that are most effectively facilitated by specific types of directives, as well as strategies the language interventionist can use:

1. Milieu approaches using follow-in directives are most effective for facilitating the acquisition of vocabulary and early semantic relations.
2. Directives that are not based on the child's focus of attention (redirectives) are not facilitative of language development.
3. Directives that change the topic or direct the child's attention to new stimuli (introductions) are not positively related to language development outcomes.
4. The responsiveness of adults is not inhibited or lessened when directives are used appropriately, as follow-in directives.
5. While the importance of follow-in directives is established in promoting language development, cultural variation is not accounted for and requires further research.
6. The use of redirectives and introductions has validity in some cases, particularly with children who have behavioral problems.

LANGUAGE AND LITERACY DEVELOPMENT

Connections between language development in young children and literacy have been more clearly documented in recent years, confirming what parents and teachers already knew. The pleasure of early book reading and the benefits for children of learning vocabulary from favorite stories are familiar to every parent, grandparent, and teacher of young children. Several studies in the past five years have demonstrated the effectiveness of joint book reading with parents/

family members because it helps children at risk of communication delays and disorders and those with identified language delays to increase their vocabularies and communication skills (Crain-Thoreson & Dale, 1999; Dale, Crain-Thoreson, Notari-Syverson, & Cole, 1996; Hess, 1999; Heubner, 2000; Mogford-Bavan & Summersall, 1997). Key features of the studies were the introduction of a structured, regular joint book-reading session with family members and young children between the ages of 1 to 5 years.

Crain-Thoreson & Dale (1999) and Huebner (2000) found that "dialogic reading" intervention improved children's vocabulary quantity and quality, their rate of response to questions, and increased the mean length of utterance. Dale, Crain-Thoreson, Notari-Syverson, and Cole (1996) found that dialogic reading in which parents maintained the child's focus in joint book reading with milieu teaching approaches was more effective for increasing the language expressiveness of children with language delays than a more general, responsive language training program. The importance of these recent studies provides additional ways for language interventionists to involve family members. For many families, book reading is a natural routine and a picture book or storybook provides a predictable language intervention activity that is repeatable and enjoyable for both partners. Further, the defined vocabulary and topics in a given book may help parents and caregivers to assess communication and language progress more easily than more open-ended and child-directed activities.

Mogford-Bavan & Summersall (1997) identified the importance of joint picture-book reading (PBR) with young children for promoting language development. The context of book reading is rich with opportunities for parent–professional partnership in early language intervention. As Mogford and Summersall point out, the context of book reading provides multiple opportunities for young children to rehearse and practice vocabulary skills, answer questions, ask questions, and form relationships between words and ideas. Emerging literacy in young children is integrally tied to language development and language intervention strategies involving joint book reading are increasing in the literature. For example, four developmental stages of book reading skills were found by Mogford and Gregory in their study of PBR that included thirty children who were typically developing over five age groups, 12, 15, 18, 24, and 30 months (1992, cited in Mogford-Bavan & Summersall):

- Stage 1: Mothers focused on encouraging preverbal children to attend visually to pictures on the page. A turn-taking structure was observed with child responses characterized by gesture, visual referencing, smiling, and a range of vocalization. The children also demonstrated basic book-handling skills (holding the book and turning pages) and attention to pictures.

- Stage 2: Children demonstrated more advanced book-handling skills, orienting the book correctly and opening it at the beginning. The interactions between parents and children continued to be highly structured, with short episodes of two to three turns. Only a few pages of the book were completed at each sitting, and the children began to respond verbally to the parent. The children showed only limited inclination to initiate the activity. Parents used a high degree of "tutorial" questions with increasing complexity, and the children responded to increasingly complex questions within the same interactions.
- Stage 3: The children increased their attention to the books and often completed them. Conversations and topics between parents and children about the pictures became more elaborated, and children demonstrated their ability to respond to requests to repair communication failures such as "Tell me again, what is he doing?" Both children and adults extended their conversations about pictures by asking and responding about the pictures and book content, for example, the children began to ask questions about simple story elements. The adults selected books with simple story development and paraphrased the stories, adjusting their language to maintain the children's attention and responsiveness.
- Stage 4: The child showed increased listening skills as the adults began to read several lines of more difficult text. Conversation about the story related events in the story to similar events in the children's lives and explained the relationship of pictures to events in the story. Child showed awareness of words in print, asking the adult to "read" the words and often "reading" the words with memorized phrases related to the story. The children demonstrated the ability to finish a book. The ability to listen and comprehend an entire book or story with pictorial support is expected when children begin preschool and kindergarten. Children without this skill may be at risk of social and educational delay.

In their study with a limited sample of 11 children 2 years 6 months and 3 years 9 months of age with language delays, Mogford-Bavan and Summersall identified a major limitation of joint book reading among parents and children. The limited attention and responsiveness of the children with language delays resulted in an unrewarding and frustrating experience for parents, a pattern found in Mongford and Gregory's (1992, cited in Mogford-Bavan & Summersall) study of joint book reading with hearing-impaired children. The difficulties and language delays exhibited by preschool children in the study appear to influence book reading and create a situation that parents may avoid. Thus, language-delayed children are at risk of limited exposure to picture books and that particular type of parent–child interaction, which may result in further delays in early language and emerging literacy skills.

FAMILY PARTNERSHIPS IN ASSESSMENT

The goal of working with families is not merely to seek their involvement in a peripheral way, but to focus all interactions toward one primary goal, to positively influence the quality of life for families and children. Based on our current understanding of the central role that families and caregivers have in the child's daily life, professionals are challenged to enhance the system of support around individual children. Dunst, Trivette, and Deal (1988) have called this process **empowerment,** a process that supports family members in gaining control over life circumstances and in providing nurturance and care for family members. Bailey and Simmeonson (1988) have defined the primary goals for early intervention professionals as being to support families to care for their children, to enhance child development outcomes, and to facilitate positive interactions between caregivers and children in the family context. In working with families, professional activities support families to understand the child and to integrate the child into the family. The primary goal for professionals in communication and language intervention is to increase positive communication between the child and other family members. Following the direction of Bailey and Simmeonson, this section of this chapter outlines several strategies language intervention professionals can use to assist families to: (1) integrate the child with communication and language delays into the family; (2) increase positive communication skills for the child and adult; and (3) enhance developmental outcomes for the child.

Based on the preceding discussion of changing policy and practices to involve families in communication and language intervention, there are multiple variables to keep in mind for effective partnerships with families. Family preferences and resources are determined by unique cultural, economic, and life-cycle stage variables that influence their degree of involvement in communication and language intervention with their children. Increasing cultural and linguistic diversity among families with young children and school-age children creates challenges for professionals in the provision of appropriate services. The remainder of this chapter is devoted to specific applications of policy and practice recommendations in several fields including speech-language pathology, special education, early childhood special education, general education, and early intervention in key steps of the assessment and intervention process.

Family Roles in Assessment

Assessment of the child's communication and language development offers the initial point of contact for building partnerships with families. The identification of concerns regarding the child's development is most appropriately in the domain of the family. In most cases, referrals for assessment are based on parental concerns, even when a professional, such as a physician, makes the referral. Through establishing a focus with family members, using the definitions and statements of their concerns, the "ownership" of the assessment process is shared by family members and professionals. Practices that place families in control of the assessment process, rather than as recipients of professional decisions, are more effective for building trust and facilitating communication between parent and professional. For example, special education practices require signed parental consent prior to assessment of children's communication and language skills. Parents are also often asked to provide written descriptions and background prior to the actual testing. These are positive steps to seek information from parents that can be used to plan more meaningful assessments with children. However, parents often provide the requested paperwork but do not hear the results and/or follow-up steps to the assessment in a timely manner. A more supportive practice would include a meeting with parents, the child's teacher, and specialists to share information and conduct informal assessment, prior to formal assessment. The purpose of initial contacts with families is to begin to build a relationship that will form a meaningful partnership through all steps of the assessment and intervention process.

Initial contacts need not be extensive to be effective. However, even a brief, focused interview with family members can communicate professional respect and reliance on information provided by family members. The roles that family members can play in initial meetings and contacts are important to professionals in the following areas:

1. family definitions of the child's apparent communication and language problem;
2. family perceptions of the child's language development in a native language other than English;
3. family relationships at home (identifying the primary caregivers, those who spend most time with the child);
4. the level of care that is required for the child at home;
5. family reports of the child's health history and efforts to date for addressing reported communication problems;
6. family preferences for information and future contacts/involvement around the child's assessment results and program planning.

Information from parents to address these areas can be gathered informally through discussion and talking with the professionals involved. Professionals can then review parents' responses and ask further questions to determine areas of emphasis in communication and language assessment. In addition to informal interviews with family members, several communication assessment tools are available for parents or other primary caregivers to use in identifying the child's current communication strengths and needs. *The Receptive-Expressive Emergent Language Scale (REEL)* (Bzoch & League, 1991) provides an interview guide to determine receptive and expressive milestones, and the results can be scored for normative purposes. Other tools appropriate at this stage of the assessment process include the *MacArthur Child Development Inventories for Infants(CDI)* (Fenson et al., 1993), and the *Infant/Toddler Checklist for Communication and Language Development* (Wetherby & Prizant, 1993). The validity of parent reports as key components in the language assessment process was demonstrated in studies using the CDI (Dale, 1991; Reznick, & Schwartz, 2001).

Family-Accessible Reports

Following assessment, the summary of information is often completed in the form of a written report. The format of assessment reports varies from handwritten notes to formal typed reports. Often in educational settings time constraints require brief reports to accompany the Individualized Educational Program (IEP) plan. Although parents' legal rights to information indicate that copies of all reports must be available to them, actual practices vary widely regarding the written reports that are routinely provided to parents. With the knowledge that parents are entitled to all information regarding their children, the preparation and presentation of assessment reports become critical. The need for information that is understandable, useful, accurate, and helpful to parents in understanding their child's communication and language problems requires that reports be written with those goals in mind. Attention to the content and format of reports is essential if the information is to be accessible to families of diverse backgrounds. Discussion of the content and format of reports follows.

Content of Reports

Traditionally, assessment reports have followed a medical model, with the presentation of background and diagnostic summary. While legislation and policy require reporting of assessment findings by a multidisciplinary team, there is flexibility within the legal requirements for designing reports that are responsive to family concerns and priorities. The key to including families in the determination of content in reporting appears to be keeping the focus on family members as the "owners" of assessment information about their child. Assessment reports typically contain data and results of formal assessment tools, as required by schools, hospitals, insurance companies, and state and federal agencies. In addition to the required information, Overbeck (1992) recommends that the content of assessment reports reflect a structure and process based on the priorities and concerns of family members, as follows:

- statement of family goals/preferences for assessment
- assessment observations
- care principles
- summary and recommendations

Each of the above components of an assessment report is found in varying sequence and format in most professional reports. A sample report format is provided in Figure 4.2.

The importance of the report components, shown in Figure 4.2, is not derived from the titles or the sequence, but from the content and integrity in representing family concerns and priorities. The following suggestions are more detailed descriptions of the recommended components for family-accessible reports. Figure 4.3 provides an example of excerpts from one team report and the inclusion of the individual family concerns throughout.

Statement of Family Concerns/Preferences for Assessment

A suggested process to identify family concerns and preferences for assessment with children was outlined and discussed in a preceding section. Following initial conversations with family members regarding referral concerns, a summary statement is made to include family/parent descriptions of the child's communication or language delays as well as the major questions that the family wishes to address in the assessment process.

Assessment Observations

A subsequent section of the report contains summary information regarding child-specific performance using formal and informal assessment methods. In addition to the assessment data, observations of individual strengths are recommended. The focus on communication or language behaviors that the child uses to communicate with family members, peers, or others can assist families and professionals to work together in the identification of both the child's current abilities and future intervention steps.

Care Principles

Care principles refer to the basic information and approaches that are needed for all professionals to interact with a particular child and family. This information is not typically contained in assessment reports, and, if present, may appear in final recommendations. The rationale for highlighting care principles separately within the report is based

FIGURE 4.2 Sample report format

COMMUNICATION/LANGUAGE DEVELOPMENT
TEAM ASSESSMENT REPORT

NAME: DATE OF ASSESSMENT:
B.D.:
C.A.:
TEAM MEMBERS:

<u>Background</u>

<u>Assessment</u> <u>Observations</u>

    <u>Family</u> <u>Preferences</u>:

    <u>Developmental</u> <u>Processes</u>:

    <u>Individual</u> <u>Differences</u>:

    <u>Communicative</u> <u>Contexts</u>:

    <u>Team</u> <u>Model</u>:

    <u>Intervention</u> <u>Principles/Strategies</u>:

<u>Summary</u> <u>and</u> <u>Recommendations</u>

on the need for continuity of services from all professionals who interact with the child and family. An individual child and family may interact with nearly a dozen professionals, including an occupational therapist, physical therapist, therapy assistant, social worker, physician, nurse, psychologist, and others. If basic care principles are stated by family members and written into reports, each of the individuals who interacts with the family will have critical information such as special health concerns, behavioral strategies, medication issues, family stressors, cultural and linguistic considerations, alternative health care practices, and so forth.

Summary and Recommendations

Summary and recommendations typically include assessment results and further referral and intervention recommendations. As a supplement to this section of traditional assessment reports, specific intervention strategies are included. The integration of the preceding information regarding family concerns/preferences, child strengths, and care principles forms the basis of intervention strategies, as illustrated in the following example:

> *Josh's family preferred that he attend a regular preschool. Although he communicated nonverbally, Josh demonstrated social responsiveness and gestures toward other children. As a primary care principle, his parents stated the need to provide Josh time to respond to new people and activities. Resulting strategies recommended by Josh's parents and team members included showing Josh new items such as foods, toys, and games before asking him to choose one item.*

In the above example, the consistency between family preferences, assessment of the child's strengths, care principles, and specific intervention strategies provides continuity for the child and family members in the development of the Individualized Family Support Plan (IFSP) and the Individualized Educational Program (IEP) plan.

FAMILY PARTNERSHIPS IN INTERVENTION

Planning Intervention

One of the requirements of Part C of IDEA is "to enhance the capacities of families to meet the special needs of their infants and toddlers." If key family members are consulted in the assessment process, the development of goals together is a natural step in the process. Developing goals with families involves reviewing assessment information, identifying the child's strengths and areas of need, prioritizing areas for further development, and deciding on methods to achieve developmental gains.

FIGURE 4.3 Sample report content

One Team's Story

Portions of the team assessment report, completed with Naomi's mother, Ann, and her team members are highlighted. This first step was to develop an *Assessment Plan.* Ann met with her team to identify her family's preferences and concerns.

Ann's first concern was her request for clarification about her own expectations and those of the team. She stated her need to continue learning about Naomi's medical care and condition, to be knowledgeable of community resources, and to share her feelings of joy and challenge in caring for Naomi. She reminded the team to be practical and realistic in making recommendations. She stated her preference that issues be perceived as concerns raised in the course of her experiences in providing care for Naomi, rather than problems.

Ann and her team members further discussed *Care Principles,* or the way that she wants all professionals to interact with her family, and especially Naomi.

Caring for a child with special health needs, like Naomi, requires a lot of time, care, love, nurturing, and especially respect for her individuality. Respecting Naomi as an individual, no matter what her special needs are, opens up opportunities in creating a more natural working relationship in meeting her needs. For example, Naomi does not verbalize any words; therefore, Ann encourages her to develop ways of communicating her needs through gestures, noises, and/or movements to indicate what she wants. This form of respect allows Naomi to develop a sense of autonomy with her world.

Provision of care for a child with special health needs ultimately falls on the child's family. Naomi's family requires support, understanding, empathy, and, most importantly, respect for their abilities and capabilities as a family unit. Ann stresses her request that professionals address, listen, and hear her family's needs rather than make assumptions based on medical and other professionals' diagnosis. She also requested respect for her family's need for confidentiality, timetables, and their rights as individuals as well as a family in building a relationship.

To complete the report, the team provided *Summary and Recommendations* for other persons who may work together with Naomi and her family in the future.

Ann is very resourceful in seeking and obtaining needed services to help Naomi live a full and happy life and to enhance her family in functioning as a unit. Recommendations are addressed to those professionals who come into contact with Naomi and her family. First, include and encourage Ann's active input in the planning. Second, utilize and incorporate the family's daily schedule, other family members, transportation resources, etc., in all interventions. Finally, Ann stated, "Just because we are parents with a child with special health needs doesn't mean we have a problem. We are dealing with Naomi's situation the best way we can and we don't see it as a problem."

Most professionals are familiar with the requirement to develop goals with families, particularly with legislated mandates for parental input to goals and objectives developed for individual program plans, through the IFSP or IEP process. The intent of the legislation—to develop goals, objectives, and intervention processes that match actual family concerns and preferences for young children with disabilities—is clear. The actual process for developing collaborative goals with families is much less straightforward. A discussion with family members and all members of the early intervention team is needed to identify goals, preferences, and needs that include family dreams, teacher expectations, and professional assessment results to build on the child's strengths and skills for participation in *natural environments.*

The concept of natural environments is compatible with naturalistic language intervention strategies, or milieu approaches, discussed earlier in this chapter. Young children typically participate in environments that center around the family, home, and community. As they progress to preschool, kindergarten, and elementary settings, school becomes an increasingly central environment in their daily lives. Communication and language intervention can be effectively implemented in the context of natural environments, where children typically participate in activities appropriate to their developmental and chronological age. Depending on the age and developmental skills of the child and family routines, natural environments may include home, relatives' homes, day care, preschool, community parks, shopping centers, school buses, church, school, and other settings. IDEA 1997 regulations for Part C require that the IFSP include a statement of how early intervention services will be implemented in natural environments or a clear justification of why separate environments are needed.

Edelman (2001) expanded the definition of natural environments to include familiar contexts, routines, and activities in which children typically participate. The development of communication and language goals, objectives, and activities within the context of the child's daily life provides the opportunity to involve all family members in determining specific routines and activities that the child enjoys. At least two approaches that are relevant for developing communication and language intervention in natural environments are the McGill Action Planning System (MAPS) and the ecological assessment approach, as outlined in Chapter 7. While detailed steps are provided in Chapter 7, the integration of the *person-centered planning* approach used in MAPS with an ecological framework that considers typical environments for individual children and families provides a practical guide for maintaining the focus on family priorities and the communicative strengths of the child. The following example with Nicole and her mother Janis illustrates the process of communication intervention in natural environments:

Nicole, a four-year old girl with many nonverbal communication skills and few words, often threw her food from her plate throughout meal time. Her mother, Janis, expressed her desire that Nicole eat with the family; choose one food at a time; and eat the food she chose, rather than throwing it on the floor. When observing the family meal time, the early childhood specialist, Tina, noted that the entire family of five sat at the table together and preferred to include Nicole in the family meal. Nicole was seated at the table in a booster chair and she showed the ability to reach and grasp her spoon and cup, but required assistance to use both. The family passed platters of food to each member and when Nicole's turn came, Janis paused to ask Nicole if she wanted some of each item. Nicole responded "yes" to each one and a large spoonful of each food was placed on her plate. After several bites of her favorite foods, macaroni and cheese, she pushed the food from the plate to the floor unless an adult intervened in time.

In order to support Janis in her goal for Nicole to eat appropriately with her family and to communicate her food choices, Tina and Janis worked together to increase Nicole's communication and participation in family mealtime.

Tina observed that Nicole watched each person and reached toward all the foods presented at the table. She identified Nicole's favorite foods with Janis's input and created a colorful placemat with pictures of each food spread out on the mat. As the family began their meal, Nicole was asked "What do you want to eat?" She touched a picture on her placemat and her mom then gave her a small spoonful of that particular food to try. After one or two bites, she was asked, "Do you want more?" Nicole responded either by nodding "yes" or touching a picture of her food choice. In either case, she was given a small amount of her choice. If she attempted to throw the food, her plate was removed and she was assisted to sign "all done." After three meals, Nicole increased her communication by choosing foods by pointing to pictures, signing, and vocalizing; and her attempts to throw food decreased significantly.

Several elements of naturalistic communication and language intervention are found in the above example. Tina, the early childhood specialist, focused on Janis's priorities for Nicole to learn to eat with her family and to communicate more effectively. The family routine, mealtime, provided multiple opportunities to build Nicole's communication skills and to expand her repertoire to request foods through pointing to pictures, signing, and vocalizing. All members of the family were engaged in the activity, giving Janis support and giving Nicole multiple practice opportunities for her new skills. The use of naturally occurring routines within the family provides rich opportunities to develop activities that follow the child's focus of attention, thus setting the stage for continued interaction, turn-taking, and expanding communication skills.

Implementing Intervention

Planning for partnership with family members in communication and language intervention includes consideration of family life in daily contexts. Naturalistic, or milieu, approaches to intervention are particularly well suited to family involvement as they are based on assumptions that children learn to communicate in the context of familiar, daily routines with responsive adults. Naturalistic approaches originated from the work of Hart and Risely (1975), who described "incidental teaching" that required a time-delay procedure to elicit communication with children with developmental delays. Since the 1970s, naturalistic or milieu intervention approaches have been elaborated to include specific steps that begin with (1) establishing joint attention with the child; (2) taking turns in communicative interactions; (3) expanding the child's communication form; and (4) providing natural consequences to reinforce communicative attempts. Several authors presented intervention models in the context of natural daily routines of children, families, and classrooms (Kaiser & Hester, 1994; MacDonald & Carroll, 1992; Noonan & McCormick, 1993; Norris & Hoffman, 1990a; Warren & Gazdag, 1990; Warren & Kaiser, 1986; Wilcox, Kouri, & Caswell, 1991). The terminology used to describe similar methods of embedding language intervention within naturally occurring activities and routines includes (1) transactional teaching; (2) pragmatic intervention; (3) child-oriented teaching; (4) interactive modeling (Wilcox, Kouri, & Caswell, 1991); (5) social partnership (MacDonald & Carroll, 1992); and (6) enhanced milieu teaching (Kaiser & Hester, 1995). A more complete review of naturalistic/milieu intervention approaches was provided by Warren and Gazdag (1990), who defined several common elements, including incidental teaching, social routines, turn-taking, and environmental arrangement. Several approaches with direct application to family involvement in communication and language intervention are summarized in Table 4.3.

The key elements of milieu intervention approaches are found in many commercially available parent language intervention programs. Baxendale, Frankham, and Hesketh (2001) demonstrated the effectiveness of the Hanen Parent Programme with children ages two to three years and found results to be comparable to clinic-based, direct intervention. The application of naturalistic communication and language intervention approaches with families requires that professionals and parents problem-solve together to determine daily routines, activities, and communication goals for the individual child. Family members (including parents, siblings, aunts, uncles, grandparents, cousins, day-care workers, and others) can share in the intervention sessions and be supported by professionals at critical points, as

TABLE 4.3 Naturalistic Communication and Language Intervention Approaches

Naturalistic Model	Description	Authors
ECO Model: Social Partnership, Conversational	Turn-taking between parent and child are "balanced" in play interactions. Parents respond to child's simplest actions and/or sounds, interpreting child's behavior as communicative. Effects have shown child's increased imitation, turns and vocal skills.	MacDonald & Carroll (1992) MacDonald & Gillette (1985) Mahoney & Powell (1985)
Responsive Interaction & Responsive Small Group	Adult interaction follows the child's lead and builds on the establishment of joint attention to expand the child's communication and turn-taking within environments that are arranged to engage the child in typical, relevant activities.	Yoder & Warren (2001)
Milieu Teaching	Milieu approaches incorporate incidental teaching strategies central to the application of naturalistic communication interventions and are based on the identification of *teachable moments* with young children. "Incidental teaching occurs when a child initiates interaction with the teacher in the form of a request, question, comment or other communicative behavior" (p. 49). Adults follow the child's bids for communication with techniques referred to as question prompt, mand, partial and full models.	Jones & Warren (1991)
Enhanced Milieu Teaching (EMT)	Strategies taken from milieu teaching include following the child's lead, environmental arrangement, and embedding modeling in routines and social interactions. Adults implement specific steps to structure and respond to the child's communication through selection of toys, expansion of child behavior, and natural consequences.	Halle, Baer, & Spradlin (1981) Norris & Hoffman (1990) Kaiser & Hester (1994)
Prelinguistic Milieu Intervention (PMT)	PMT is implemented in a play setting while adults employ time delay, joint-attention, and environmental arrangement to elicit requesting behaviors with young children. In addition, linguistic mapping is used to label the child's actions and focus of attention. As children increased in their intentional communication behaviors, adults increased responsive communication toward the children.	Norris & Hoffman (1990) McDonald & Carroll (1992) Yoder, Warren, Kyoungram, & Gazdag (1994a) Yoder & Warren (1999)

Adapted from Robinson & Robb (2001).

adapted from a three-step process recommended by Norris & Hoffman (1990).

1. Family members organize the play environment with developmentally appropriate toys and activities.
2. Family members provide communication opportunities for the child through interpretation of child behavior, response, and expansion of child-initiated behavior. Suggested strategies include procedures referred to as: cloze, gestures and pantomime, relational terms, binary choices, turn-taking cues, and phonemic cues.
3. Family members provide natural consequences to extend communication in the forms of acknowledgment, nonverbal response, verbatim repetition, rewording, recounting physical actions/events, modeled dialogue, semantic contingency, personal reactions, questions/comments, and predictions/projections.

While short-term effects of naturalistic interventions described are promising, long-term effects are not yet reported. The benefits of naturalistic approaches for families are the informal implementation strategies and "goodness of fit" that is possible based on actual family environments and routines. Limitations are found in the use of naturalistic interventions with older children and those with severe disabilities in cognitive, behavioral, and sensory domains.

Language and Literacy Interventions

The opportunities to apply recent research and findings of the effective approaches shown in naturalistic language intervention and early literacy development are clearly complementary methodologies. The techniques described in studies of joint book reading with a mediated dialogue designed to maintain the child's focus of attention and facilitate expanded communication and language skills are directly applicable to professional and family partnerships discussed so far. Challenges in the application of joint book reading include the need to consider family preferences, culture, language, and literacy background. The importance of finding books in the family's preferred language and/or the use of narratives that are familiar to each family is key to successful implementation in the family context. Chang, Lai, and Shimizu (1995) reported that their study of inner-city families of Cantonese background showed that little time at home was devoted to reading activities between parent and child. These authors recommend that professionals work with families to identify alternative literacy development opportunities that build on family routines, such as talking about a TV show or movie to review main characters and events and emphasizing language concepts in daily chores at home. Another example may include telling traditional family stories and teacher follow-up at school to assist children in creating pictures to display around the house with vocabulary words for practice. The challenge for language interventionists is to support families in early book reading experiences in order to create success for both parent and child. Possible strategies include:

1. Select books that are within the child's visual and cognitive developmental level.
2. Coach parents in methods to maintain the child's attention, based on milieu teaching procedures.
3. Identify question forms within the child's receptive language level that elicit frequent and appropriate responses such as "Where's the birdie?" and "What is the birdie eating?"
4. Encourage parents to accept any communicative response that the child is capable of and that keeps the interaction going, such as patting the picture to answer parents' questions and looking at the appropriate picture.
5. Encourage parents to also follow the child's lead in picture-book reading by allowing children to choose a book each time they read and comment on the sounds, gestures, words that they make while looking at pictures.
6. For children who are verbal, encourage parents to use incidental teaching techniques to model, expand, and request increasingly complex language with the child.
7. Remember that book reading is a more abstract form of communication than playing with toys and other concrete objects and so is more challenging to the child's visual and auditory processing skills.
8. Make book reading a regular routine when the child is most likely to be responsive, such as after a bath at night or after breakfast in the morning.
9. Keep a comfortable and calm place for joint book reading. Above all, make this an enjoyable time for both parent and child.

Family Partnerships in Communication and Language Assessment and Intervention

Up to this point, we have discussed and demonstrated strategies to support family members in playing a central role in communication assessment and intervention and outlined and described the process for developing partnerships. The underlying assumption of the methods described is that families have choices to determine the level and type of involvement that fits individual needs. In order for professionals to be effective in establishing partnerships with families of diverse backgrounds at all levels of assessment, intervention, structuring activities, and progress evaluation, a range of skills and resources is needed. Key questions for professionals to address in working with each family are:

1. What is the level of daily physical care involved for family members to assist the individual with a disability?
2. Who is home during the day?
3. Who is the primary caregiver?
4. What cultural values and preferences are expressed regarding communication patterns in the family at home and in community settings?
5. What are family expectations and estimations of child skills and needs?
6. Who are communication partners for the child at home?
7. What is the English reading ability and language used by primary caregivers?
8. What are family goals and expectations for the child?
9. How will the family observe and keep track of progress in a way that fits into its daily routines?
10. What are services provided and what is the frequency of parent contact?
11. What is the parent's (or other family members') preference for involvement in language intervention with the child?

SUMMARY

This chapter presented perspectives and strategies to build partnerships with families in communication and language assessment and intervention with young children. The central role of families in providing care and influence throughout the developmental years was emphasized. The point of view that family members are the primary context and that family life is the natural context to begin and implement communication assessment and intervention is supported in research and legislation. The practice of family-centered care is complex for professionals, requiring flexible attitudes and excellence within and across disciplines. The challenges to professionals in communication and language intervention include the need to implement clinical excellence in family environments, particularly in culturally and linguistic diverse settings. In an era of cost containment for health, human services, and education, the time for building partnerships with families is extremely limited. However, policies and practice guidelines for professionals to support family members and to work together effectively are established and demonstrated nationally. It is this author's hope that professional development for the reader will lead toward greater self-awareness and responsiveness to families with diverse cultures, strengths, and needs.

The effectiveness of involving family members in communication and language intervention with young children has been demonstrated repeatedly. Recent publications support the role of family members in increasing children's communication and language skills and improving early academic and language abilities in the early school years. There are assistive technologies, professional resources, parent guides, children's books, and toys available to assist family members in becoming effective communication partners in the facilitation of communication development with young children with communication delays and disorders. With the wealth of resources available, it may be tempting for busy professionals to require all parents to participate in similar ways to enrich language and learning environments for their children. The guidelines for family-centered and culturally competent practices, however, empower professionals to adapt interventions to meet unique family strengths and needs. For example, providing children's storybooks in the family's primary language may provide a critical bridge for joint book reading and storytelling activities. More complex challenges and opportunities blur the traditional lines between the roles of "parent/family member" and "professional" in the creation of partnerships to meet shared goals for communication intervention.

REFERENCES

Adler, S. (1990). Multicultural clients: Implications for the SLP. *Language, Speech, and Hearing Services in the Schools, 21,* 135–139.

Anderson, N. B. (1991). Understanding cultural diversity. *American Journal of Speech and Language Pathology, 1,* 9–10.

Bailey, D. B., & Simeonsson, R. J. (1988). *Family assessment in early intervention.* Columbus, OH: Merrill.

Baxendale, J., Frankham, J., & Hesketh, A. (2001). The Hanen Parent Programme: A parent's perspective. *International Journal of Language & Communication Disorders, 36,* 511–516.

Bricker, D., & Gripe, J. J. (1992) *An activity-based approach to early intervention.* Baltimore: Brookes.

Bruner, J. (1983). *Child's talk: Learning to use language.* New York: Norton.

Bzoch, K., & League, R. (1991). *Receptive-Expressive-Emergent-Language Test (REEL-2).* Austin, TX: PRO-ED.

Carson, D. K., Perry, C. K., Diefenderfer, A., & Klee, T. (1999). Differences in family characteristics and parenting behavior in families with language-delayed and language-normal toddlers. *Infant-Toddler Intervention, 9,* 259–279.

Chang, J. M., Lai, A. J., & Shimizu, W. (1995). LEP parents as resources: Generating opportunity to learn beyond schools through parental involvement. In L. R. L. Cheng (Ed.), *Integrating language and learning inclusion: An Asian American focus* (pp. 265–290). San Diego, CA: Singular.

Crain-Thoreson, C., & Dale, P. S. (1999). Enhancing linguistic performance: Parents and teachers as book reading partners for children with language delays. *Topics in Early Childhood Special Education, 62,* 28–39.

Crais, E. (1991). Moving from "parent involvement to family-centered services." *American Journal of Speech-Language Pathology, 1,* 5–8.

Cross, T., Bazron, B., Dennis, K., & Isaacs, M. (1989). *Towards a Culturally Competent System of Care* (Vol. I). Washington, DC: Georgetown University Child Development Center, CASSP Technical Assistance Center.

Dale, P. S. (1991). The validity of a parent report of measures of vocabulary and syntax at 24 months. *Journal of Speech and Hearing Research, 34,* 565–571.

Dale, P. S. (1995). The value of good distinction. *Journal of Early Intervention, 19,* 102–103.

Dale, P. S., Crain-Thoreson, C., Notari-Syverson, A., & Cole, K. (1996). Parent-child book reading as an intervention technique for young children with language delays. *Topics in Early Childhood Special Education, 16,* 213–235.

Damico, J. S., & Damico, S. K. (1993). Language and social skills from a diversity perspective: Considerations for the speech-language pathologist. *Language, Speech, and Hearing Services in the Schools, 24,* 236–243.

Developmental Disabilities Assistance and Bill of Rights Act, 1994 Amendments to P.L. 103-230. Administration on Developmental Disabilities, Administration for Children and Families, United States Department of Health and Human Services.

Dunst, C. J., Trivette, C., & Deal, A. (1988). *Enabling and empowering families: Principles and guidelines for practice.* Cambridge, MA: Brookline Books.

Early Intervention Program for Infants and Toddlers with Disabilities. Part C of the Individuals with Disabilities Education Act (IDEA), 1997 Amendments to P.L. 105-17. 20 USC Chapter 33, Sections 1431–1445.

Edelman, L. (2001). *Just being kids.* JFK Partners, Project Enrich, and the Colorado Department of Education, CO: Western Media Products.

Eiserman, W. D., Weber, C., & McCoun, M. (1995). Parent and professional roles in early intervention: A longitudinal comparison of the effects of two intervention configurations. *Journal of Special Education, 29,* 20–44.

Elder, J. H. (1995). In-home communication intervention training for parents of multiply-handicapped children. *Scholarly Inquiry for Nursing Practice, 9,* 71–92.

Erickson, M. F., & Kurz-Riemer, K. (1999). *Infants, toddlers, and families: A framework for support and intervention.* New York: Guilford.

Fenson, L., Dale, R., Reznick, S., Thal, D., Bates, E., Hartung, J., Pethick, S., & Reilly, J. (1993). *MacArthur Communicative Development Inventories.* San Diego: Singular.

Field, T. (1983). High risk infants "have less fun" during early interactions. *Topics in Early Childhood Special Education, 3,* 77–87.

Girolametto, L. (1995). Reflections on the origins of directiveness: Implications for intervention. *Journal of Early Intervention, 19,* 104–106.

Girolametto, L., Pearce, P. S., Stieg, R., & Weitzman, E. (1996). Interactive focused stimulation for toddlers with expressive vocabulary delays. *Journal of Speech & Hearing Research, 39,* 1274–1283.

Girolametto, L., & Tannock, R. (1994). Correlates of directiveness in the interactions of fathers and mothers of children with developmental delays. *Journal of Speech and Hearing Research, 37,* 1178–1191.

Goode, T. D. (2001). *Getting started, planning, implementing and evaluating culturally competent service delivery systems for children with special health needs and their families.* Georgetown University Child Development Center, DC: National Center for Cultural Competence. [On-line]. Available at: http://gucdc.georgetown.edu/nccc

Grieser, D. L., & Kuhl, P. K. (1988). Maternal speech to infants in a tonal language: Support for universal prosodic features in motherese. *Developmental Psychology, 24,* 14–20.

Halle, J. W., Baer, D., & Spradlin, J. E. (1981). Teacher's generalized use of delay as a stimulus control procedure to increase language use in handicapped children. *Journal of Applied Behavior Analysis, 14,* 389–411.

Hampson, J., & Nelson, K. (1990). Early relations between mother talk and language development: Masked and unmasked. *Papers and Reports on Child Language Development, 29,* 781–785.

Hanson, M. J., Lynch, E. W., & Wayman, K. (1990). Honoring the cultural diversity of the family when gathering data. *Topics in Early Childhood Special Education, 10,* 112–131.

Hart, B., & Risely, T. (1975). Incidental teaching of language in the preschool. *Journal of Applied Behavioral Analysis, 8,* 411–420.

Hart, B. & Risely, T. (1995). *Meaningful differences in the everyday experiences of young American children.* Baltimore: Brookes.

Hess, L. J. (1999). Let's talk and play: A study of poverty mothers and toddler daughters. *Infant-Toddler Intervention, 9,* 1–16.

Heubner, C. E. (2000). Promoting toddlers' language development through community-based intervention. *Journal of Applied Developmental Psychology, 21,* 513–535.

Iacono, T. A., Chan, J. B., & Waring, R. E. (1998). Efficacy of parent-implemented early language intervention based on collaborative consultation. *International Journal of Language & Communication Disorders, 33,* 281–303.

Jamison, C., & Robinson, N. (2000). Cultural competence outcomes for speech-language pathology graduates. Poster presentation at *American Speech-Language and Hearing Annual Conference.* Washington, DC, November 15–18.

Johnson, B., Jeppson, E., & Redburn, L. (1992). *Caring for children and families: Guidelines for hospitals.* Bethesda, MD: Association for the Care of Children's Health.

Johnston, J. R., Miller, J. F., Curtiss, S., & Tallal, P. (1993). Conversations with children who are language impaired: Asking questions. *Journal of Speech and Hearing Research, 36,* 973–978.

Jones, H., & Warren, S. (1991). Enhancing engagement in early language teaching. *Teaching Exceptional Children, 23,* 48–50.

Kaiser, A. P., Hancock, T. B., & Nietfeld, J. P. (2000). The effects of parent-implemented enhanced milieu teaching on the social communication of children who have autism. *Early Education & Development, 11,* 423–446.

Kaiser, A. P., Hemmeter, M. L., Ostrosky, M. M., & Fischer, R. (1996). The effects of teaching parents to use responsive interaction strategies. *Topics in Early Childhood Education, 16,* 375–406.

Kaiser, A. P. & Hester, P. P. (1994) Generalized effects of enhanced milieu teaching. *Journal of Speech and Hearing Research, 37,* 1320–1340.

Kaiser, A. P., Hester, P. P., Alpert, C. L., & Whiteman, B. C. (1995). Preparing parent trainers: An experimental analysis of effects on trainers, parents, and children. *Topics in Early Childhood Special Education, 15,* 385–414.

Kemler-Nelson, D. G. (1989). How the prosodic cues in motherese might assist language learning. *Journal of Child Language, 16,* 55–68.

Kennedy, M. D., Sheridan, M. K., Radlinshi, S. H., & Beeghly, J. (1991). Play-language relationships in young children with developmental delays: Implications for assessment. *Journal of Speech and Hearing Research, 34,* 112–122.

Lee, S., & Kahn, J. V. (2000). A survival analysis of parent–child interaction in early intervention. *Infant-Toddler Intervention, 10,* 137–156.

MacDonald, J., & Gillette, Y. (1985). *Social play: A program for developing a social play habit for communication development.* Columbus, OH: Merrill.

MacDonald, J. D., & Carroll, J. Y. (1992). A social partnership model for assessment of early communication development: An intervention model for preconversational children. *Language, Speech, and Hearing Services in the Schools, 23,* 113–124.

Mahoney, G., O'Sullivan, P., & Dennebaum, J. (1990). Maternal perceptions of early intervention services: A scale for assessing family-focused intervention. *Topics in Early Childhood Special Education, 10,* 1–15.

Mahoney, G., & Powell, A. (1985). *The transactional intervention program: Preliminary teachers' guide.* Unpublished manuscript, School of Education, University of Michigan.

McCathren, R. B., Yoder, P. J., & Warren, S. F. (1999) The relationship between prelinguistic vocalization and later expressive vocabulary in young children with developmental delay. *Journal of Speech, Language, and Hearing Research, 42,* 915–924.

Mogford-Bavan, K. P., & Summersall, J. (1997). Emerging literacy in children with delayed speech and language development: Assessment and intervention. *Child Language Teaching and Therapy,* 143–159.

National Commission on Children. (1991). *Speaking of kids: A national survey of children and parents.*

Noonan, M. J., & McCormick, L. P. (1993). *Early intervention in natural environments: Methods and procedures.* Pacific Grove, CA: Brooks/Cole.

Norris, J. A., & Hoffman, P. (1990). Language intervention within naturalistic environments. *Language, Speech, and Hearing Services in the Schools, 21,* 72–84.

Overbeck, D. (1992). *Transdisciplinary conjoint assessment with young children with special needs*. Honolulu, Hawaii: Lanakila Infant Development Program.

Paul, J. L., Porter, P. B., & Falk, G. D. (1993). Families of children with disabling conditions. In J. L. Paul & R. Simeonsson (Eds.), *Children with special needs: Family, culture, and society* (2nd ed., pp. 3–24). New York: Harcourt Brace, Jovanovich.

Paul, J. L., & Simeonson, R. (1993). *Children with special needs: Family, culture, and society* (2nd ed.). New York: Harcourt, Brace, Janovich College Publishers.

Ramey, C. T., Campbell, F. A., Ramey, S. L. (1999). Early intervention: Successful pathways to improving intellectual development. *Developmental Neuropsychology, 16,* 385–392.

Reznick, J. S., Schwartz, B. B. (2001). When is an assessment an intervention? Parent perception of infant intentionality and language. *Journal of the American Academy of Child and Adolescent Psychiatry, 40,* 11–17.

Robinson, N., & Robb, M. (2001). Early communication assessment and intervention: A dynamic process. In D. Bernstein & E. Tiegerman (Eds.), *Language and communication disorders in children.* (5th ed., pp. 155–196). Boston: Allyn & Bacon.

Shelton, T., Jeppson, E., & Johnson, B. (1987). *Family-centered care for children with special health care needs*. Washington, DC: Association for the Care of Children's Health.

Snow, C. (1979). The role of social interaction and the development of communicative ability. In A. Collins (Ed.), *Children's language and communication*. Hillsdale, NJ: Lawrence Erlbaum.

Snow, C. (1984). Parent–child interaction and the development of communicative ability. In R. Schiefelbusch & J. Pickar (Eds.), *Infants and their acquisition of communicative competence.* pp. 69–107. Baltimore, MD: University Park Press.

Snow, C., & Ratner, N. (1984). *Talking to children: Therapy is also social interaction*. Paper presented at the annual meeting of the American Speech, Language and Hearing Association. November, 1984, San Francisco, CA.

Terrell, B., & Hale, J. E. (1992). Serving a multicultural population: Different learning styles. *American Journal of Speech-Language Pathology, 1,* 5–8.

Turnbull, A. P., & Summers, J. A. (1985, April). *From parent to family support: Evaluation to revolution*. Paper presented at the Down Syndrome State-of-the-Art Conference, Boston, MA.

Turnbull, A. P. & Turnbull, R. (1990). *Families, professionals, and exceptionality: A special partnership* (2nd ed.). Columbus, OH: Merrill.

Warren, S. F., Yoder, P. J., Gazdag, G., Kim, K., & Jones, H. (1993). Facilitating communication skills in young children with developmental delay. *Journal of Speech and Hearing Research, 36,* 83–97.

Warren, S. R., & Gazdag, G. (1990). Facilitating early language development with milieu intervention procedures. *Journal of Early Intervention, 14,* 62.

Warren, S. R. & Kaiser, A. (1986). Incidental language teaching: A critical review. *Journal of Speech and Hearing Disorders, 51,* 291–299.

Weber-Olsen, M. (1984). Motherese: The language of parent to child. *Journal of Education, 11,* 123–141.

Wetherby, A., & Prizant, B. (1993). *Communication and symbolic behavior scales.* Chicago: Riverside.

Wilcox, M. J., Kouri, T. A., & Caswell, S. (1990). Partner sensitivity to communication behavior of young children with developmental disabilities. *Journal of Speech and Hearing Disorders, 55,* 679–693.

Yoder, P. J., & Warren, S. (1999). Prelinguistic communication intervention may be one way to help children with developmental delays learn to talk. *Augmentative and Alternative Communication, 8,* 11–12.

Yoder, P. J., & Warren, S. F. (2001). Relative treatment effects of two prelinguistic communication interventions on language development in toddlers with developmental delays vary by maternal characteristics. *Journal of Speech, Language, & Hearing Research, 44,* 224–237.

Yoder, P. J., Warren, S., Kyoungram, K., & Gazdag, G. E. (1994). Facilitating prelinguistic communication skills in young children with developmental delay II: Systematic replication and extension. *Journal of Speech and Hearing Research, 37,* 841–851.

CHAPTER 5

Policies and Practices

Linda McCormick

This chapter provides an introduction to key regulations of the Individuals with Disabilities Education Act (IDEA): nondiscriminatory assessment, the Individual Family Services Plan (IFSP), the Individual Education Plan (IEP), the least restrictive environment mandate, and related services. Then we consider paradigm shifts, specifically those in the area of language intervention that have contributed to new service delivery practices. Finally, the remainder of the chapter provides a rationale for collaboration and suggestions for putting the "collaboration imperative" into practice.

IDEA REGULATIONS

In 1975, Congress enacted a law governing educational provisions for students with disabilities. This 1975 law was Public Law (P.L.) 94-142, the Education of All Handicapped Children's Act. Since 1975, there have been a number of changes and amendments to that law. In 1990, it was renamed the Individuals with Disabilities Education Act (IDEA) and amended to include (1) provisions for transition and assistive technology, and (2) two new disability categories (autism and traumatic brain injury). The reauthorization of IDEA in 1997 (P.L. 105-17) recognized that the law had been successful in ensuring free appropriate public education and improved education results for students with disabilities. However, Congress also acknowledged the need for some improvements. In 1997, Congress made changes to key parts of the legislation to improve educational opportunities for students with disabilities. Among the most important of these changes were:

- giving students greater access to the general education curriculum;
- strengthening roles and opportunities of parents as participants in their children's education;

- providing special education and related services, aids, and supports in the general education classroom "whenever appropriate";
- supporting high quality professional preparation and in-service education;
- providing incentives to help children before they become labeled;
- focusing resources on teaching and learning; and
- reducing paperwork requirements that do not improve educational results.

Congress also reduced the number of sections in the law from nine to four. Part A describes the purposes and policies underlying the legislation (e.g., the goals of equal opportunity, full participation or inclusion, independent living, and economic self-sufficiency). Part B sets out and provides for the obligations of the States, requirements for States' participation in IDEA, procedural safeguards, and monitoring and enforcement. Part C contains provisions for the identification and provision of early intervention services for infants and toddlers with disabilities and their families (and procedural safeguards). Part D includes provisions for research, teacher training, resource centers, parent training, information centers, and state improvement grants.

IDEA regulations have an important and direct impact on assessment, planning, and special instruction. This section provides a brief description of the regulations specifically related to these activities.

Nondiscriminatory Assessment

IDEA guarantees all students with disabilities the right to an unbiased evaluation of their educational strengths and needs. This evaluation has three purposes: (1) to determine whether a student has a disability; (2) to determine whether the student needs special education and related services (because of the disability); and (3) to determine the kind of special education and related services the student will receive.

IDEA sets forth the following guidelines to ensure that the assessment process is unbiased and nondiscriminatory:

- No single instrument or assessment strategy may be used as the sole criterion for placement and planning;
- All areas related to the suspected disability must be considered, including health, vision, hearing, social and emotional status, general intelligence, academic performance, communication, and motor abilities;
- Assessment instruments and strategies must not discriminate on racial or cultural bases;
- Assessment instruments and strategies must be valid for the specific purposes for which they are used;

- Assessment instruments and procedures must not reflect the student's sensory, manual, or speaking impairments unless skills in these areas are being measured;
- Tests must be administered in the student's native language or other mode of communication;
- Procedures must be administered by personnel in conformance with test instructions;
- Assessment must consider all available evaluation data as well as information provided by parents, current classroom-based assessments and observations, and information provided by teachers and related service providers.

After eligibility has been determined and the child's strengths and needs have been identified, the next step is to develop an individualized intervention plan. IDEA provides for two types of individualized plans: the **individualized family services plan** (IFSP) and the **individualized educational plan** (IEP). Which plan is developed depends on the age of the child.

The Individual Family Service Plan (IFSP)

Part C of IDEA requires development of an IFSP for each eligible infant or toddler and his or her family. The IFSP specifies desired outcomes for the child based on the child's development and needs. There is also an option for families to identify their resources, priorities, and concerns related to enhancing their child's development.

The IFSP is a process of continuously gathering, sharing, and exchanging information. In addition to specifying services needed by the child and family, it provides a context for establishing professional–family relationships. The IFSP may be frequently expanded and modified as the family makes decisions about what early intervention services they want and need for their child and themselves. The IFSP process continues throughout intervention.

Although the form used for the IFSP is relatively unimportant, there are very specific guidelines as to the information that needs to be assembled *in the course of the IFSP process*. Table 5.1 lists the types of information to include on the IFSP.

Some programs begin the IFSP process with blank sheets of paper rather than using a preprinted form (which can be intimidating to parents). Others use a simple form such as the IFSP form shown in Figure 5. 1, which was developed by staff of the Zero-to-Three Hawaii Project. Note that Hawaii chooses to call the IFSP the Individual Family Support Plan. Like many other programs in the nation, the Zero-to-Three Hawaii Project encourages parents to write their own IFSP. This IFSP was written by the child's parents.

TABLE 5.1   Required IFSP information

The IFSP should include:
- a statement based on objective criteria of the child's present functioning in cognitive, communication, social/emotional, physical, and adaptive development;
- the family's concerns, priorities, and resources related to enhancing their child's development;
- expected intervention outcomes, including criteria, procedures, and time lines for determining whether the outcomes are achieved and whether modifications will be necessary;
- specific intervention services to be provided to the child and family, and their frequency, intensity, and method of delivery;
- the natural environments where services will be provided and why they will not be provided in those environments if the plan so provides;
- projected dates for initiation of services and expected duration of services;
- the name of a service coordinator(s) who will coordinate with other agencies and facilitate planning and intervention processes; and
- procedures to ensure successful transition from infant services to preschool services.

The Individual Education Plan (IEP)

The purpose of the IEP is to ensure that each eligible child receives appropriate and individualized special education and related services. It is an agreement between the parents and the school about what the child needs and what the school system will do to address the child's needs. The major components of the 1EP are: (1) evaluation information indicating whether the student has a disability and needs special education services and related services; (2) appropriate annual goals and short-term objectives, with criteria, procedures, and schedules that will be used to determine whether the objectives are met; (3) a statement of the appropriate special education placement and the specific related services that the student will receive; (4) the amount of time the student will be in the general classroom with supplementary aids and services. Table 5.2 lists these IEP requirements.

The members of a student's IEP team (sometimes called the IEP *committee*) are the same people who served on the evaluation committee: the student's parents, the student (when appropriate), at least one of the student's general education teachers (if the student is or may be participating in general education settings), at least one special education teacher, a representative of the local education agency knowledgeable about curriculum and resources, an individual capa-

Figure 5.1a

INDIVIDUAL FAMILY SUPPORT PLAN

Zero-to-Three Hawaii Project
Hawai'i Department of Health

Child's Name Nathan Takumoto

Prepared with Family By SELINA FLORES

DOB 7-18-92

Date 7-18-94

- Interim
- ✓ Initial
- Review

1. INFORMATION ABOUT THE CHILD

A. My Child Nathan _____ has the following strengths, qualities & needs:

He is able to communicate through gestures. He knows what he wants and when he wants to do it. He is independent. He has good attention span and listening skills.

As Nathan's parents we would like more information on what Nathan is doing, compared to other children his age, so we can determine if he has any needs.

B. Screening/Evaluation Tool: _____ Date: _____

Explanation/Notes:

C. Family strengths and resources related to enhancing the development of the child (optional):

As parents we understand Nathan's gestures and needs. We try to look at what he is doing through his eyes. We keep communication open with his sitter and she provides a nurturing environment. He has many relatives who cater to his every whim and are willing to do anything for him.

FIGURE 5.1b

INDIVIDUAL FAMILY SUPPORT PLAN

Zero-to-Three Hawaii Project
Hawai'i Department of Health

Child's Name __Nathan Takemito__

Prepared with Family By __Selina Flores__   Date __7-18-94__

I/WE WANT:	WAYS TO GET IT & WHO CAN HELP:	TIME IT MAY TAKE:	WHAT HAPPENED:
1 Want Nathan to be able to communicate (talk) with us, to tell us what he wants, what's bothering him, or what he doesn't want.	1a. Mike/Patty can call Kapiolani Medical Center. 973-8235 and speak with Julia Tobin who will schedule Nathan's appt. 1b. Mike/Patty will share information regarding Nathan's behavior with strengths, to promote a positive meeting.	by end of week — Friday 4/22/94 prior to Evaluation date	
2 Want to have Nathan's hearing tested to rule out any problems.	2a. Mike/Patty can call Kapiolani Medical center (973-8235), tell the receptionist they would like to schedule an audiology appt. for their son Nathan. 2b. Mike/Patty will call Selina (942-8245) with appointment dates & times for the authorization for services form (to ensure free services).	by end of week — Friday, 4/22/94 As soon as the appts. are made.	
3 Want Nathan to interact with other kids (play, talk, defend himself).	3a. with Mike & Patty's permission Selina will write up their description of Nathan's behavior and their concerns for 0-3 Child psychologist M. Kapin, Ph.D. for a telephone consult. 3b. M. Kapin will contact family directly to schedule phone consult.	by end of day Wed. 4/20/94 one week, ending 4/25/94	

Child Enrolled in __Zero-to-Three Hawaii Proj.__ (Program)

Parent Signature: __Patty Takemoto__   Date: __7/18/94__

Co-Care Coordinator: __Selina Flores__   Date: __7-18-94__

TABLE 5.2   Required IEP information

The IEP (for students ages three through twenty-one) should include:
- The student's present levels of education performance, including (1) how the disability of the student affects his or her involvement and progress in the general curriculum (if ages of six through twenty-one), and (2) how the disability affects his or her participation in appropriate activities (if ages three through five);
- Measurable annual goals, with short-term objectives, related to (1) meeting needs resulting from the disability in order to progress in the general education curriculum, and (2) meeting the student's other disability-related needs;
- The special education and related services and supplementary aids and services that will be provided and the program modifications or supports for school personnel so that the student can (1) meet annual goals, (2) progress through the general curriculum and participated in extracurricular activities, and (3) be educated and participate with other students (with and without disabilities) in general education;
- The extent to which student will *not* participate with students without disabilities in general education classes and extracurricular activities;
- Modifications in state-or district-wide assessments that will enable the student to participate in those assessments;
- Projected date for beginning the services and program modifications and the anticipated frequency, location, and duration of each;
- Transition plans, including:
  - a statement of the student's needs related to transition services (beginning age fourteen and each year thereafter);
  - a statement of needed transition services, including interagency responsibilities for needed linkages (beginning age sixteen);
  - a statement that the student has been informed of his or her rights that will transfer to the student from the parents when the student becomes of age (beginning at age eighteen);
- How the student's progress toward annual goals will be measured and how the parents will be informed of the student's progress.

ble of interpreting the results of the assessment process, and other individuals who have knowledge or special expertise (at the parents' or agency's discretion). Other professionals on the team may include a language interventionist, a nurse, a school psychologist, a physical therapist, and/or occupational therapists.

IDEA stipulates that the IEP must be finalized and signed prior to actual placement. This can be a problem when the child is not yet in his placement because members of the IEP team do not yet know what the child's strengths and needs are relative to the expectations of that specific placement. Bateman (1992) and others have commented on this, noting that the IEP is written at the wrong time and for the wrong purpose. It can be argued that the validity and appropriateness of the goals and objectives on a child's *first* IEP should be questioned *if* assessment focused exclusively on establishing eligibility for services and the type of services needed (rather than the child's specific instruction and support needs); *if* the goals and objectives were developed by people unfamiliar with the child's daily functioning *in natural environments;* and *if* the goals and objectives were generated by people other than those responsible for the child's daily instructional activities.

The Least Restrictive Environment (LRE) Mandate

The next concern after the IEP has been developed is identifying the least restrictive environment (LRE). IDEA creates what is termed a "presumption" in favor of educating student with disabilities with their peers who do not have disabilities. The LRE mandate of IDEA states that a school system must educate a student with a disability with students who do not have disabilities *to the maximum extent appropriate* for the student and that the school must not remove the student from the regular education environment unless, because of the nature or severity of the student's disability, he or she cannot be educated there successfully even after the school provides supplementary aids and support services for the student.

The only way that this presumption in favor of inclusion can be set aside is if it can be demonstrated that the student cannot benefit from being educated with peers who do not have disabilities, even with the provision of supplementary aids and services. The student cannot be placed in a more specialized and less inclusive program unless this "failure to benefit with supplementary aids and services" is documented.

Schools also have to ensure that students with disabilities may participate in extracurricular and other general education activities. These include meals, recess, and such services as counseling, athletics, transportation, health services, recreational activities, special interest clubs, and school social activities.

The term *inclusion* has generally replaced the term *integration* in the educational arena. Stainback, Stainback, and Jackson (1992) prefer the term *inclusion* because it

> *more accurately and clearly communicates what is needed—all children need to be included in the educational and social life of their neighborhood schools and classrooms, not merely placed in the mainstream (p. 3).*

Integration and mainstreaming attempted to help children fit into the mainstream of their schools. Inclusion is different. Inclusion is not about changing students so that they will fit into the mainstream: Rather, it is about changing the mainstream to support and nurture individual differences and about supporting and nurturing professionals to work together in ways that they have not had much opportunity to do in the past. Inclusion is a shift from helping only those children identified as having a disability to addressing the needs of every member of the school (school personnel and children alike) to be successful, secure, and welcome in the educational mainstream.

Inclusion begins with the assumption that the mainstream is where *all* children belong. This is very different from integration and mainstreaming, which focused on preparing excluded children for the mainstream. Inclusion focuses on how the mainstream environment can accommodate children's needs, *not* how children can accommodate to the mainstream environment. Mainstreaming often involved episodic visits to the general education classroom for art, music, and/or circle time and joining the general education class for special activities (e.g., field trips). Inclusion is *not* visiting: inclusion is *belonging*.

In inclusive general education classrooms there is unconditional acceptance of *all* children and teachers are provided with whatever supports and resources are needed to enable them to provide beneficial and successful educational experiences. In inclusive classrooms, the emphasis is on what children *can* do, rather than what they *cannot* do. The needs of children with disabilities are not promoted over those of children without disabilities and support services are never sacrificed or compromised in any way. *Every* child has whatever resources and supports she needs *and* a challenging educational program geared to her abilities, needs, and interests. *All* (children and adults alike) are welcomed and their abilities as well as their disabilities are valued. The inclusive general education classroom is a place where children learn to respect and depend on one another.

Over the past two decades the extraordinary progress toward including students with disabilities in schools and in the general education program has been heartening. There is now a substantial and growing research documenting the progress that teachers and parents have made as they have worked together to move from mainstreaming to inclusion (Lipsky & Gartner, 1997). This progress requires the collaborative practices that will be addressed later in this chapter.

Related Services

Supplementary aids and services are defined as aids, services, and other supports that are provided in regular education classes and other education-related settings to enable children with disabilities to be educated with nondisabled children to the maximum extent appropriate. Related services are speech pathology and audiology, psychological services, physical and occupational therapy, recreation, rehabilitation counseling services, social work services, medical services (for diagnosis and evaluation), school health services, transportation, transition services, and assistive technology services and devices. Also subsumed under the heading of supplementary aids and services are curricular or instructional adaptations and staff supports such as instructional assistants and volunteers.

PARADIGM SHIFTS

A paradigm is an overall philosophy or a conceptual framework. Because these frameworks determine what we value and, thus, view as relevant, the paradigms of service fields influence decisions having to do with (1) *what* types of services are provided; (2) *how* services are provided; and (3) *where* services are provided.

The inclusion movement has had the most far-reaching impact in special education in the last two decades. Paralleling that shift have been major paradigm shifts in the area of language intervention (Westby & Erickson, 1992):

1. from standardized testing to naturalistic assessment;
2. from exclusive concern for children's needs to concern for the child's social systems;
3. from viewing children as much alike to awareness and concern for cultural and linguistic diversity;
4. from focus on spoken language to focus on literacy; and
5. from working with individual students and small groups in a therapy setting to working in natural environments (e.g., classroom, homes, community settings).

Not surprisingly, these trends have contributed to widespread changes in the services provided for children with language and communication difficulties (whether as a primary or a secondary disability) and service delivery systems.

Naturalistic Assessment

Westby and Erickson (1992) describe the shift in assessment as a shift from "discrete point, decontextualized, standardized testing to integrative, descriptive, naturalistic assessment" (p. v). This shift reflects new conceptualizations about the nature of language and language learning: that, although standardized (psychometric) language tests permit comparison of the performance of students with one another on some language-related skills, they do not provide information about children's use of language in natural environments or why language is not developing at the expected rate.

Naturalistic assessment complements the information provided by psychometric testing. Chapter 7 describes naturalistic assessment procedures—ecological assessment and planning—to develop and implement appropriate and effective language/communication intervention.

Social Systems Intervention

Social systems intervention reflects the premise that language and communication problems reside not within the child but, rather, in the child's interactions with family members and peers. This view of the child as part of many social systems is a primary thesis of the ecological theory of development discussed in Chapter 7 (Belsky, 1981; Bronfenbrenner, 1986).

Social systems assessment and intervention challenges traditional child-focused approaches. Social systems assessment identifies (1) the social communicative difficulties that the child is likely to encounter in daily interactions in natural environments (school, home, and community settings), (2) roles and functions in her particular social systems, and (3) the specific environmental supports and disincentives for language and communication efforts in those systems. Social systems intervention focuses on mobilizing and strengthening competency-enhancing supports and resources in the social systems and teaching the child a variety of positive social and communication strategies.

Cultural and Linguistic Diversity

The term *culture* refers to the many different factors that shape our sense of group identity—race, ethnicity, religion, geographical location, income status, gender, and occupation. Everyone thinks of himself as belonging to a family. We also belong to a cultural group. The ways we think, feel, perceive, and behave reflect our cultural group membership.

Teaching for diversity must be the norm because diversity is the norm. It is estimated that at least one in every three persons in the United States belongs to a linguistically or culturally diverse group. As would be expected, the population in our schools mirrors this diversity. The paradigm shift from a focus on student similarities to focus on student diversity acknowledges (1) the rapidly changing population demographics, and (2) the essential role that language plays in the socialization of children to their culture.

Some minority children are quite competent in English when they enter school; others have had only minimal exposure to English. They may speak Spanish, the second most common language in the United States, one of the Asian languages, a native American dialect (e.g.,

Hawaiian pidgin), or some less common language, such as Arabic or Tongan. Faced with the reality of working with increasing numbers of children and families whose languages, beliefs, and practices differ in important ways from their own, professionals are working to develop cultural competence.

Cultural competence is "respect for differences, eagerness to learn, and a willingness to accept that there are many ways of viewing the world" (Lynch & Hanson, 1992, p. 356). Cultural competence depends on a complex and subtle interaction between feelings and understanding of cultural and linguistic differences and similarities. It requires professionals to recognize and acknowledge the influence of their culture on their concepts, perceptions, and language.

Acknowledging our own cultural beliefs leads to appreciation of the relativity of our judgments. As professionals come to understand their own socialization they are able to see how it affects their views about family roles and relationships, child-rearing practices, what is proper and appropriate social behavior, life expectations and aspirations, time and space, health, food, dress and personal appearance, and religion.

Cultural competence has been achieved when people are able to

- acknowledge and step outside their own cultural framework;
- understand how each family's cultural background influences its relationships, daily functioning, and values, beliefs, and practices regarding a child's disability;
- see strength in behaviors that reflect beliefs and assumptions that are different from their own; and
- understand that the very same functioning styles and behaviors that may appear at first glance to be problems are very often among the families' (and children's) greatest resources.

Meeting the instructional and support needs of children from linguistically and culturally diverse backgrounds requires professionals to go beyond the surface features of culture, such as food and holidays, to understanding the communication style of the cultural group (Kayser, 1995). A study by Kayser (1989) provides an example of this "closer look" at culture. Kayser observed the interactions of three Anglo and three Hispanic language interventionists during language screening sessions. The verbal and nonverbal behaviors of the two groups of professionals with the Hispanic children they were screening were strikingly different. The Anglo language interventionists kept a social distance of 48 to 60 inches from the children and they did not touch them. The Hispanic language interventionists sat much closer (a range of 18 to 48 inches), and they used touch to control the children's behavior and to get their attention. Verbal communication was also very different, The Anglo interventionists used verbal reinforcements, questions, permission statements, statements of need, hints, explanations concerning a task, and "if–then" statements (e.g., "if you show me the car, then we can play with the toys") to coax the child to complete a task. The Hispanic clinicians were more directive: They used primarily performatives, such as *say, show me,* and *do this* (in Spanish). When clarification was necessary, the Anglo professionals tended to rephrase the utterance, whereas the Hispanic professionals repeated the utterance.

Focus on Literacy

Literacy is not simply an accumulation of the specific skills related to reading and writing. Beginning in infancy, it evolves through social and cognitive processes, gradually developing as a function of exposure to and interaction with print materials and children and adults who are *using* print (called "literary events"). Mere exposure to literacy materials and experiences is not sufficient for the development of literacy: It is the adult–child interaction centered around such events that is important.

A growing recognition of the interdependency of literacy and overall language abilities has precipitated the shift from exclusive attention to spoken language to a focus on "whole language." The "whole" in *whole language* emphasizes the integrity of language and the language process. It also recognizes the importance of language in the acquisition of literacy: that each area aids in the development of other areas (Goodman, 1986).

Ultimately, adherence to whole language principles affects the way we view language, language learning, and curriculum (including instruction, materials, and evaluation). Oral and written language are no longer viewed as separate skill and instructional domains, with literacy "assigned" to teachers and language "assigned" to language interventionists. Recognition that oral and written language abilities are interdependent, that language abilities are a frequent and powerful contributor to academic success and failure, and, finally, that literacy is, in fact, a fundamental dimension of normal language development in our culture and vice versa, has led to collaboration toward the shared goal of facilitating language and literacy (Westby & Erickson, 1992).

Intervention in Natural Environments

It is not generally recognized that, if it is to be effective, intervention for language and communication difficulties must be provided when and where the child needs to understand and use language. Moving from traditional service delivery methods that adhered to a clinical model of one-to-one or small-group therapy provided in a separate setting (the isolated therapy model) to integrated methods of service delivery, which focus on providing therapy in context and in collaboration with families and other professionals (integrated therapy), is a dramatic change. The shift from one-to-one instruction provided in a separate setting to language and communication instruction provided in the context of daily activities in the classroom, the home, and other natural environments reflects recognition that language cannot be separated from other aspects of a child's daily life. It was prompted by research in both special education and language-communication development.

THE COLLABORATION IMPERATIVE

The rate at which the professional literature in the area has grown over the last two decades is an indication of the importance of interdisciplinary collaboration, coordination, and teaming to provide services for students with disabilities. From the first days and weeks of inclusion in the early eighties it was readily apparent that collaboration among everyone concerned with students with disabilities—families, professionals and paraprofessionals in general and special education, early intervention, and related services disciplines (e.g., speech-language pathology, psychology, occupational therapy, physical therapy)—was imperative. Failure to attend to the collaboration imperative seriously threatens the quality and effectiveness of services for children and families. The remainder of this chapter discusses the challenges faced by professionals as they work to integrate their work with students with disabilities and their families and some possible solutions to these challenges.

Teaming Models

When researchers first began to look for teaming models that would make it possible to combine resources to meet the multifaceted needs of children with disabilities, they considered the multidisciplinary, interdisciplinary, and transdisciplinary team models (e.g., Lyon & Lyon, 1980; McCormick & Goldman, 1979; Sternat, Messina, Nietupski, Lyon, & Brown, 1977). The **multidisciplinary team model** was judged the least desirable where collaboration is concerned. In this model, there is little, if any, information sharing, joint planning, or team accountability. Professionals (typically from different disciplines) implement separate assessment procedures and function separately when providing services. Both the **interdisciplinary team model** and the **transdisciplinary team model** initially evolved in response to dissatisfaction with the lack of communication and the fragmented services associated with the multidisciplinary model. In an interdisciplinary team model, team members work together to develop joint intervention goals and intervention strategies. In a transdisciplinary team model, team interactions and activities go beyond collaboration for planning, and professionals work closely together to implement and evaluate intervention. In a transdisciplinary model, in addition to collaborating on mutual goals, professionals and parents are consultants and trainers for one another.

The transdisciplinary team model offered solutions to many of the problems inherent in traditional service delivery configurations. However, initial conceptualizations of this model lacked guidelines concerning *where* and precisely *how* assessment and intervention/ instruction should be provided. Even though team members tried to plan and implement joint assessment, there was some overlap and redundancy across assessment activities. Moreover, because special instruction (including language intervention) was not provided in natural environments, there continued to be problems related to lack of generalization of newly trained skills. Arena assessment and integrated intervention were a response to these concerns.

Arena assessment (also called joint assessment) takes its name from the way the team members (including the parents) arrange themselves for the assessment sessions. They usually sit on the floor in a circle or semicircle around the child. One person, designated as an assessment facilitator, engages the child in targeted activities in a physical environment adapted to the physical needs of the child. Other team members record their observations. The point of this arrangement is to elicit optimal behavior from the child.

Arena assessment has a number of advantages over traditional individual assessment (Wolery & Dyk, 1984). One advantage is avoiding the redundancy that comes about because the same test items often appear in the assessment protocol of different disciplines. The effect of this redundancy is that the different professionals tend to present many of the same tasks to the child and they ask parents almost identical questions. With arena assessment all of the professionals on the team can observe and score the overlapping items at the same time.

A second major advantage of arena assessment is that, rather than seeing the child only from the perspective of their own discipline, team members get a more holistic view. Finally, a third advantage of arena assessment is the opportunity for collaboration among professionals and with parents and other family members and the opportunity to achieve consensus because everyone present observes the same constellation of behaviors. Professionals and parents can talk to one another about what they are seeing, and parents can add information concerning the child's performance in other contexts and whether behavior observed in the assessment situation reflects his or her best efforts.

Transdisciplinary play-based assessment (TPBA) is the most well-known example of arena assessment (Linder's, 1993). TPBA uses play (a normal activity for young children) in a natural environment (e.g., preschool classroom, home) as the assessment context. It provides guidelines for planning and implementing observations in four domains: social/adaptive, cognitive, communication/language, and sensorimotor. The guidelines are easy to use because they are stated in the form of questions to encourage observations of the qualitative aspects of "how" the child performs—not just "if" the child performs—the task.

Integrated intervention is special instruction, facilitation, and support provided in the general education classroom or some other natural environment in the context of ongoing activities and routines and usually with other students present. Other terms for this type of service are *integrated therapy* or *integrated services*. Integrated intervention is a radical departure from the traditional service delivery model in which language interventionists (and other therapists) provided therapy services in separate clinic or therapy rooms. The rationale underlying this isolated therapy model was that children acquire skills most efficiently when taught in a highly structured, distraction-free environment where there is access to specialized equipment.

Cirrin and Penner (1995) discuss how the isolated therapy model emerged and why it persisted for so long. One explanation for the growth of this model has to do with the fact that services to children with language disorders were typically provided in speech clinics where individual children or small groups of children received therapy in separate therapy rooms. A second explanation had to do with the advantages inherent in being able to control the environment. Being able to control the communication context makes it possible for therapists to maximize opportunities to practice production of specific linguistic targets. Auditory and visual distractions are eliminated so that the child's attention and production capacities are easily managed. Third, in the past it was perfectly reasonable and sound to focus intervention on effecting change in discrete linguistic units such as vocabulary or length or type of sentence because most descriptions of language emphasized phonology and syntax. At that time there was less attention to the functions and uses that language serves for the child in social contexts or the relationship between language and learning in school contexts.

The past decade has seen a shift away from the isolated therapy model. Factors contributing to this shift in practices are:

- *Lack of generalization of newly acquired language skills from the clinic room to natural settings:* Many students, particularly those with severe disabilities, do not apply the skills that they have learned in one-to-one therapy settings at appropriate and necessary times in natural environments.
- *Persuasive arguments concerning the role that language plays in social interactions and literacy:* There was grow-

ing recognition that systematic, highly specialized, adult-directed instruction that characterizes traditional isolated therapy is not compatible with holistic theories of language learning that stress adult–child interactions and active engagement with the environment.

- ***The potential negative effects of removing children from their classrooms (i.e., missing the general education curriculum):*** There was growing consensus that removing children from the classroom to receive therapy has negative consequences: it deprives them of whatever instruction is in process and it marks them as different (in the eyes of their peers).
- ***Growing consensus that providing more intensive therapy does not necessarily affect proportionately greater gains:*** Professionals and families alike were dissatisfied with the tendency to confound successful intervention with numbers of hours of therapy (the idea that "more is better").
- ***Fragmentation and overlap of services:*** In addition to fragmentation of services, there is the potential for inadvertently sabotaging one another when the language interventionist (or other therapist) and the teacher do not know what the other is working on with a particular child.
- ***The LRE mandate:*** IDEA specifies that related services are to be provided as needed to make it possible for the child to benefit from instruction in the least restrictive environment.

In practice, integrated intervention is substantially more complicated than simply relocating services from separate settings to natural environments, and the benefits are much broader than increased generalization. It has required professionals to redefine both their responsibilities and their goals. However, the many advantages associated with integrated intervention make the effort well worthwhile. Table 5.3 lists some advantages of integrated therapy.

As the integrated delivery of related services in natural environments has become accepted, it has been repeatedly praised by frontline professionals and endorsed by the professional organizations of the disciplines that work in school settings. Freagon and Kachur (1993) note in advocating for integrated therapy:

> It is possible for a child's speech and language goals to be carried out all day long by each person who works with the child instead of three times a week for twenty minutes as was done in traditional therapy designs. This allows for the implementation of all therapy goals throughout the school day (p. 19).

The professional organizations of special education, occupational therapy, physical therapy, and speech-language pathology have all set forth guidelines promoting the tenets of integrated intervention in educational environments (American Occupational Therapy Association,

TABLE 5.3   Advantages of integrated intervention

- The student gains and maintains access to "regular" educational opportunities and learning outcomes.
- Opportunities for team collaboration are maximized and fragmentation (gaps, overlaps, and/or contradictions) in services are avoided.
- The input and methods of all team members are synthesized as they address a shared vision for the student's participation in social, educational, and vocational settings.
- Skills taught through integrated intervention are likely to generalize because they were learned and practiced in the integrated, natural environments where they need to be used.

1989; American Physical Therapy Association, 1990; American Speech-Language-Hearing Association, 1989, 1991, 1993; Association for Persons with Severe Handicaps, 1986).

Collaborative Teams

A team is "a group of persons who have a shared goal and required actions to perform in order to achieve that goal" (McCormick, 1990, p. 262). When team members share responsibilities and accountability and pool their skills and resources, they are a collaborative team (sometimes cooperative team) (Rainforth et al., 1992). The collaborative team model is basically an evolved version of the interdisciplinary and transdisciplinary team models. As set forth by Thousand and Villa (1992), a collaborative team is a group of people who:

- agree to coordinate their work to achieve common, agreed-on goals; hold a belief system that all members of the team have unique and needed expertise;
- demonstrate their belief in parity by alternately engaging in the dual roles of teacher and learner, expert and recipient, consultant and consultee;
- use a distributed functions theory of leadership wherein the task and relationship functions of the leader are distributed among all members of the group; and
- use a collaborative teaming process that involves face-to-face interaction; positive interdependence; the performance, monitoring and processing of interpersonal skills; and individual accountability.

Thousand and Villa discuss a sixth aspect which, in their opinion, is most important: The team must be an effective cooperative learning group. When the team functions as a cooperative learning group, the other five aspects tend to occur automatically. Drawing from Johnson and Johnson's (1987) definition of the requirements to be an effective cooperative learning group, the first is that members must interact face-to-face on a frequent basis. Second, they must have a mutual, "we are all in this together" feeling of positive interdependence. Third, they must be committed to developing small-group interpersonal skills (e.g., trust building, communication, leadership, creative problem solving, decision making, conflict management). Fourth, they must agree to setting aside time regularly to assess and discuss the team's functioning and set goals for improving relationships and accomplishing tasks more effectively. Finally, members must agree on methods for holding one another accountable for agreed-on responsibilities.

Forming a Collaborative Team

The size and the composition of collaborative teams vary. There may be as few as two or as many as six professionals from different fields and the parents. Ideally there is agreement that all services (including assessment) will be provided in the classroom and other natural environments.

Following are the steps to form a collaborative team (D. W. Johnson & F. P. Johnson, 1975, 1987). (When people are already working together, these steps can be used to restructure the team to function as collaboratively.)

1. **Spend the time necessary to get well acquainted.** Share expectations about team activities and goals and talk about individual needs and desires that the group might help meet. One activity that helps to get people started talking about this is to ask them to complete sentences such as "When I first enter a new group I feel . . . or "What I hope this team will be able to accomplish is. . . ."

2. **Decide on operating ground rules.** Formulate procedures concerning (1) how decisions are going to be made, and (2) how goals and objectives will be addressed. Talk about possible barriers to maximum effectiveness and consider ways of avoiding and/or working through these barriers.

3. **Visualize ideal outcomes.** Visualize desired outcomes and discuss strengths and resources of the team as a whole and those of the various team members as they contribute to these outcomes. Then develop team goals and objectives. These are examples of one team's goals:
   - Implement collaborative assessment and generate a collaborative assessment report.
   - Use a consensual decision-making process to develop a prioritized list of skills and environments for each student with disabilities.
   - Ensure that IEP goals integrate instruction strategies from the teachers, the language interventionist, and the therapists.

- Develop IEP goals that specify priority skills, priority environments, and activities.
- Provide all intervention in the context of activities routines in the classroom and other school environments.

4. **List and analyze potential supports and barriers.** Discuss specific forces that will support and those that might hinder accomplishing team goals. Consider all types of positive and negative forces, for example, political, theoretical, attitudinal, logistical, that could conceivably affect the team's accomplishments.

5. **Develop a plan.** This is the point at which to discuss instructional procedures. Brainstorm different action plans, select a first choice, and work out procedures for implementing the plan. Among the instruction design issues that need to be considered are how often and where instruction will occur, how children will be prepared for instruction, what type of prompts will be used to elicit desired performance, what adaptations will be used to enhance performance, and how performance will be evaluated. Rainforth, York, and MacDonald (1992) urge collaborative teams to become informed as to the specific instructional philosophies and current best practices for school environments.

6. **Plan monitoring procedures.** Determine how progress toward goals will be monitored and develop specific criteria for goal attainment. This step is particularly important. Talk about ways for members to exchange feedback with one another as a means of continually improving individual effectiveness and team effectiveness. The collaborative team becomes an interdependent support system for obtaining the feedback essential to continued improvement of individual skills and group skills. Ultimately, the functioning of the students with disabilities for whom the team is responsible is the most valid indicator of the team's effectiveness.

Roles and Responsibilities

Rainforth and others (1992) distinguish between core team members and support team members. ***Core team members*** are those team members who are directly involved in the design and implementation of the student's educational program. These are the child's key decision makers who need to be in frequent contact with one another. At the very least, the core team includes the student, family members, teachers (special and general educators), and one or more related services professional (e.g., language interventionist, physical and/or occupational therapist, vision or hearing specialist, nurse) and possibly a paraprofessional or classroom aide who helps to support the student in the classroom. Composition of the team depends on the child's needs.

Support team members are individuals who are not as closely involved with day-to-day programming. They may only participate in planning and decision making once or twice a year. Physical and occupational therapists are support team members for many children with mild disabilities. Other professionals who are often support team members include psychologists, social workers, nurses, dietitians, and orientation and mobility specialists.

Some roles and responsibilities are shared by all team members, core team members and support team members alike. Rainforth and others (1992) call these *generic team member roles.* They include: (1) helping to set priorities and plan interventions, (2) participating in problem solving across all aspects of programming; (3) sharing discipline-specific information and competencies that will enhance the student's participation and progress; (4) supporting the contributions and efforts of fellow team members; and (5) continuing education about general practices to support and facilitate quality of life for all persons with disabilities in all aspects of family, school, and community life.

Other roles and responsibilities are specific to the different disciplines involved with children with disabilities. Tables 5.4, 5.5, and 5.6 present roles and responsibilities of the language interventionist, the special educator, and the general education teacher. Because each person's training, experiences, and interests are different, there are many differences among professionals in a discipline. However, all

TABLE 5.4   Major roles and responsibilities of the language interventionist

1. Provide information about normal speech and language development.
2. Provide information about delays and disorders of speech, language, or communication.
3. Collect information about speech, language, and communication strengths and intervention needs to maximize participation in the classroom and other school settings.
4. Interpret assessment information to others and help to develop intervention goals and objectives, plan activities, and select appropriate methods and materials.
5. Provide direct instruction for specific speech, language, and communication skills to individuals and small groups.
6. Demonstrate for, teach, and assist others (i.e., teachers, parents) to implement language and communication intervention procedures.
7. Participate in decision making related to provision of augmentative and alternative communication devices.
8. Evaluate and monitor student progress and program effectiveness.
9. Work collaboratively with others to promote student participation in age-appropriate activities and natural environments.

TABLE 5.5 Major roles and responsibilities of the special education teacher

1. Provide information about exceptional learners (students with disabilities and gifted students).
2. Provide information about special education laws and accompanying rules and regulations.
3. Develop and provide information to others about adapting curriculum, instructional materials, and equipment.
4. Implement assessment of abilities and disabilities or delays in cognitive, social, academic, and vocational skills and assist assessment of language and communication.
5. Provide direct instruction for a broad range of functional and academic skills (including language and communication) to individuals and small groups.
6. Demonstrate for, teach, and assist others (i.e., teachers, parents) to provide individualized instruction.
7. Manage, and assist others to manage, serious behavior problems.
8. Plan and implement environmental modifications to promote learning and generalization.
9. Evaluate and monitor student progress and program effectiveness.
10. Work collaboratively with others to promote participation of students with disabilities in normal activities and natural environments.

TABLE 5.6 Major roles and responsibilities of the general education teacher

1. Provide information about the curriculum philosophy, scope, and sequence.
2. Provide information about the classroom schedule and expectations for participation in routine activities.
3. Provide suggestions for adapting curriculum, instructional materials, and equipment.
4. Assist the language interventionist and the special educator to learn the skills for managing group activities.
5. Arrange peer interactions to teach social and communication skills.
6. Assist individual instruction.
7. Schedule planning time with support professionals and parents.
8. Implement environmental modifications to promote learning and generalization.
9. Co-teach with the special educator and the language interventionist.
10. Work collaboratively with others to promote participation of students with disabilities in normal activities and natural environments.

professionals in speech-language pathology/communication disorders and special education who work in the schools should have the skills necessary for the roles and responsibilities shown in Tables 5.4, 5.5, and 5.6.

Collaborative teams are effective to the extent that members are focused and committed to positive child outcomes more than to the specific concepts and methods and skills of their discipline. To be effective as a team, members must cooperate with one another, share information, and plan together to minimize the effects of the child's limitations on her functioning in natural environments.

Characteristics of Effective Collaborative Teams

Recognition of the importance of working together is clearly a prerequisite for collaborative teaming, but collaboration is more than an attitude. Groups who aspire to becoming collaborative teams should begin by studying and discussing characteristics of effective teams as well as guidelines for teaming skills and procedures (as presented in this section). Sources for this information include the group process literature (e.g., D. W. Johnson & F. P. Johnson, 1987; Napier & Gershenfeld, 1993; Parker, 1990), and theory and research in cooperative learning (D. W. Johnson & R. T. Johnson, 1989). These sources suggest the following as key characteristics of effective collaborative teams:

1. **Commitment to a shared vision.** Effective teams agree on the reasons for their existence and the parameters of their activities. There is discussion and acceptance of ground rules (including how barriers and conflicts will be handled) and logistics of meeting times and locations. These ground rules and conflict resolution strategies are periodically reviewed and revised (if needed).

2. **Clear goals.** Effective teams formulate and agree on a set of measurable and observable goals. All team members recognize that they must work together if the goals are to be accomplished and use the goals to guide the team's activities.

3. **Open communication and active listening.** The members of effective teams trust one another. They communicate openly and honestly about where they stand and how they feel. Ideas and feelings are shared in an atmosphere of nonjudgmental acceptance so that team members feel that their contributions are valued. Equally importantly, they listen to one another (Parker, 1990). It is not sufficient to listen to hear; team members must learn to listen to understand. Active listening procedures can minimize misunderstandings and distortions about ideas and feelings. Active listening is a series of techniques developed by Gordon (1980) to ensure that messages are accurately received. Table 5.7 shows examples of the most common active listening strategies: clarification and "I" messages.

TABLE 5.7 Active listening strategies for collaborative teams

1. ***Use Clarification*** When a team member makes a declarative statement, this is a way to request feedback to ensure that you understood what was said and the way the message was meant. Use one or another of the following phrases to request clarification (in a nonconfrontational way). Begin the request for clarification by saying

   "Do you mean . . . "
   "Am I hearing you say that . . . "

2. ***Use an "I" Message*** "I" messages are a way for team members to communicate the issue that needs to be addressed and resolved in a nonthreatening way. The message includes your feeling about an action within the team, the consequence of the action, and a decision to resolve it.

Affect (feeling, wondering)	*"I feel frustrated" or "I feel uncomfortable"*
Behavior (action)	*"When we start the meeting late" or "When people come late"*
Consequence(s)	*"Because we aren't able to finish what we need to get done"*
Decision(s)	*"We need to talk about meeting times and time constraints."*

4. **Shared leadership and consensual decision making.** In effective teams, team members share leadership responsibilities as well as decision making. Who the leader is on different occasions depends on the particular concern that the team is addressing. One important benefit of distributing and rotating leadership and decision-making powers among team members is that it encourages feelings of positive interdependence. While it may be unrealistic for all members on the team to agree on all decisions, consensual decision making is most desirable. The greater the agreement on a decision, the greater the commitment to its implementation. Table 5.8 shows the steps in consensual decision making.

5. **Constructive conflict resolution.** Effective teams practice constructive conflict resolution to manage disagreements. When members disagree, the discussion takes place in a positive and cooperative atmosphere with a focus on generating creative and productive solutions. All ideas and feelings are listened to enthusiastically and uncritically. They are respected and valued. Members paraphrase one another's ideas and feelings as accurately as they can and without making value judgments about them. They try to view the messages of other members from their perspective, and negotiate the meaning of their colleagues'

TABLE 5.8 Steps in consensual decision making

Steps for joint Decision Making and Problem Solving

1. *Clearly define the problem.* Separate relevant from irrelevant details, clarify vague or ambiguous terms, and assemble all the available information. Then write a consensus definition/description of the problem on the chalkboard or chart paper.

2. *Analyze the issue.* Clarify the problem and relationships among events that are associated with the problem situation as clearly as possible. Gather supporting evidence on the nature of the problem. Then use all available information to restate the problem in terms of a condition that exists and that, to some extent, needs to be modified. Then isolate specific causal factors. Finally, when all available data have been gathered, the problem has been stated as a condition to be changed, and various causal factors have been isolated, make a determination as to whether the team has the ability to solve the problem. If not, work to state the problem more realistically, bring others into the process (e.g., other professionals, other family members), or determine who does have the resources to solve the problem.

3. *Generate possible alternatives.* Brainstorm and list ideas for solutions. (Avoid any tendency to think about the "best" solution at this point.) Integrate and synthesize the ideas into a smaller number. Discuss and weigh the possible alternatives. Consider the consequences of each alternative. Then rank the solutions with the "most preferred" as 1. There should then be decision by consensus that the group will support and try the first-ranked alternative.

4. *Select specific implementation strategies.* Discuss the solution and decide how it can be implemented. Write this on the chalkboard or chart paper: "What will we do? How will we do it? Who will do what? When will we do it?" Plan the sequence of steps for implementation of the solution and assign roles and responsibilities. Decide how much will be completed by the next meeting. Decide (and note) what part of the progress each team member will report on.

5. *Begin implementation of the agreed-on steps.*

6. *Reassess the situation and make modifications (if needed).* Use objective information to determine whether the strategy is producing the desired outcomes. If the intervention is not producing the desired outcomes, either modify it or reenter the problem-solving loop and select the next-highest-ranked solution to try.

messages. The issue is not to establish who is "right" or "wrong" or who has the best answer but, rather, to get as much information as possible and explore different perspectives to come up with the best team decision possible.

6. **Shared accountability.** On effective teams, accountability is shared. Shared accountability is an important principle of collaborative teams. Working as a team clearly reduces the autonomy and freedom that teachers and support personnel have traditionally enjoyed when they have operated independently (Skrtic, 1991), but shared accountability relieves them of the onus of being (or at least feeling) solely responsible for programming decisions. Effective teams also keep records of and monitor the effectiveness of all team decisions and activities.

Collaborative Consultation

Consultation is a triadic relationship involving a consultant, a consultee or mediator of change, and a person seeking change (Tharp & Wetzell, 1969). There are two major types of consultation models: **collaborative models** and **expert models.** Collaborative consultation differs from expert consultation in that the consultant is not viewed (and does not view herself) as having more expertise than the consultee. The triadic model relies on parity between the partners: The consultant has the knowledge or skills to mobilize the mediator's influence and the mediator has the data to influence and inform the consultant. Both the consultant and the mediator "own" the problem and both are accountable for the success or failure of whatever instructional practices they decide to implement.

Collaborative consultation is more than just planning and problem solving; it is the essential relationship between people from different backgrounds that makes the process possible. The collaborative consultation model stresses reciprocity and mutuality (Tharp, 1975; Tharp & Wetzell, 1969). In educational applications, the mediator is typically the general educator: The consultant may be the language interventionist, special educator, physical therapist, occupational therapist, or another support professional (e.g., a remedial reading teacher). Collaborative consultation is more than two professionals working together to provide special instruction or intervention in the general education classroom. It involves joint planning, shared responsibility, shared resources, shared accountability, and a willingness to invest the time and energy necessary to become familiar with one another's viewpoints, values, and vocabulary. Both participants must truly believe that "two heads are better than one" and that sharing will increase the probability for optimal outcomes (Thousand & Villa, 1992). Table 5.9, which reflects a synthesis of work by Idol, Paolucci-Whitcomb, and Novin (1987), Thousand and Villa (1992), and West and Cannon (1988), provides some guidelines for a successful collaborative consultation relationship.

Collaborative consultation may be direct or indirect. Which approach is used will depend on the classroom, students' needs, and

TABLE 5.9   Guidelines for a successful collaborative consultation relationship

- Behave in ways showing respect for and trust of one another's opinions, skills, and abilities.
- Share ownership of the problem as well as the proposed solutions.
- Learn from one another by regularly exchanging roles (shifting from consultant to consultee and vice versa).
- Use active listening and responding techniques (paraphrasing, perception checks, questions, acknowledging feelings) to facilitate communication.
- Give credit for each other's ideas and provide immediate positive feedback for one another when mutually agreed-on goals are achieved.
- Avoid professional jargon.
- Be available for one another.

teacher preferences. There are several possible direct contact collaborative consultation arrangements. The special educator and/or the language interventionist may work with the general education teacher to provide classroom-based individual or small-group special instruction, using modified classroom materials or special materials, with content drawn from the curriculum and/or the results of ecological assessment as described in Chapters 7 and 8. A second possible arrangement is co-teaching, in which the language interventionist and/or the special education teacher share responsibility for instruction (for the entire class) with the general education teacher.

There are also two possible indirect contact collaborative consultation arrangements. One is a collaborative support arrangement in which the language interventionist and/or the special educator provide minimal classroom-based services, occasionally teaching or demonstrating language activities and providing materials to the teacher. In this arrangement, the primary role of the language interventionist and the special educator is as support team members. They provide technical assistance, consultation, and in-service training. The second possibility is actually an expert support arrangement in which the language interventionist and/or the special educator provide only technical assistance and/or in-service training for the general education teacher. Staffing arrangements for both direct and indirect contact are discussed at more length in Chapters 8.

Based on five years' experience with collaborative consultation in 11 schools in California, Montgomery (1992) points out that no two applications of the collaborative consultation models will look and operate exactly the same because of differences in students' needs and differences in teaching styles. Montgomery argues that development of collaborative goals and objectives with the teacher must be a priority. She contends that all goals and objectives should be "shared by at least one other adult on the campus, such as the teacher, teacher's aide, bus driver, cafeteria worker, or resource teacher" (p. 363), so that there are opportunities for reinforcement throughout the day in different settings. The greatest challenge, according to Montgomery (and many others), is finding adequate time for planning and preparation. Over time, however, scheduling for planning and preparation becomes less a problem because consultation partners gradually become more informed and more efficient: The language interventionists come to know the curriculum in several subject areas and teachers become more adept at embedding language instruction in the curriculum activities.

Another example of collaborative consultation in practice is provided by Roller, Rodriguez, Warner, and Lindahl (1992). They describe an elementary school in Denver where there are teacher and language interventionist teams for classes at all grade levels. All classes include children who are developing language at an expected rate and students with severe language disabilities. The teacher–language interventionist teams share space, materials, resources, and responsibilities. As Roller and colleagues put it:

> *Depending on the teams, responsibilities are divided in various ways. As speech-language pathologists and regular educators in the same room, we are responsible for teaching the appropriate grade-level curriculum to the entire group of students. We modify and adapt the curriculum as needed to ensure that Individual Education Plan (IEP) goals are met for the learners with disabilities and that school and district level goals are met for the typical students. We also share responsibility for parent conferences, evening programs, and decisions concerning report cards for all the students (p. 23).*

The previous reports of successful collaboration highlight the importance of sharing information and joint training. The special educator and the language interventionist must schedule time with the teacher to plan how to learn about the curriculum with special attention to the vocabulary, the language skill expectations, the complexity of instructions, and the materials. (In addition to the teacher, another source for this information is teachers' manuals.) Additionally, they should arrange to analyze examples of the student's written language, assignments, and classroom tests and to observe in the classroom. Classroom observations should focus on (1) how well the student attends to tasks and instruction; (2) how the student's communicative attempts are responded to; (3) whether the student asks for help; (4) whether the student seems to understand directions; (5) the student's participation in discussions; and

(6) whether the student communicates appropriately with the teacher and with peers.

Creating time and opportunity for collaboration requires the most creativity. West and Idol (1990) offer some suggestions for freeing up teacher time. One idea is to schedule special experiences (e.g., films, plays, guest speakers) that bring students together in a large group. Because fewer staff are needed to oversee large-group experiences, some teachers can use this time for collaborative planning or make arrangements for students to work on group projects in a setting in which they require minimal supervision. Another idea is for the principal or other support staff to teach a period a day on a regular basis. Having aides, student teachers, and/or volunteers guide and supervise transitions, lunch, and recess routines frees up teachers at those times. Finally, the faculty may vote to extend their instructional day for twenty minutes two days per week to provide time for planning meetings.

SUMMARY

Development and maintenance of effective partnerships and successful team functioning are extremely difficult and time-consuming, and they require constant vigilance, but they are worth the effort for all involved (students, parents, and professionals). As discussed in Chapter 10, collaborative consultation and teaming in early intervention programs may be most challenging because professionals from different agencies (as well as from different disciplines) are involved. The challenges are both logistical and conceptual. Foremost among the logistical challenges are (1) resource management (specifically allocation of financial and time resources), and (2) division of responsibilities (for example, who will be responsible for developing the Individual Family Service Plan [IFSP]?). Conceptual challenges include difficulties establishing a parity relationship when professionals come from different agencies, and lack of familiarity with the vocabulary and procedures of one another's fields.

The basic reason for collaboration is pooling of staff expertise so that the needs of all students can be met. One method for continuing professional growth and support, suggested by Johnson and F. P. Johnson (1987), is networking with other collaborative teams. Developing a schoolwide team support network in which teams can share ideas, lessons, and successes is a way to ensure continued support for and improvement of collaborative methods. Collaborative teaming empowers teaching staff, support personnel, parents, and students alike. They are enfranchised through their participation in decision-making processes. Regardless of the arrangement, special instruction and intervention can be embedded in the general education curriculum, and students with language and communication difficulties (whether the difficulties are primary or secondary) can remain in the general education classroom if a collaborative team model is implemented.

Discussion Questions

1. Discuss the reasoning behind the IDEA assessment guidelines and what might occur if the law did not provide them.
2. Discuss how the LRE mandate, the regular education initiate (REI), and inclusion are related to one another.
3. Discuss the major paradigm shifts in language intervention and how they influence decisions about what *types* of services are provided; *how* services are provided; and *where* services are provided.
4. Discuss how the "collaboration imperative" affects the amount and quality of services provided to students with disabilities.
5. Discuss similarities and differences between the roles and responsibilities of the special education teacher and the language interventionist.

Activities/Projects

1. Invite parents of children with disabilities to share their experiences with assessment, inclusion, and working with professionals. After the parents have shared their experiences, they could be asked to participate with the class (as a whole or in teams) in developing a list of suggestions for more effective partnerships with families.
2. Invite professionals who have experience with developing IFSPs and/or IEPs to discuss how they are developed and provide copies of the forms.

References

American Occupational Therapy Association. (1989). *Guidelines for occupational therapy services in the public schools* (2nd ed.). Rockville, MD: Author.

American Physical Therapy Association. (1990). *Physical therapy practice in educational environments*. Alexandria, VA: Author.

American Speech-Language-Hearing Association. (1989). Competencies for speech-language pathologists providing services in augmentation communication. *ASHA, 31,* 107–110.

American Speech-Language-Hearing Association, Committee on Language Learning Disorders. (1991). A model for collaborative service delivery for students with language-learning disorders in the public schools. *ASHA, 3,* 33–35.

American Speech-Language-Hearing Association. (1993). Guidelines for caseload size and speech-language service delivery in the schools. *ASHA, 35* (Suppl. 10), 33–38.

Association for Persons with Severe Handicaps. (1986). *Position statement on the provision of related services.* Seattle, WA: Author.

Belsky, J. (1981). Early human experience: A family perspective. *Developmental Psychology, 17,* 3–23.

Bronfenbrenner, U. (1986). Ecology of the family as a context for human development: Research perspectives. *Developmental Psychology, 22,* 723–742.

Cirrin, F. M., & Penner, S. G. (1995). Classroom-based and consultative service delivery—models for language intervention. In M. E. Fey, J. Windsor, & S. F. Warren, (Eds.), *Language intervention: Preschool through the elementary years* (pp. 333–362). Baltimore: Brookes.

Freagon, S., & Kachur, D. S. (1993). *Thoughts, perspectives, and ideas presented at the Illinois Deans of Colleges of Education symposium on inclusive education of students with disabilities.* Springfield: Illinois Planning Council on Developmental Disabilities.

Goodman, K. (1986). *What's whole in whole language?* Portsmouth, NH: Heinemann.

Gordon, T. (1980). *Leadership effectiveness training (LET).* New York: Wyden Books.

Hoerr, T. R. (1996). Collegiality: A new way to define instructional leadership. *Phi Delta Kappan, 77,* 380–381.

Idol, L., Paolucci-Whitcomb, P., & Nevin, A. (1987). *Collaborative consultation.* Austin, TX: PRO-ED.

Johnson, D. W., & Johnson, F. P. (1975). *Joining together: Group theory and skills.* Englewood Cliffs, NJ: Prentice-Hall.

Johnson, D. W., & Johnson, F. P. (1987). *Joining together: Group theory and skills* (3rd ed.). Englewood Cliffs, NJ: Prentice-Hall.

Johnson, D. W., & Johnson, R. T. (1989). *Cooperation and competition: Theory and research.* Edina, MN: Interaction.

Kayser, H. (1989, November). Communication strategies of Anglo and Hispanic clinicians with Hispanic preschoolers. Paper presented at the American Speech-Language-Hearing Association and Convention, St. Louis.

Kayser, H. (1995). Intervention with children with linguistically and culturally diverse backgrounds. In M. E. Fay, J. Windsor, & S. F. Warren (Eds.), *Language intervention: Preschool through the elementary years* (pp. 315–33). Baltimore: Paul H. Brookes.

Linder, T. W. (1993). *Transdisciplinary play-based assessment: A functional approach to working with young children,* Revised Edition. Baltimore: Paul H. Brookes.

Lipsky, D. K., & Gartner, A. (1997). *Inclusion and school reform.* Baltimore: Paul H. Brookes.

Lynch, E. W., & Hanson, M. J. (1992). *Developing cross-cultural competence*. Baltimore: Brookes Publishing.

Lyons, S., & Lyon, G. (1980). Team functioning and staff development: A role release approach to providing integrated educational services for severely handicapped students. *Journal of the Association for the Severely Handicapped, 9*(2), 125–135.

McCormick, L., & Goldman, R. (1979). The transdisciplinary model: Implications for service delivery and personnel preparation. *AAESPH Review, 4*(2), 152–161.

Montgomery, J. K. (1992). Perspectives from the field: Language, speech, and hearing services in schools. *Language, Speech and Hearing Services in Schools, 23,* 363–364.

Napier, R. W., & Gershenfeld, M. K. (1993). *Groups: Theory and experience* (5th ed.). Boston: Houghton Mifflin.

Parker, G. M. (1990). *Team players and teamwork*. San Francisco: Jossey-Bass Publishers.

Rainforth, B., York, J., & MacDonald, C. (1992). *Collaborative teams for students with severe disabilities*. Baltimore: Paul H. Brookes.

Roller, E., Rodriguez, T., Warner, J., & Lindahl, P. (1992). Integration of self-contained children with severe speech-language needs into the regular education classrooms. *Language, Speech, and Hearing Services in Schools, 23,* 365–366.

Skrtic, T. (1991). *Beyond special education: A critical analysis of professional culture and school organization*. Denver, CO: Love.

Stainback, S., Stainback, W., & Jackson, H. J. (1992). Toward inclusive classrooms. In S. Stainback and W. Stainback (Eds.), *Curriculum considerations in inclusive classrooms* (pp. 2–17). Baltimore: Brookes.

Sternat, J., Messina, R., Nietupski, J., Lyon, S., & Brown, L. (1977). Occupational and physical therapy services for severely handicapped students: Towards a naturalized public school service delivery model. In E. Sontag, J. Smith, & N. Certo (Eds.), *Educational programming for the severely and profoundly handicapped* (pp. 263–287). Reston, VA: Council for Exceptional Children.

Tharp, R. G. (1975). The triadic model of consultation. In C. Patter (Ed.), *Psychological consultation in the schools: Helping teachers meet special needs* (pp. 133–151). Reston, VA: Council for Exceptional Children.

Tharp, R. G., & Wetzel, R. J. (1969). *Behavior modification in the natural environment*. New York: Academic Press.

Thousand, J. S., & Villa, R. A. (1992). Collaborative teams: A powerful tool in school restructuring. In R. A. Villa, J. A. Thousand, W. Stainback, & S. Stainback (Eds.), *Restructuring for caring and effective education* (pp. 73–108). Baltimore: Brookes.

Thousand, J. S., & Villa, R. A. (2000). Collaborative teaming: A powerful tool in school restructuring. In R. A. & J. S. Thousand (Eds.), *Restructuring for caring and effective education: Piecing the puzzle.* (pp. 254–292). Baltimore: Brookes.

West, J. F., & Cannon, G. S. (1988). Essential collaborative consultation competencies for regular and special educators. *Journal of Learning Disabilities, 21*(1), 56–63.

West, J. F., & Idol, L. (1990). Collaborative consultation in the education of mildly handicapped and at-risk students. *Remedial and Special Education, 11*(1), 22–31.

Westby, C., & Erickson, G. (1992). Prologue. *Topics in Language Disorders, 12*(3), p. v–viii.

Wolery, M., & Dyk, L. (1984). Arena assessment: Description and preliminary social validation data. *Journal of the Association for the Severely Handicapped, 9*(3), 231–235.

CHAPTER 6

Diagnostic and Descriptive Assessment

Diane Frome Loeb

Assessment is a process, not a single procedure. It is "a multilevel process, beginning with screening procedures and continuing through diagnosis, planning of intervention, and program monitoring and evaluation" (Richard & Schiefelbusch, 1991). Assessment involves multiple observations of the child over a period of time in many contexts. The processes of assessment parallel the multiple purposes for assessment. This chapter will examine five purposes of assessment: (1) screening and identification, (2) diagnosis, (3) eligibility determination, (4) intervention planning, and (5) evaluating intervention progress. Diagnosis of a language impairment entails the use of both formal and informal methods. The purposes of assessment will be discussed at length in the following sections, with an emphasis on traditional methods of assessment.

SCREENING AND IDENTIFICATION

The goal of screening in the schools is to identify children who may have language and/or communication delays and disorders that place them at risk for social and/or academic problems. Screening tools may be comprehensive (covering motor, cognition, speech, language, and other areas of development) or may be specific to speech and language. Screening may be provided individually or through mass screening. Individual or selective screening occurs when children are referred by a parent or teacher because of concern about their communication development. Preschool and kindergarten programs may have large-scale screening programs in place to identify children who may need special assistance. In mass screening, a large number of children are screened at one time. Klee,

Carson, Hall, and Muskina (1994) found that mass-screening by mail to parents was an efficient and cost-effective measure for screening two-year-olds. They sent the Language Development Survey (LDS; Rescorla, 1989) to parents who had contacted them requesting a speech-language evaluation. The parents completed the survey, which asks for parents' report of a child's vocabulary and early word combinations, then mailed the completed LDS back to the clinic. Those children who did not meet the LDS criteria were seen for further speech-language assessment.

Screening involves a quick look to see if the child's language skills are adequate or whether there are deviations from normal expectations that warrant further assessment. The screening procedure may last anywhere from three to fifteen minutes. The results of a screening do not satisfy the objective of determining whether or not a child has a language disorder. Children who do not pass a screening are referred for a complete speech and language evaluation. Some children who need services may be missed (under-referral), and sometimes children who do not need services are referred for evaluation (over-referral). A screening tool's rate of over- and under-referral is related to its specificity and sensitivity. Tests that are sensitive appropriately identify children needing additional assessment. A test that is specific will not refer children who do not require further assessment. The less sensitive a screening test is, the greater the number of under-referrals. Losses in specificity result in an increased number of over-referrals. The levels of specificity and sensitivity are related to a screening tool's validity. Validity tells us the extent that a test measures what it says it measures. Unfortunately, a survey of preschool speech and language screening tests by Sturner, Layton, Evans, Heller, Funk, and Machon (1994) indicates that only a few screening tools contained the information necessary to make computation of validity possible. This finding highlights the importance of taking great care when selecting screening tools and interpreting screening results.

Screening tools typically use observations, parent report, or some combination of the two. Parental report is a valid method most commonly used with very young children and children with very limited language abilities (Dale, 1991; Glascoe, 1991; Rescorla, 1989). Parents may be asked to: (1) complete a checklist of words the child understands and/or produces; (2) indicate the types of word combinations the child uses; and/or (3) report verbal and nonverbal communication attempts.

A summary of screening tools is provided in Table 6.1. Children who have an established risk for communication problems generally forgo the screening process. The category "established risk" includes children who have a diagnosed medical condition that is known to have a negative impact on development (e.g., Down syndrome,

TABLE 6.1   Summary of Screening Tools

Name of Test	Authors	Age Range	Areas Assessed	Method*
Birth to Three Developmental Survey	Bangs & Dobson (1986)	0–36 months	language	DO
Early Language Milestone Scale-2	Coplan (1993)	0–36 months	auditory expressive, auditory receptive, visual	DO, PR
Early Screening Profiles	Harrison, Kaufman, Kaufman, Bruininks, Rynders, Ilmer, Sparrow, & Cicchetti (1990)	2–6; 11 years	cognitive, language, motor, self-help/social	DO, PR
Denver-II	Frakenburg et al. (1992)	0–6 years	personal–social, fine motor-adaptive, language, gross motor	DO, PR
Mother–Infant Communication Screening	Raack (1989)	Infancy	mother–infant interaction including language and synchrony, play and neutral state, distress, feeding, and rest	DO
Language Development Survey	Rescorla (1989)	2 years	expressive language	PR
The Screening Kit of Language Development	Bliss & Allen (1982)	2–5 years	receptive and expressive language	DO
Fluharty Preschool Speech–Language Screening Test-2	Fluharty (2000)	3–6; 11 years	receptive and expressive language	DO
Bankson Language Screening Test (BLT-2)	Bankson (1990)	3–6; 11 years	receptive and expressive language	DO
Compton Speech & Language Screening Evaluation	Compton (1978)	3–6 years	language, articulation	DO
Northwest Syntax Screening Test	Lee (1969, 1971)	3–7 years	receptive and expressive language	DO
Patterned Elicitation Syntax Screening Test	Young & Perachio (1981, 1983)	3–7; 6 years	expressive syntax	DO

(continued)

TABLE 6.1   Continued

Name of Test	Authors	Age Range	Areas Assessed	Method*
Pragmatic Screening Test	Prinz & Wenir (1987)	3; 5–8; 5 years	expressive pragmatics	DO
Screening Children for Related Early Education Needs	Hresko, Reid, Hammill, Ginsburg, & Baroody (1988)	3–7 years	multiple academic areas	DO
Test of Early Language Development-3	Hresko, Reid, & Hammill (1999)	2–7; 11 years	receptive and expressive language	DO
Kindergarten Language Screening Test, 2nd edition	Gauthier & Madison (1998)	3; 6–6; 11 years	receptive and expressive language	DO
Language Identification Screening Test for Kindergarten	Illerbrun, McLeod, Greenough, & Haines (1984)	Kindergarten	receptive and expressive language	DO

*Method is parent report (PR) or direct observation (DO).

hearing impairment, cerebral palsy) (Tjossem, 1976). Children who have established risks should receive comprehensive evaluation of their abilities in multiple domains.

DIAGNOSIS

An evaluation of the child's speech and language skills is conducted in order to make a diagnosis. The first step in a speech-language evaluation is to determine the concerns of caregivers, teachers, and significant others. Next, procedures are implemented to collect as much descriptive information as possible about the child's language, speech and communication abilities. Diagnostic information may come from a case history provided by caregivers, reports from other professionals, and direct observation of the child. Following a collection of information about a child's communication skills, a diagnosis is made that describes the nature of the problem, severity of the problem, and possible causes and maintaining factors. The diagnosis has direct implications for the type and intensity of intervention. In order to provide a diagnosis, the language interventionist must perform a range of informal and formal procedures to determine the child's current level of functioning.

Formal and Informal Language Assessment

Assessment activities extend over a continuum of "formal" to "informal" procedures. Formal procedures typically are more structured and norm-referenced. Informal procedures tend to be more naturalistic; however, the naturalness of an informal procedure will depend on the specific measure.

Formal Procedures

Formal procedures are commercially available tests that are standardized and/or norm-referenced (Table 6.2 provides examples of norm-referenced, standardized tests). A standardized test is one that must be administered in a prescribed manner. A norm-referenced test compares one child's behavior with other children's behavior. Typically, such tests include mean and standard deviation scores that tell the extent a child deviates from same-age peers. The mean is the average performance of the normative group. The standard deviation gives the range of the variance or diverse range of scores in a population. Scores that fall within one standard deviation of the mean are generally considered within normal limits and account for 68 percent of the population. The standard deviation to indicate language impairment varies from 1 standard deviation to greater than 2 standard deviations. Percentiles are also used as a way to describe development. Percentiles indicate how a child performs relative to same-age peers. For example, if a child scores at the 10th percentile, 90 percent of the children performed better than he or she did.

Tests are only as good as the psychometric criteria on which they are based. Psychometric criteria reflect the reliability and validity of the test instruments. Reliability refers to the consistency of a test. The more stable a test is, the more one can trust the results. Validity is how well a test measures what it says it measures. McCauley and Swisher (1984a) evaluated preschool speech and language tests for their psychometric properties and found that less than 20 percent of the thirty tests evaluated met half of the psychometric criteria (Table 6.3). This finding indicates that the validity and reliability of many speech and language tools are questionable.

More recently, Plante and Vance (1994) reported that the validity and reliability of preschool language tests continues to be a major problem. They found that only 38 percent of the twenty-one tests evaluated met half of the same psychometric criteria set forth by McCauley and Swisher. Plante and Vance further studied four of the tests that met half of the psychometric criteria by administering them to a group of children with normal language development and a group identified as language impaired. The tests were unable to differentiate normally developing children from children with language impairment.

TABLE 6.2   Examples of Formal Tools for Speech-Language Assessment

Name of Test	Authors	Areas Assessed	Expressive	Receptive	Ages
Assessing Semantic Skills through Everyday Language	Barrett, Zachman, & Huisingh (1988)	Semantics	XXX	XXX	3–9 years 11 months
Comprehensive Receptive and Expressive Vocabulary Test, 2nd Edition	Wallace & Hammill (2002)	Semantics	XXX	XXX	4–89 years 11 months
Expressive One-Word Picture Vocabulary Test	Brownell (2000)	Semantics	XXX		2–18 years 11 months
Full-Range Picture Vocabulary Test	Ammons & Ammons (1948)	Semantics			2-adult
Illinois Test of Psycholinguistic Abilities, 3rd Edition	Hammill, Mather, & Roberts (2001)	Semantics, Grammar, Phonology, Reading Comprehension, Word Identification, Spelling	XXX		5–12 years 11 months
Receptive One-Word Picture Vocabulary Test	Brownell (2000)	Semantics		XXX	2 years 10 months– 18 years; 11 months
Peabody Picture Vocabulary Test, Revised	Dunn & Dunn (1981)	Semantics		XXX	2–40 years
Test for Auditory Comprehension and Language, 3rd Edition	Carrow-Woolfolk (1999)	Semantics Morphology Syntax		XXX	3–9 years 11 months
Test of Relational Concepts	Edmonston & Thane	Semantics		XXX	3–8 years
Test of Word Finding, 2nd Edition	German (2000)	Semantics	XXX	XXX	6–12 years 11 months
Test of Word Finding in Discourse	German (1991)	Semantics	XXX		6 years 6 months– 12 years; 11 months
The Word Test-Elementary, Revised	Huisingh, Barrett, Zachman, Blagden, & Orman (1990)	Semantics	XXX		7–11 years

TABLE 6.2   Examples of Formal Tools for Speech-Language Assessment (*continued*)

*Miller-Yoder Test of Language Comprehension	Miller & Yoder (1984)	Syntax, morphology		XXX	3–8 years
Structured Photographic Expressive Language-Preschool	Werner & Kresheck (1993)	Syntax, morphology	XXX		3–5; 11 years
Structured Photographic Expressive Language Test-II	Werner & Kresheck (1983)	Syntax, morphology	XXX		4–9; 5 years
Test for Examining Expressive Morphology	Shipley, Stone, & Sue (1983)	Morphology	XXX		3–8 years
Assessment of Phonological Processes-R	Hodson (1986)	Phonology	XXX		Preschool
Arizona Articulation Proficiency Scale	Fudala (1978)	Articulation	XXX		3-adult
Bankson-Bernthal Phonological Process Survey Test	Bankson & Bernthal (1990)	Phonology	XXX		
Fisher-Logemann Test of Articulation Competence	Fisher & Logemann (1971)	Articulation	XXX		
Goldman-Fristoe Test of Articulation-2	Goldman & Fristoe (2000)	Articulation	XXX		2–21 years
Khan-Lewis Phonological Analysis	Khan & Lewis (1986)	Phonology	XXX		2; 6–adults
Phonological Process Analysis	Weiner (1979)	Phonology	XXX		
Photo Articulation Test, 3rd Edition	Lippke, Dickey, Selmar, & Soder (1997)	Articulation	XXX		3–8; 11 years
Smit-Hand Articulation and Phonology Evaluation	Smit & Hand	Articulation, Phonology	XXX		3–9 years
Structured Photographic Articulation Test II	Dawson & Tattersall (0000)	Articulation, Phonological processes	XXX		3–9 years
Templin-Darley Test of Articulation	Templin & Darley (1969)	Articulation	XXX		3–8 years

(*continued*)

TABLE 6.2   Examples of Formal Tools for Speech-Language Assessment (*continued*)

Name of Test	Authors	Areas Assessed	Expressive	Receptive	Ages
Communication & Symbolic Behavior Scales	Wetherby & Prizant (1993)	Pragmatics	XXX		8–24 months
Test of Pragmatic Language	Phelps-Terasaki & Phelps-Gunn (1992)	Pragmatics	XXX		5–13; 11 years
Test of Pragmatic Skills	Shulman (1985)	Pragmatics	XXX		3–8; 11 years
Bankson Language Test-2	Bankson (1990)	Language	XXX	XXX	3–6; 11 years
Basic Language Concepts Test	Engelman, Ross, & Bingham (1986)	Language	XXX	XXX	4–6; 5 years
Boehm Test of Basic Concepts-3	Boehm (1986)	Language		XXX	3–5 years
Comprehensive Test of Phonological Processing	Torgesen, Wagner, & Rashotte (1999)	Phonological awareness, memory and rapid naming			5–24; 11 years
Communication Abilities Diagnostic Test	Johnston & Johnston (1990)	Language			3–8 years
Clark-Madison Test of Oral Language	Clark & Madison (1986)	Language	XXX		4–8 years
*Criterion-Referenced Inventory of Language	Wiig (1990)	Language	XXX		
Language Processing Test, Revised	Richard & Hanner (1995)	Language	XXX		5–11 years
MacArthur Inventory of Language Development	Fenson, Dale, Reznick, Thal, Bates, Hartung, Pethick, & Reilly (1993)	Language	XXX		8–30 months
Preschool Language Assessment Instrument	Blank, Rose, & Berline (1978)	Language	XXX	XXX	3–8 years
Preschool Language Scale-3	Zimmerman, Steiner, & Pond (1991)	Language	XXX	XXX	18 mo.– 17 years

TABLE 6.2 Examples of Formal Tools for Speech-Language Assessment (*continued*)

Receptive-Expressive Emergent Language Test-2	Bzoch & League (1991)	Language	XXX	XXX	0–3 years
Reynell Developmental Language Scales (U.S. Edition)	Reynell & Gruber (1990)	Language	XXX	XXX	1–6; 11 years
Sequenced Inventory of Communication Development	Hedrick, Prather, & Tobin (1984)	Language	XXX	XXX	4–48 months
Structured Photographic Expressive Language Test-II		Language	XXX		4–9; 5 years
Structured Photographic Expressive Language Test-Preschool		Language	XXX		3–5; 11 years
Test of Problem Solving	Zachman, Barrett, Huisingh, & Jorgensen (1995)	Problem Solving	XXX	XXX	6–11 years*
Test for Auditory Comprehension of Language, 3rd edition	Carrow-Woolfolk (1999)	Language		XXX	3–9; 11 years
Test of Children's Language	Barenbaum & Newcomer (1996)	Language, reading, writing	XXX		5–8; 11 years
Test of Language Development-Primary, 3rd Edition	Newcomer & Hammill (1997)	Language	XXX	XXX	4–8; 11 years
Test of Language Development-Intermediate, 3rd Edition	Hammill & Newcomer (1997)	Language	XXX	XXX	8–12; 11 years
Token Test for Children	DiSimoni (1978)	Language		XXX	3–12 years
Utah Test of Language Development-3	Mecham (1989)	Language	XXX	XXX	3–9: 11 years

*Indicates a criterion-referenced assessment tool.

TABLE 6.3   Properties of Norm-referenced Tests

Psychometric Criteria

1. *Information about the standardization sample that includes geographic, socioeconomic, and normalcy should be present in the test manual.
2. Adequate sample size should be present for the subgroups of the standardization (100 or more per subgroup).
3. Systematic item analysis should be reported.
4. Measures of central tendency and variability of the test results should be present.
5. *Evidence of concurrent validity.
6. *Evidence of predictive validity.
7. *Estimate of test re-test reliability (.90 or better significant at the .05 level).
8. *Evidence of inter-examiner reliability (.90 or better at the .05 level).
9. Description of test administration, scoring, and interpretation should be described in detail and be consistent with the standardization procedures.
10. Information about test administrator or scorer qualifications.

*Asterisk indicates which criteria were not achieved frequently.

The implications of these findings are that language interventionists need to carefully evaluate the tests they administer in terms of validity and reliability. Plante and Vance's findings emphasize the importance of comparing the test's population characteristics with those of the child being assessed. When tests do not include children with various language abilities in their normative sample, the variation is decreased. This reduction in variation makes it more likely that children with language impairment will appear very different from the normed population. Plante and Vance (1994) further suggest that language interventionists need to evaluate the test manual for evidence of discriminant analysis. Such an analysis will report the accuracy of a test in identifying language-impaired children and give an empirically derived cutoff score at each age level.

Another disadvantage of formal tests is that they often lack ecological validity. That is, they fail to take into account the child's ability to use language in functional or everyday contexts. Many formats place the child as the "responder" in question–answer situations that are unlike any found in real-life situations. Thus, the artificial nature of the testing environment fails to measure the child's use of language as he or she would interact in everyday situations. Placing the child in the role of a responder who provides information already known by both the child and examiner is unusual in some cultures. For example, some Native American children are raised in a culture that does not require them to answer questions when the answer is known. Further, with the exception of a few specially designed tests (cf. Shulman, 1985; Wetherby & Prizant, 1993), it is difficult to assess a child's pragmatic skills using formal procedures.

Another concern about using standardized tests is related to their lack of cultural sensitivity. School-based speech-language pathologists indicate that tests that could not be appropriately applied to different cultures were a significant problem in their practice (Huang, Hopkins, & Nippold, 1997). Possible solutions to this problem include collecting normative data or conducting more informal measures of language assessment such as an authentic assessment. An authentic assessment involves developing a criterion-referenced protocol for a given group of individuals. Schraeder, Quinn, Stockman and Miller (1999) provide data that support using authentic assessment with three-year-old children from multicultural and low-income homes.

A final weakness of standardized tests is their restricted usefulness beyond the purpose of identifying a problem. Formal procedures have limited application to intervention planning and monitoring intervention progress. Because most tests are designed to assess fairly broad areas of skills, it is not appropriate to derive specific intervention targets from the tests (McCauley & Swisher, 1984b). This same reason has been used in arguing that formal tests should not be relied on solely for evaluating the progress made during intervention. McCauley and Swisher warn against using norm-referenced tests to assess progress because they may over- or underestimate change observed as a result of intervention. With respect to overestimation, children who show improvement on a norm-referenced test show a "gain score." For example, a pre-intervention score of 70 compared with a post-intervention score of 80 would yield a gain score of 10. The significance of a gain score is difficult to interpret because the gain score can be a result of chance or a test's imperfect reliability. Thus, a child who makes no discernable progress in therapy, yet shows a gain score, may not have made the progress indicated by the gain score. Underestimation occurs when a child does not show gains on a norm-referenced test, yet has clearly made gains in intervention. In this instance, the norm-referenced test is too broad to measure the specific changes observed.

Despite these many inadequacies, formal procedures are relied on to diagnose children with language impairment and, in school districts, to establish eligibility criteria for intervention. Speech-language pathologists (language interventionists) and others concerned with the limitations of formal procedures can use clinical judgment and informal procedures to guide decision making. Clinical judgment is a belief statement(s) about a client's abilities. The belief statement is derived from the professional's clinical experience, intuition, and knowledge of language development and language impairment. The best approach for making diagnoses and eligibility determination is to use a combination of formal procedures, informal procedures, and clinical judgment.

Informal Procedures

Informal procedures include developmental scales, parent interviews, criterion-referenced tests (commercially available or self-constructed probes), and language sampling (see Table 6.2), procedures that allow a level of flexibility and in-depth testing not afforded by standardized tests. Developmental scales are checklists of speech-language behaviors or milestones that occur in children with normally developing speech and language. These might be administered by observing the child or through a caregiver's report. A developmental scale provides information about the child's overall development. In contrast, criterion-referenced tests probe one specific area of language learning.

Criterion-referenced tests typically evaluate a very specific area, such as pronouns, speech acts, or meaning relations in sentences (such as patient or agent). Criterion-referenced tests evaluate a child's performance on certain items and a number correct score is derived. Criteria are set at an arbitrary level, for instance, 80 percent success in order for the child to succeed. Criterion-referenced tests are thought to be more appropriate measures of change that occur during intervention because of their specific focus. Unfortunately, with the exception of a few (e.g., the Criterion Referenced Inventory of Language (Wiig, 1990) and the Miller-Yoder Test of Language Comprehension (Miller & Yoder, 1984), there are a limited number of criterion-referenced tests available. Thus, language interventionists rely on constructing their own probes to evaluate specific areas of language ability. An example of an informal probe would involve assessing production of word final *s* and *z* in nonmorphophonemic contexts such as *bus* or *fuzz* (i.e., words that do not have morphology expressed phonemically such as *bats* or *goes*). This type of probe might be used to determine if a child who is not producing some grammatical morphemes, such as plural *-s* or possessive *-s*, has a problem learning morphemes exclusively, or if there is a phonological component to the problem and the child has difficulty producing these sounds at the end of words that are not marked with grammatical morphemes (e.g., *house* or *rose*). This is an important thing to know because the child who cannot produce s or z in either morphological or nonmorphological contexts presents a different problem than the child who can produce final s and z in phonological, but not morphological, contexts. The information derived from this probe would greatly influence whether grammatical or phonological goals were targeted for intervention.

Language Sampling

A very rich source of information about a child's expressive language can be derived from language sampling. Language sampling is the collection of the child's language during play, telling stories, or everyday conversational exchanges. The advantage of this procedure is that it provides a detailed picture of the child's communication in a fairly naturalistic context. A drawback is that transcription and analyses of samples are time-consuming. However, the gains in information derived from language sampling and the increase in computerized programs to assist with language analysis (Miller, Freiberg, Rolland, & Reeves, 1992) make this procedure a worthwhile investment.

The most important consideration when eliciting a language sample from a child is that it be representative. That is, the language the child produces should accurately represent how the child interacts with others. Thus, like our concerns regarding validity and reliability for formal assessment procedures, we must also be concerned about the validity and reliability of language sampling by obtaining a representative sample. Miller (1981) suggests several factors to be taken into consideration to ensure a representative sample. These include:

1. the nature of the interaction;
2. the setting where the interaction takes place;
3. the materials used to elicit the language sample;
4. the methods of recording the sample;
5. the size of the language sample.

The nature of the interaction concerns not only who interacts with the child, but also how the stage is set so that the child feels comfortable to talk. Speech-language pathologists, teachers, peers, and parents are excellent candidates for interactional partners. If the interactant is unfamiliar to the child, or if the child is placed in a new situation, he or she may be reticent to interact for the first few minutes of play. Rather than ask a series of closed questions that will elicit a minimal response, such as "What's that?" or yes/no questions, "Do you like dolls?" it is recommended that the child be given time to warm up to the environment with a short period of silent play. The danger with asking too many questions is that it could result in many one-word responses from the child, which, in turn, will negatively influence the representativeness of the sample. An alternative to a short silent period would be to have the individual who is interacting with the child produce "self-talk" or "parallel play." The technique of "self-talk" involves the interactor playing with some of the materials and talking about what he or she is doing. "Parallel play" means to play alongside the child, either doing similar things as the child or a variation of the same theme. During parallel play, the interactant can talk about what the child is doing by using "description." Complying with the child's play agenda is referred to as "following the child's lead." The ability to follow the child's lead relies on the language interventionist's willingness to let the child control the pace and topic of play. Even with artful use of all the techniques available, the person collecting the language sample will not be successful if he or she is not enjoying him-or herself or is not truly interested in the child and play. These types of procedures are illustrated in the following example.

(Erik and the language interventionist are playing with a set of toys)

> ERIK: (moves a truck up a street ramp)
> LI: (**follows his lead** by doing the same thing with a motorcycle)
> LI: "You're going up the hill. (description of child's play) I'm coming too. (**self-talk**)
> I hope I can make it. (**self-talk**)
> Uh oh. I stopped! (**self-talk**)
> I need gas. (**Self-talk**)
> Someone, help me!"
> ERIK: (pretends to give the language interventionist's car gas)
> LI: (gives the child's car some gas [parallel play])

Language samples can be obtained in many places, including the home, classroom, or clinic setting, but there may be certain limitations on communication in some settings. The language interventionist should be aware of what these are and take them into account when determining representativeness. For example, there may be times in a child-care setting, such as group reading, when it is inappropriate to take a language sample because the teacher is the main speaker and interaction is not encouraged.

Materials that are used to elicit a language sample should be interesting to the child. The child's developmental level and interests, as well as his or her physical and sensory abilities, should be taken into consideration when selecting toys. The use of familiar books and games may elicit more routinized language. Puzzles may elicit locatives such as *on* and *in*. Introduction of unfamiliar toys or toys with band-aids or other unusual characteristics (broken leg, pink hair, etc.) are novel and lead to child-initiated topics. Another common procedure is to use a play theme, such as a farm with many people and animals or a schoolhouse with children and teachers.

During the sampling, the language interventionist will audiotape or transcribe on-line what the child says (i.e., write down what is said as it is being said). In many cases it is not feasible to transcribe every word produced by the child on-line. Instead, the language interventionist can write down utterances on a time basis that would involve five minutes of transcribing and five minutes of rest, until a predetermined time or number of utterances had been attained. Regardless of whether on-line recording or audio recording is used, it is beneficial to make notes of the ongoing context (i.e., nonverbal occurrences or explanations) or to repeat what the child says when he or she is not understood.

The size of the language sample will vary, depending on the child's willingness and ability to interact. Time sampling or a specified number of utterances can be used as guidelines for how many utterances to analyze or transcribe from a language sample. Miller (1981) recommends a thirty-minute sample if the time sample format is used. The alternative is to set a number of utterances to be collected. The sample should have a minimum of fifty child utterances in order to be representative. The larger the sample, the more representative it is. However, because of time constraints, fifty–one-hundred utterances samples are common.

Once a language sample has been collected and transcribed, analyses deemed relevant to the child's needs can be initiated. All areas of language (syntax, phonology, morphology, semantics, pragmatics, and interactions thereof) can be analyzed in any language sample if careful attention is given to recording the verbal and nonverbal contexts of interaction. Videotaping is often necessary if one is analyzing the pragmatic aspects of an interaction.

Informal procedures will be relied on more when the purpose of the assessment is to plan intervention or to monitor the progress of an intervention program. Procedures such as specific probes or language sampling provide a more detailed look at the child's skills. It is for this reason that they are appropriate for determining intervention goals. Additionally, informal procedures may be more effective at measuring gains observed during intervention because they can be tailored to elicit the child's speech and language targets.

Specific Informal Assessment Procedures

Assessment must determine not only *if* a problem exists, but also *the nature* and *extent of the problem*. Typically, both receptive and expressive language functioning are assessed in multiple domains of language (i.e., form, content, and use). Following are a number of potential analyses for several areas of language, with an emphasis on analyses that can be performed on language sample data.

Form

Form is divided into phonology, morphology, and syntax. When evaluating form, one will ask the following questions:

1. Does the child understand sentences of varying complexity?
2. Does the child have difficulty formulating grammatical sentences? If so, in what respect are they ungrammatical? Do they lack appropriate noun phrase marking or elaboration? Are negation and question formation skills at the appropriate developmental level?

3. Is age-appropriate morphology present? Is noun–verb agreement appropriate for the child's age?
4. Does the child produce grammatical sentences, yet produce short utterances that lack grammatical complexity? If so, what is the level of complexity used? What levels of complexity are absent?
5. Does the child produce sentences that are difficult to understand (i.e., unintelligible)? Is the unintelligibility due to a problem producing speech sounds or production of phonological processes?
6. Does the child have difficulty producing some sounds you would expect them to be able to make or is he/she using phonological processes that you would predict to be absent at this point in the child's development?

Although there are several formal or standardized procedures available for assessing syntax, morphology, and phonology (see Table 6.2), the above questions can also be explored using informal procedures. One commonly used index of syntax derived from a language sample is mean length of utterance or MLU. MLU is the average length of a child's utterance. It is a gross measure of complexity. It is computed by counting the number of morphemes per utterance, adding the morphemes, and dividing by the number of utterances. An example is given below for a child who is three-and-a-half years old. The child (C) is playing with a McDonald's toyhouse with an adult examiner (E). The morphemes per utterance are in parentheses. Chapman (1981a) provides guidelines for counting morphemes to compute MLU based on Brown (1973), provided in Table 6.4.

> E: I almost sat on it.
> 1. C: Yeah. (1)
> 2. C: These go here. (3)
> 3. C: That my fry. (3)
> E: That's right.
> E: That's your french fry.
> 4. C: Open these me. (3)
> E: Open that for you?
> 5. C: Yeah. (1)
> 6. C: Me not do. (3)
> E: There you go.
> 7. C: That up? (2)
> E: Yep, that goes anywhere you want.
> 8. C: Me go. (2)
> E: You can go in there.
> 9. C: Put this on. (3)
> E: I'll put the lid on.
> 10. C: Where this go? (3)
> E: Where does that go?
> E: It goes up here.

TABLE 6.4   Guidelines for MLU Computation

Do Count:

1. Each meaningful morpheme is counted.
Example: Dog = 1, Dog/s = 2

Count as Only One Morpheme:

2. Words that are repeated for emphasis.
"No!" "No!" "No!" = 1 morpheme per utterance in 3 utterances
3. Compound words (2 or more free morphemes), proper names, and ritualized or routinized forms.
"Bye bye" "choo choo" "oopsadaisy" "snowman" "Big Bird"
4. Irregular past tense verbs count as one morpheme.
fell, saw, ran, etc.
5. Count only the first instance of a disfluency.
Example: "My, my, my baby is cry/ing." Count only one of the *my*s.
6. Words such as *yeah, nuuh, no, yes, ok, hi.*
7. Semi-auxiliaries or catenatives such as *gonna, wanna, gotta.*
8. Diminutive forms (-*y*) *daddy, mommy, puppy, rainy.*

Don't Count:

1. Fillers such as *oh* or *um*. These forms serve to hold the conversational floor, but should not be counted as adding meaningful content or complexity to the child's message.
2. Counting, alphabet recitals, singing, nursery rhymes. Utterances that appear to be memorized strings of information should be excluded.
3. Conjunctions at the beginning of sentences that appear repeatedly throughout the language sample. Some children begin many sentences with *and* or *but.*
4. Imitations of the adult utterances that exceed 20 percent of the entire sample and/or if their inclusion leads to an unrepresentative sample.
5. Frequent self-repetitions. Miller & Chapman recommend two analyses be conducted, one with and one without the self-repetitions. Self-repetitions should be excluded when their inclusions leads to an overall increase or decrease of MLU.

Based on Miller & Chapman (1979).

Total morphemes = 24
Divide 24 by 10 utterances= an MLU of 2.4 morphemes

If this MLU value had been derived from fifty utterances and from a representative sample, it could be compared to normative guidelines to determine if this child was within normal limits for his or her age (Miller, 1981; Table 6.5). An MLU of 2.4 would be in Brown's Stage II

TABLE 6.5   Mean Length of Utterance Normative Data

Early Stage I

	1.01	1.10	1.20	1.30	1.40	1.50
Predicted Age* (+ 1 SD)	19.1 (16.4–21.8)	19.8 (17.1–22.5)	20.6 (17.9–23.3)	21.4 (18.7–24.1)	22.2 (19.5–24.9)	23 (18.5–27.5)

Late Stage I

	1.60	1.70	1.80	1.90	2.00	
Predicted Age (+ 1 SD)	23.8 (19.3–28.3)	24.6 (20.1–29.1)	25.3 (20.8–29.8)	26.1 (21.6–30.6)	26.9 (21.5–32.3)	

Stage II

	2.10	2.20	2.30	2.40	2.50	
Predicted Age (+ 1 SD)	27.7 (22.3–33.1)	28.5 (23.1–33.9)	29.3 (23.9–34.7)	30.1 (24.7–35.5)	30.8 (23.9–37.7)	

Stage III

	2.60	2.70	2.80	2.90	3.00	
Predicted Age (+ 1 SD)	31.6 (24.7–38.5)	32.4 (25.5–39.3)	33.2 (26.3–40.1)	34 (27.1–40.9)	34.8 (28–41.6)	

Early Stage IV

	3.10	3.20	3.30	3.40	3.50	
Predicted Age (+ 1 SD)	35.6 (28.8–42.4)	36.3 (29.5–43.1)	37.1 (30.3–43.9)	37.9 (31.1–44.7)	38.7 (30.8–46.6)	

Late Stage IV–Early Stage V

	3.60	3.70	3.80	3.90	4.00	
Predicted Age (+ 1 SD)	39.5 (31.6–47.4)	40.3 (32.4–48.2)	41.1 (33.2–49)	41.8 (33.9–49.7)	42.6 (36.7–48.5)	

Late Stage V

	4.10	4.20	4.30	4.40	4.50	
Predicted Age (+ 1 SD)	43.4 (37.5–49.3)	44.2 (38.8–50.1)	45 (39.1–50.9)	45.8 (39.9–51.7)	46.6 (40.3–52.9)	

*Age is in months.

Based on Miller (1981).

of language development, with a predicted chronological age of 30.1 months (+ 1 standard deviation of 24.7–35.5 months). The child that we elicited the language sample from was 42 months of age. Thus, the MLU was below age-level expectations by at least one standard deviation. It is critical to remember that MLU is a gross measure of syntax. It cannot be used by itself to indicate the presence or absence of an expressive syntax impairment. Klee (1992) found that Mean Syntactic Length (MSL), a measure similar to MLU that excludes one word utterances, was a good diagnostic indicator to differentiate between children with typical language and those with specific language impairment.

Additional informal analyses such as Assigning Structural Stage (Miller, 1981), Developmental Sentence Scoring (Hughes, Fey, & Long, 1992; Lee, 1974), or Language Assessment, Remediation, and Screening Procedure (LARSP; Crystal, 1979) are available to evaluate the use of sentence constituents and their relationships more precisely. These procedures allow a much closer examination of expressive syntax. Most of these procedures can be computed by hand or via computer analysis programs (Long, Fey, & Channell, 2000; Miller & Chapman, 2001).

With respect to morphology, a grammatical morpheme analysis also can be performed on a child's language sample. This analysis evaluates the child's production of Brown's fourteen grammatical morphemes in terms of percentage of correct usage in obligatory contexts. An obligatory context is the presence of a morpheme where it is required in adult language use. For example, a child who says "That mine" has omitted the copula *is* in an obligatory context. The copula can be contracted, so it is an omission of a contractible copula. A contractible copula or morpheme does not have to be contracted to be contract*ible*. For instance, in the sentence "She is happy" the *is* is contractible, because you could say "She's happy" Uncontractible copulas (and auxiliaries) are those that cannot be contracted, such as "There he is," which cannot be stated as "There he's." The following example shows the computation of the percentage of correct use of the contractible auxiliary in obligatory contexts.

1. C: Here's my hat.
2. C: I'*m* going home now.
3. C: My mom says it's cold outside.
4. C: But she *is fixing dinner.
5. C: She *is* making macaroni and cheese.
6. C: That's my favorite in the whole world.
7. C: I'*m* gonna eat my broccoli too.
8. C: It gives me muscles.
9. C: There's father.
10. C: He'*s* driving the Volvo.

The occasions when the child produced the contractible auxiliary are underlined. The times that the child should have used an auxiliary, but omitted it, are indicated by an asterisk before the missing morpheme. Thus, utterance #4 was produced as "But she fixing dinner."

Percentage use in obligatory contexts is computed by counting the number of times the morpheme is used correctly divided by the number of times that it was obligated (present + omitted + used incorrectly). The ratio in the example presented would be 4/5 or 80 percent correct use in obligatory contexts. This data is then compared with developmental data, which tell us that the contractible auxiliary would be predicted to be mastered (90 percent correct use) at Post Stage V language stage.

Because children with language impairments have been found to have difficulty with verb morphology related to marking finiteness (see Chapter 3 for more information), Goffman & Leonard (2000) have suggested that a finite verb morphology composite be computed from a child's language sample. This would entail determining the combined percentage of correct use in obligatory contexts of the following grammatical morphemes: regular past tense-*ed*, third person singular-*s* (e.g., *walks*), copula *is*, *am* and *are*, and auxiliary *is*, *am* and *are*.

Phonological disorders often occur in children who display a language impairment. These children may be described as being hard to understand or as not saying their sounds right. Crucial steps during assessment include understanding which sounds the child can produce, the contexts of correct and incorrect sound production, and the child's use or overuse of phonological processes. At this point, it is important to consider whether a child displays an articulation disorder or a phonological disorder or a combination of the two. Articulation disorders can be of a functional (i.e., of unknown origin) or organic etiology. A distorted *s* sound, often referred to as a lisp, or a *w* for *r* substitution, such as saying *wing* for *ring,* are common examples of functional articulation disorders. An organic articulation disorder is one for which there is a structural reason for the child's difficulty in making the sound(s), such as a child with a cleft palate or weakness and inarticulate movements due to damage of the central nervous system. The key to why these are articulation disorders and not associated with phonological disorders is that a phonological disorder reveals a pattern of responses and is therefore a rule-based phenomenon. These patterns of responses have been called *phonological processes.* One example of a phonological process that is common among children with and without language impairment is final consonant deletion. The child leaves off the end of a closed syllable (e.g., consonant-vowel-consonant) and says /d' / ("daw") for *dog* and /kae/ ("cah") for *cat.* In this case, a child will leave off many final consonants regardless of his or her ability to produce the sound itself. Thus, in the example given, it is not that the child cannot produce a *g* or a *t,* but that the child has not learned to put a final consonant on CVC structures. However, it is important to note that, oftentimes, even in the case of speech problems of an organic origin, phonological processes do occur. Thus, articulation and phonological problems may coexist in cases of functional or organic etiology. Finally, a small number of children have been described as having developmental verbal apraxia. These children have difficulties with the sequencing of motor movements needed for speech production. Their speech is characterized as very difficult to understand and effortful. In such cases, evaluation of the child's oral motor structures and functions as well as prosody is warranted. A thorough understanding of the sounds and contexts that a child can and cannot produce assists in determining the nature of the problem. This can be accomplished by generating a phonetic inventory for the child. A phonetic inventory consists of all the phones the child makes according to manner and placement. Syllable and word-shape abilities of children also provide valuable information on a child's developing phonological system.

Phonological abilities can be assessed using a variety of formal or informal procedures. Some tests assess articulation abilities on a sound-by-sound basis, others assess phonological processes, and others provide evaluation of both. Further, analysis of spontaneous speech sound use from a language sample is often helpful for children with limited language skills. (Refer to Table 6.2 for a summary of these available procedures.)

Content

Content includes understanding and production of vocabulary, semantic relations of meanings found in one-, two-, and three-word utterances, and case relations in sentences. Content also refers to the propositions or ideas within utterances. The language interventionist may ask the following questions with respect to age-appropriateness:

1. Does this child understand and produce a number of words and a variety of word types?
2. Does the child understand and express words to convey different meanings?
3. Is the child able to understand and express a variety of ideas at the sentence level?
4. Does the child have difficulty retrieving words to express his or her ideas?

Although there are numerous tests available to assess vocabulary understanding and production, fewer formal instruments are available to assess word type and relational meaning in utterances. In the past, the variety of words a child used was evaluated using the language sample with a measure called the type–token ratio (TTR; Templin, 1957). The TTR is used to determine the diversity of words spoken, and is computed by dividing the number of different words (types) used by the total number of words used (tokens) in a fifty utterance sample. A TTR of .50 is within normal limits. The usefulness of the TTR to determine language-impaired from nonimpaired populations has been challenged

(Klee, 1992; Watkins, Kelly, Harbers, & Hollis, 1994). Instead of using the TTR, some clinical researchers have begun to look more closely at the types of words that children produce in their samples. Klee (1992) found that a child's total number of words (TNW) and number of different words (NDW) are two measures that differentiated children with specific language impairment from those without language impairment. Additional detailed information about a child's semantic diversity can be gained by examining the TTRs of individual parts of speech. For instance, Watkins, Rice, and Moltz, (1993) have examined verb type–token ratios in children. The same can be done with nouns, adjectives, or adverbs to provide clinically relevant information. Watkins et al. (1994) suggest evaluating the child's total number of different words (NDW) as well as NDW for specific form classes such as nouns, verbs, adjectives, pronouns, and copula/auxiliary/modal verbs.

The evaluation of the relational meaning of the words involves a semantic relations analysis, which details the meaning expressed by words. This type of analysis can be performed when children are producing one-, two-, and three-word combinations. For example, a child who says "daddy go," "mommy kiss," and "doggy jump" is expressing the meaning relation of "agent + action." During the language sampling, the language interventionist needs to be careful to note the contexts in which the child produces utterances in order to derive the child's intended meaning. The utterances are then coded according to their meaning. Categories for one-, two-, and three-word semantic relations are presented in Table 6.6.

Many children who display language impairments in their first five years of life are later identified as having word-finding problems. That is, children may know a word, but be unable to retrieve the word when they want to use it. There are only a few standardized tests available for assessing these difficulties (refer to Table 6.2). Evaluating a language sample for excessive use of nondescript terms (i.e., using *this* instead of the referent label) and a low NDW may be indications of problems in this area. In addition, McGregor & Apel (1994) provide three nonstandard probes to assess word-finding problems. These include repeated confrontation naming (i.e., asking the child to label a picture three times in a row), story retelling and drawings, and cued naming (i.e., giving the child semantic, syntactic, or phonological cues to assist in retrieving the word).

Use

How children use language to communicate their needs and their ability to regulate conversation may be determined by asking the following basic questions:

1. Does the child understand and express a variety of intentions?
2. Does the child express a variety of intentions in appropriate ways? Is the child responding and initiating with a variety of in-

TABLE 6.6 Semantic Relation Analysis

Semantic Relation	Level		
	One word	**Two word**	**Three word**
Nomination *that,* "that ball"			
Recurrence "more pie"			
Rejection "no juice"			
Disappearance "no bear"			
Denial "no boy"			
Notice "hi mommy"			
Agent + Action "daddy go"	*********		
Action (+ Object) "ride bike"			
Agent + Object "doggy ball"	*********		
Action + Location "sit blankie"	*********		
Locative State "me bed"			
Possession "sissy duck"			
Attribution "big frog"			
Instrument + Action "hammer nail"	*********		
Experience + Experiencer "baby sad"	*********		
Classificatory "toby boy"	*********		
Comitative "walk mommy"	*********		
Conjunction "daddy mommy"	*********		
Total			

Based on Bloom & Lahey (1978) and Brown (1973).

teractional partners? Does the child follow the topic of conversation and contribute appropriately?

3. Does the child participate in conversation in ways that lead to continued successful interactions? Can the child monitor interactions and repair conversations when they break down?

4. Is the child able to formulate and produce an appropriate narrative that is cohesive, free of communication breakdowns, with sufficiently complex syntax?

Several methods exist for evaluating language use in young children. Because of the need for functional contexts, assessment usually involves informal procedures such as language samples or setting up situations to elicit specific speech acts. However, a few formal assessment tools for very young children have emerged that assess functional language use (cf. Wetherby & Prizant, 1993). Brinton & Fujiki (1994) detail an assessment approach that uses conversation as the context of choice for assessment. Their approach focuses on three essential components of conversation: turn exchange, topic manipulation, and conversational repairs. Brinton & Fujiki provide a list of screening questions to ask the child who may be experiencing difficulty conveying his or her message to others (Table 6.7).

Speech Act & Conversational Participation

Informal procedures for evaluating language use include determining the types of communication intents children are expressing. Several types of pragmatic analyses can be performed on language samples that vary depending on the age of the child and the area of language use of interest. Speech acts for children at the one-word level can be identified using Dore's (1978) conversational acts (see Table 6.8).

TABLE 6.7   Questions to Ask to Screen Conversation Skills

Question	Not Observed	Sometimes Present	Frequently Observed
The child hesitates to interact with peers and adults.			
The child interrupts other speakers.			
The child does not introduce referents when a new topic begins.			
The child does not contribute to topics introduced by others.			
The child continues to persist with one topic, when the topic has been changed.			
The child focuses on tangential elements of the topic, not the "big picture" of the topic.			
The child is late in responding to questions.			
You have to work hard to interact with the child.			
The child does not respond appropriately to requests for clarification such as "huh?" "what?" or "Which one?"			
The child does not ask for help if they do not follow the conversation.			
Certain aspects of the child's communication distract from the interaction process.			

Adapted from Brinton & Fujiki (1994)

TABLE 6.8   Dore's Speech Acts

Speech Act	Example
Label	Child points to teacher and says "teacher".
Repeat	Adult: "That's a nice puppy." Child: "Puppy." All or part of the adult sentence is repeated.
Answer	Adult: Where's your bear?" Child: "Room".
Request Action	Child: Tries to button coat but can't do it. Child says or gestures for "Help".
Request	Child: Hears car door and says "Daddy?"
Calling	Child: Yells to other "Sister!"
Greeting	Child: "Hi" and "bye" at appropriate times.
Protesting	Child: Cries when parent washes hair (word may be produced).
Practicing	Child: "Book" is said when a book is not present.

Based on Chapman (1981)

Fey (1986) provides another useful system for evaluating the communication intents of children at various levels of language development. Fey's system involves analyzing children's utterances in terms of assertiveness and responsiveness (Table 6.9). The child's utterances are analyzed at fairly specific levels, allowing the language interventionist to evaluate production of speech acts. This analysis leads to a determination of the child's overall social–conversational participation. Social–conversational participation can fall along a continuum of assertiveness and responsiveness that results in four possible styles: passive, inactive, active, or nonverbal communicator (Figure 6.1). Intervention goals may be established based on these social–conversational profiles. For example, children who are inactive communicators may need to increase assertive acts. Alternatively, the intervention plan for a child who is a passive communicator may be to increase responding.

Another procedure for coding children's responsiveness and assertiveness is the Social Interactive Coding System (SICS) (Rice, Sell, & Hadley, 1990). SICS is an on-line procedure that codes a child's initiations and responses according to: (1) the play activity (e.g., art table, block area, etc.); (2) the interactional partner (e.g., teacher or child); (3) whether the interaction is an initiation or a response and whether it was verbal or nonverbal; (4) the play level (e.g., solitary, adjacent, or social interactive); and (5) the language (e.g., English, other). The language interventionist follows a child for five minutes and codes his or her interactions (see Table 6.10 for the definitions used to code behaviors). After a five-minute rest, the language interventionist begins again, until a specified amount of sampling is completed. This procedure has been used in classroom settings and has the advantage of being less time-consuming than those that rely on contextually-laden language samples or videotape analyses. As with all of

TABLE 6.9 Fey's Codes for Conversational Assertiveness and Responsiveness

Utterance Level

Assertive Conversational Acts

Requests	Assertives	Performatives
Request for Information: Questions used to elicit new information. "Where baby?" "What that?"	Comments: Statements that describe observable events. "I'm at school." "You look pretty."	Stakes, jokes, teasing, protesting, and warnings. "Watch out!" "Mine!" "Nana nana boo boo"
Request for Action: Statements that ask the other interactant to perform an action. "You do it." "Put it there."	Statements: Expressions of rules, explanations, and feelings not directly observable. "It's supposed to be a circle." "Those are dangerous."	
Request for Clarification: Questions used to clarify a previous utterance. "Huh?" "What did you say?" "The red one?"	Disagreements: Comments or statements that are in conflict with a previous assertion or that indicate noncompliance to requests. "I don't think so." "Nope." "Forget it."	
Request for Attention: Statements used to gain the attention of or acknowledgment of the other interactant. These statements do not add new information to the interaction. "Look at this!" "Mom!" "Guess!"		

Responsive Conversational Acts

Response to Requests for Information: Statements that give new information in response to an interactant's request. "That's a cow," in response to "What's that?"

Response to Requests for Action: Statements that occur along with an action in response to interactant's request. "I did it," while drawing a star as requested by "You do it."

TABLE 6.9   Fey's Codes for Conversational Assertiveness and Responsiveness (*continued*)

Response to Request for Clarification: Statements that attempt to clarify a previous utterance through repetition or some form of revision. "I said no more," in response to "What did you say?"

Response to Assertives and Performatives: Statements that provide acknowledgment or agreement with no new information added to previous sentence. "Yep" or "Mhm" in response to an assertive or performative. When these statements occur along with an assertive, they are coded in an assertive category.

Imitations: Statements that repeat part or all of the prior sentence, with no new information added.

Others: Statements or questions that do not fit into one of the previous categories.

Discourse Level

Topic Initiation: Utterances that present new information unrelated to prior utterance.

Topic Maintenance: Utterances with no new unsolicited information, but that continue to be related to previous utterances.

Topic Extension: Utterances that continue previous utterances and add new information.

Topic Extension-Tangential: Extensions of one aspect of the topic, but in an adequate fashion.

Based on Fey (1986)

FIGURE 6.1   Fey's social–conversational system

+ Assertive + Responsive **Active Communicators**	+ Assertive − Responsive **Verbal Noncommunicators**
− Assertive + Responsive **Passive Communicators**	− Assertive − Responsive **Inactive Communicators**

Based on Fey (1986).

TABLE 6.10   SICS Definitions

SICS Definitions: Verbal Interaction Status & Play Level

Verbal Interactive Status

Initiations (I): a verbal attempt by the child to begin an interaction with another.

Repeat (Rep): repetition of child's utterance if an initial initiation attempt is not successful

Response: the verbal, nonverbal, or ignoring by the child in response to an individual.

Verbal:	(R-V-1) one-word verbal response
	(R-V) multiword verbal response
Nonverbal:	(R-NV) nonverbal response including head nods, smiles, gestures, pointing, etc.
Ignore:	(ignore) child ignores interaction partner

Play Level

Play level is coded for the child's interactions with other children. There are 3 categories:

Solitary (sol):	the child is playing by him- or herself one minute or longer.
Adjacent (adj):	the child is playing by him- or herself but there is a child close by in the same area.
Social–Interactive (SI):	the child is playing with another child.

these analyses, practice is required at identifying behaviors to ensure reliable and valid results.

A hypothetical transcript and an analysis form are presented in Table 6.11. In this hypothetical case the child tends to initiate to the adult and peer Y in the classroom. These initiations are verbal. Child

TABLE 6.11A   Hypothetical Case Application of SICS

Child A is the target child, B is the classroom teacher, and Y & Z are two other children. The activity is dramatic play.

1.1	A: My dress pretty.
1.2	B: Yes. You look very nice.
1.3	A: (tugs on dress)
1.4	B: Do you want that off?
1.5	A: (nods head yes)
1.6	B: (assists child) There you go.
1.7	Y: Can I play with that now?
1.8	A: (shakes head no)
1.9	Z: You're supposed to share.
1.10	B: Maybe you can find something else to wear.
1.11	A: Here my dress. (hands dress to Y)
1.12	B: Oh you're sharing.
1.13	Y: Now it's my turn.
2.1	A: What that? (points to feather boa)
2.2	Y: You put it on your neck.
2.3	Y: Like a scarf.
2.4	A: Pretty.

TABLE 6.11B

SICS coding sheet
Form-LAP

Child's name _____ Date _____ Time _____ Observer: _____

Play Activity	Addressee	Verbal Interactive Status		Play level	Language Used
Dramatic Play	B	(1.1)	I		English
		(1.3)	R-NV		
		(1.5)	R-NV		
			X		
	Y	(1.8)	R-NV	SI	English
		(1.11)	R-V	SI	
			X		
	Y	(2.1)	I	SI	English
		(2.4)	R-V-1	SI	
			X		

A also responds to both interactants. Responses are at the verbal one-word level when interacting with a normally developing peer (Child Y). However, note that verbal responses are longer than one word when the interactant is the adult (B). Because the sampling took place during one activity, art, it is unclear if initiations or responses would vary under slightly different conditions, such as snack or dramatic play. Importantly, SICS illustrates the child's abilities under different interaction conditions. In the hypothetical case given here, the SICS supports a tentative hypothesis that this child could benefit from being encouraged to expand verbal responses to peers with the help of the adult in the classroom. The use of one SICS analysis may not be sufficient to assess the child's interactional skills. The child's interactions during other activities and with a range of interactants should be further confirmed with continued analysis.

Another procedure that takes a different approach to coding pragmatic behaviors has been proposed by Prutting & Kirchner (1987). Their procedure involves videotaping an interaction for fifteen minutes and rating the interaction on several variables including speech acts, topic maintenance and change, turn-taking, repairs, cohesion, fluency, physical proximity, and eye gaze. The language interventionist judges whether the observed individual performs inappropriately in any of the variables rated. An inappropriate behavior is one that is distracting to the overall interaction. For example, if a child is interacting with a peer and makes no eye contact whatsoever during the interaction, it is likely that the interaction will suffer as a result. In this instance, the variable of "eye gaze" would be marked as inappropriate. The beauty of this coding system is that it rates several verbal, nonverbal, and paralinguistic behaviors. Prutting & Kirchner field-tested their procedure with children five years and older who had either Down syndrome, autism, or specific language impairment. Their results suggest interesting pragmatic profiles that may help to distinguish the groups of children. This procedure would seem particularly helpful in determining which areas of language use (i.e., physical proximity, turn-taking, or prosody) might benefit from intervention. Thus far, the pragmatic analyses presented have required the observer to code naturally occurring contexts. However, for infrequently occurring acts, it is advantageous to set up situations to assess the child's abilities. Margulies, Creaghead, and Rolph (1980) provide several helpful guidelines for eliciting speech acts with their pragmatic checklist (Table 6.12).

Narratives

The narrative requires the language interventionist to evaluate the child's formulation of sentences, selection of words, and connection of ideas to convey a story. The narrative analysis provides valuable information about how children bring these areas of language together

TABLE 6.12   Pragmatic Behavior Checklist

Pragmatic Behavior	Elicitation Condition	Mode[1]
Greeting	Check as the child enters the room.	
Request for Object[2]	Have crackers in jar within child's view, but out of reach.	
Summoning, Request for Action	Give the child the jar with the cracker. The lid should be on too tight. Tell the child to open the jar and turn away from the child.	
Request for Information	Put peanut butter and jelly on the table and tell the child to get the knife.	
Commenting on Objects	Get the knife, come back to the table and present a novel object (i.e., giant sunglasses).	
Making Choices	Ask the child if s/he wants peanut butter or jelly on his/her cracker.	
Denial	Hand the child the opposite of what s/he asked for.	
Request for Clarification	Mumble at some point during conversation with the child.	
Response to Request for Clarification	The examiner should request clarification, ask "What?" or "Huh?" at an appropriate time during the conversation.	
Commenting on Action	Drop the knife while spreading peanut butter on the cracker.	
Protesting	Eat the child's cracker (instead of your own).	
Closing	Check as the child leaves the room.	
Maintaining Topic	Check all of the remaining areas on the checklist during conversation with the child.	
Changing Topic		
Initiating a Conversation		
Volunteering to Communicate		
Attending to Speaker		
Taking Turns		
Acknowledging		

[1]Mode is Verbal (V), Nonverbal (N), or Not Observed (O).

[2]Materials needed: Crackers, jar with lid, peanut butter, jelly, knife, and novel objects.

Based on Margulies, Creaghead, & Rolph (1980).

as early as three years of age. Two types of analysis include: (1) retelling a story (Paul & Smith, 1993), and (2) telling a personal story (McCabe & Rollins, 1994).

Paul & Smith (1993) used a story retelling task designed by Renfrew (1977) (i.e., "The Bus Story Language Test") to determine differences between "late bloomers," children with normal language skills, and children with specific expressive language impairment at four years of age. The "Bus Story" is accompanied with pictures that the language interventionist uses as she or he tells the story to the child. The child is then asked to retell the story. The child's narrative is analyzed using an information score, MLU per T-unit, cohesion adequacy, and lexical diversity. The information score is a measure of relevant information provided by the child. There are normative data provided to evaluate the information score in Renfrew (1977). Analyses such as MLU per T-unit determine the average length of the child's clauses. Cohesion adequacy refers to how well the child links events within the narrative in a manner that logically keeps things together (Liles, 1985). Finally, lexical diversity is the number of word roots spoken by the child. Readers should refer to Paul & Smith for a report of normative data from a small sampling of children.

Another method of analyzing narrative skills is to ask the child to describe a personal experience. Peterson & McCabe (1983) use a protocol called the "Conversational Map" to elicit such narratives. This protocol involves using a story prompt, collecting a minimum of three narratives from each child, using neutral subprompts during the storytelling, minimizing the child's self-consciousness, and giving the child enough time to tell the story. The story prompt is the event or thing that the examiner will ask the child to talk about. McCabe & Rollins (1994) point out that young children are likely to tell stories about being scared or hurt. However, they caution against using narratives that are about experiences with death because such narratives may have more confusion and be structured differently compared to other narratives. Story prompts might include a trip to the dentist's, a ride at an amusement park, a fight with a friend or sibling, and so on. Prompts about trips and birthday parties are discouraged because they might elicit a generic-type story, rather than a specific narrative.

Three narratives are elicited from the child; however, usually only one will be analyzed. The multiple-story prompts are used because not all children will be interested in telling a story about the same thing. Thus, eliciting three narratives provides some assurance that the child will be interested in talking about one of the topics. While the child is telling the story, the language interventionist is encouraged to use neutral subprompts. These subprompts keep the child going with his or her story without too much interruption or interpretation on the part of the language interventionist. They include responses such as acknowledgments ("Oh"), open-ended statements

("Tell me more"), questions ("Then what?"), and imitating in part or whole the child's last utterance (Child: "She was the prettiest princess of all"; Language interventionist: "She was the prettiest").

After eliciting the narratives, the language interventionist selects the longest narrative for analysis because narrative length has been found to be related to its complexity (McCabe & Peterson, 1990). Only narratives when the child was present should be used. The narrative macrostructure can be analyzed by using the definitions from McCabe & Rollins (1994; Table 6.13). A small set of normative data is available with which to analyze the child's narrative structure (see Peterson & McCabe, 1983, and McCabe & Rollins, 1994). It should be kept in mind that these data were derived from a small group of Caucasian, middle-class children and are not readily applied to children from a different cultural background.

McCabe & Rollins (1994) indicate that children who are African American often use a "topic-associating narrative" (Michaels, 1981). This type of narrative combines things that happened at various times into one narrative event. In contrast, McCabe & Rollins describe a narrative by a child of Japanese culture who produced very short narratives that may not contain the same level of details compared to Caucasian, North American, English-speaking children. Stories from

TABLE 6.13 Hierarchy of Narrative Structure

Structure Type	Components
One-event narratives	A story that does not contain two past tense events.
Two-event narratives	A story that has no more than two past tense events.
Miscellaneous narratives	A story that has two or more past tense events, but does not match the real-world logical or casual sequence of events.
Leap-Frog narrative	A story that has two or more past tense events, but the order of events does not match the logical event sequence.
Chronological narrative	A story that has two or more past tense events, matches real-world sequence, has an order that matches a logical sequence of events, but no high point (i.e., concentrated evaluation comments).
End-at-High-Point narrative	A story that has two or more past tense events, matches real-world sequence, has an order that matches a logical sequence of events, has a high point, but no resolution following the high point.
Classic narrative	A story that has two or more past tense events, matches real-world sequence, has an order that matches a logical sequence of events, has a high point, and a resolution.

Based on McCabe & Rollins (1994).

Native American cultures tend to be purposeful and reflect on lessons to be learned in everyday life. When asking a Native American child to tell a story, one may have to give a reason for telling the story. Narrative structure is nonlinear and oriented toward the community rather than the individual. Background information is assumed and may not be explicitly provided by the teller of the story (Westby & Vining, 2002).

Teachers may have a particular expectation for narrative production that may be appropriate for a child from a non-Caucasian cultural background. For example, in discourse-based classroom events, such as sharing time, Micheals & Cazden (1986) found that Caucasian teachers with a middle-class background rated oral narratives that had a single topic, high cohesion, clear organization (with beginning, midpoint, and finish that has no time shifts), and clear vocabulary (including time and space concepts) more highly than those that did not contain these features.

SUMMARY

The preceding section has provided a wide sampling of the types of analyses that can be performed with young children to better understand their language abilities. The reader will need to read more about and practice each procedure before using it. The decision of which procedures to use and what areas to focus on will depend on the observation of the child and reports from the caregiver and significant others in the child's environment. In many cases, these young children will need to be seen for multiple assessment visits before a diagnosis or plan for intervention can be determined. Young children also may need to participate in a period of "diagnostic therapy" during which the child is enrolled in an intervention setting while data is collected on his or her speech and language abilities.

Classroom Assessment Procedures

The speech-language pathologist (language interventionist) traditionally has taken full responsibility for speech and language assessment. However, within school-based programs, current emphasis on meeting the Least Restrictive Environment mandate of IDEA (Individuals with Disabilities Education Act) has resulted in service delivery shifts that have modified the language interventionist's role in assessment and intervention. The parents, the special education teacher, the regular education teacher, the language interventionist, the psychologist, and the physical therapist work closely together. The language interventionist still has primary legal and ethical responsibility but is likely to share many assessment functions. The language interventionist needs to understand not only the speech and language development and disorders issues associated with a given child, but also how to view the whole child. This requires an understanding of motor development, cognitive development (in a particular learning style), self-help skills, and play abilities. Some teams use a transdisciplinary assessment in order to learn about the child's skills from a wholistic perspective (Linder, 1993). (See Chapter 5 for a complete description of collaboration and teaming.)

In best practice circumstances, the teachers, parents, language interventionist, and other professionals will determine the best intervention context given the needs of the participants, the nature of the disorder, and the desired outcome of intervention (Coufal, 1993). Movements toward working with the child within educational and child-care settings indicate increased collaboration between the language interventionist and the caregiver, the regular educator, the special educator, and/or other professionals. This collaboration should be initiated early in the identification stage following the principles of the collaborative/consultative model (Coufal, 1993). Recall that the purposes of assessment are multifaceted. Classroom assessment can be used to document a child's strengths and weaknesses within a classroom environment, determine eligibility (i.e., relevant educational outcomes), as well as assist in planning intervention. It should be noted that classroom assessment can take place not only in school settings, but also in child-care settings.

Cirrin (1994) poses three questions to ask when conducting classroom assessment:

1. What is the child's ability to use language in the classroom or child care setting with respect to spoken and listening tasks?
2. What are the characteristics of the teacher's or child-care provider's language in the classroom or child care setting?
3. What concepts, vocabulary, sentence structures, scripts, and pragmatic skills does the child need to be successful in the classroom or child-care setting?

These same questions can also be modified to include assessment of younger children in center-based preschools or home child care.

Cirrin (1994) provides an excellent array of checklists for collecting data on the three questions above. Answering the first question requires observation by the regular education teacher or child-care provider. Information about the child's form and content, listening skills, ability to share information and receive information, use of language in the classroom, and knowledge of scripts used in the classroom are all necessary. After the teacher has completed the observation checklists, the language interventionist will need to observe the child within the instructional setting while reviewing the forms completed by the teacher.

In order to answer the second question, a good collaborative or consultation relationship needs to be established. The assessment of teacher talk is voluntary on the part of the teacher, just as family assessment with the infant-toddler population is voluntary. This voluntariness is a key factor in the collaborative/consultation model (Coufal, 1993). If the teacher agrees to participate, the language interventionist will collect data regarding the length and rate of teacher instruction, the complexity of classroom language, and the effectiveness of questions, directions, and explanations. These data will be collected through direct observation or video-or audiotape recording.

The final question addresses the complexity of the sentence structures and vocabulary of the curriculum materials that the student encounters. The teacher will need to guide the language interventionist with respect to which materials are the most appropriate to examine at any given time. This type of assessment will need to be conducted many times throughout the school year if the student is to successfully link communication with educational outcome.

In addition to classroom demands, it is important to remember that the child's social use of language plays a role in the classroom. For example, many classrooms have group times or group collaboration efforts when certain communication behaviors are expected of the students. Gallagher (1991) suggests that priority should be given to assessing those areas of socialization that have been noticed as problematic by parents, teachers, and peers. Social tasks that may prove difficult for young children include: (1) entering into peer groups; (2) responding to ambiguous messages of peers; (3) responding to their own failures; (4) responding to their own successes; (4) responding to group norms and expectations; (5) and responding to teacher expectations (Dodge, 1985). Children with language impairment may also have difficulty initiating with peers, despite being able to initiate conversation with adults (Hadley & Rice, 1991). Thus, the level of support that children need from adults relative to their participation with peer interactions should be evaluated.

The classroom environments of children from diverse cultures frequently conflicts with their cultural upbringing. There are major differences between Native American cultures and Western culture in today's educational settings. In mainstream culture, boys and girls are often combined in large groups whereas some Native American children prefer small groups of the same gender. Some Native American students may need more time to answer questions, believe that direct eye contact with authority figures is disrespectful, and may benefit from visual learning cues (Westby & Vining, in 2002). These differences have clear and obvious implications for the language interventionist.

Children's abilities in all of the previously mentioned areas can be assessed systematically through observation of the classroom and by interviewing the child, teacher, parent, and peers. The answers to these questions should begin to provide a picture of how the child interacts within the classroom setting. Asking these questions should be helpful in determining not only how intervention might be implemented in the classroom environment, but also potential goals for the child's participation within that environment.

ELIGIBILITY CRITERIA

Public policy at the federal, state, and local level is instrumental in detailing the rights of children with special needs. At the federal level, several important pieces of legislation provide guidance for appropriate services within the school setting. (Chapter 5 details this legislation.) State policies implement federal policy by detailing the methods of identifying children for services and providing guidelines for eligibility of services. Certification and/or licensure requirements are also established on a state-by-state basis. Local school policies may further interpret state guidelines.

Some children may be diagnosed with a language and/or communication impairment; however, they may or may not qualify for special services in the schools. To a great extent, eligibility determination is agreed on by the state education department and local school district systems. Often such criteria are based on severity ratings and discrepancy scores. Severity ratings are rank orderings of the severity of a child's communication needs and their impact on educational needs. In some school districts, children need to have a moderate or severe disorder in order to qualify for services.

Discrepancy scores involve comparing the child with other children of the same age or may include a comparison of skills within a particular child. Comparing the child with other children is referred to as inter-referencing (Fey, 1986). This is done when children are compared to other children in the population samples of standardized tests. Inter-referencing typically makes use of chronological age (CA) comparisons. When children score below their peers on particular measures of speech and language they will qualify for services if that score is at the level prescribed by the state.

In contrast, intra-referencing allows evaluation of differences within the child's language system and/or cognitive abilities. For example, a child may have receptive language skills that are within normal limits but display expressive language skills below his or her receptive abilities. Further, a child may have particular difficulty with language form but not pragmatics or vice versa.

Another type of intra-referencing is known as cognitive referencing or MA (Mental Age) referencing. In cognitive referencing, the child's language abilities are compared with his or her nonverbal mental age. For instance, child A might have a mental age within normal limits but a language age below normal limits. According to the cognitive hypothesis, when the mental age is greater than the language age, a gap exists between what the child might be able to attain with respect to language and the child's current level of functioning. Child B, whose nonverbal cognitive functioning is at the same level as language functioning, might show no such gap, yet both might be below the child's chronological age. Children who exhibit the largest gap are oftentimes those who are given priority for intervention.

Casby (1992) reports that as many as 60 percent of the special education professionals in state departments use cognitive referencing to establish speech-language eligibility criteria. The assumption is that the children with these gaps will make the most progress because of the belief that cognition drives language development and, thus, those children whose language development is below their cognitive development will benefit the most from intervention. However, there are numerous studies that challenge this view, indicating that language might drive improvement in cognition (see Rice, 1983 for a review). In an effort to determine if cognitive referencing was a reliable procedure, Cole, Mills, and Kelley (1994) administered three commonly used nonverbal tests and three commonly used language tests to children who were identified as having language–cognition gaps. The results indicated poor agreement amongst the measures with respect to which children would receive services based on cognitive referencing criteria. Cole et al. suggest that the poor agreement might be due to the assessment tool's level of reliability and validity. As a result, some children might be denied services because of the poor psychometric characteristics of the tests that were selected for assessment. At issue is not the inclusion of children with gaps in abilities, but the exclusion of children who do not show a gap. As an option, Cole et al. suggest that the child's "unmet communication needs" be used to qualify him or her for intervention. In addition, Olswang & Bain (1991) suggest that a child should be considered for intervention if the child improves in deficient areas when given some support during assessment.

INTERVENTION PLANNING

The results obtained from assessment should provide information regarding a child's strengths and weaknesses, and emerging areas of ability. The language interventionist needs to take this information and analyze it with respect to her or his knowledge of the process of normal language acquisition, hypothesize why the child has not progressed in the normal fashion, and develop interventions to assist the child in learning language in the most effective and efficient manner possible. In some cases, intervention planning is in part determined by the method of service delivery. (Chapter 7 discusses intervention planning in inclusive settings in detail.) However, the philosophy of intervention held by the language interventionist will also affect intervention planning.

   Three philosophies to planning intervention are: developmental logic, remedial logic, and theoretical logic. The language interventionist who uses developmental logic determines the next area of development a child should master and proceeds to intervene in this area (Guess, Sailor, & Baer, 1978). In contrast, "remedial logic" (Guess, Sailor, & Baer, 1974, 1978) focuses on the child's functional communication needs in the present environment. Remedial logic is supported by individuals working within the behavioral paradigm, particularly those working with children who display severe physical and mental disabilities. Another type of logic, "theoretical logic," uses theory to predict which area(s) should be focused on during intervention. For instance, language interventionists adhering to the Principles and Parameters theory will focus on areas of grammar associated with specific parameters. In contrast, language interventionists who give more credence to the social–interactionalist models will build on what the child is producing by using recasts. Olswang and Bain (1991) follow Vygotskian theory by using dynamic assessment to provide information as to what the child is ready to learn next. Dynamic assessment is akin to the notion of "stimulability" whereby one determines if the child can imitate or produce a previously modeled target. Those areas that the child shows potential for producing are targeted before those areas that are not stimulable. Children who show a readiness to learn certain areas of language have been regarded as having a more positive prognosis or better outcome than children who do not show such an emergence. Regardless of which type of logic is used to plan intervention—developmental, remedial, or theoretical—an in-depth understanding of the child's abilities is necessary prior to intervention planning.

EVALUATING INTERVENTION PROGRESS

Assessment for the purposes of evaluating an intervention program is called *treatment efficacy*. The effectiveness of intervention can be determined by measuring the child's performance prior to intervention and then measuring it again after the intervention and comparing the two results. It also may involve evaluating changes in a caregiver's, peer's, or teacher's language interaction with the child who has language impairment. One method that has been used in the past to measure change is a multiple baseline design. The idea behind this assessment of change is to choose a goal other than the target goal and leave that goal untreated. This procedure enables the language interventionist to determine whether change has occurred in one goal but not the other. Such a result would indicate that the intervention was responsible for change in the target goal and not some other factor such as maturation. This type of procedure is rarely used in practice, however. Instead, many language interventionists rely on pre- and post-test measure comparisons. Although such a procedure lacks control from outside variables, if the intervention procedure is based on positive results derived from previous experimental studies it may be the most realistic measure of accountability available (Fey & Johnson, 1998). One way to evaluate change using a pre- and post-intervention comparison with standardized measures is to compare standard scores pre- and post-intervention, taking into consideration the standard error of measurement associated with the test. For example, if a child had a standard score of 70 on a language subtest before intervention and a standard score of 85 following intervention, it might appear that the child had made tremendous progress. However, if the standard error of measurement for this subtest was greater than 15, a score of 85 would be within the range of the child's true score (70+16=86). In contrast, if the standard error of measurement was 5, the estimated true score might lie anywhere between 65 and 75. The true score for 85 would be 80 to 90. Thus, the latter case would confirm that the child had improved.

Another method of evaluating intervention is through social validity measures. Social validity is the relevance of the child's advances in relation to his or her social system as determined by individuals other than the language interventionist (Goldstein, 1990; Wolf, 1978). Teachers, parents, and peers are all potential sources for social validity assessment of a child's intervention program. This might be accomplished by preparing a set of questions concerning the child's speech and language skills and the importance of these skills in view of the child's eventual language functioning. This set of questions could be administered before and after intervention to assess the parents' (and others') opinion about the value of a child's success in the intervention program. Olswang and Bain (1994) suggest that both types of data, qualitative data that addresses social validity issues and quantitative data, which is more objective in nature, should be used to evaluate treatment outcome.

Dismissal from Intervention

Olswang (1993) suggests that there are both short- and long-term objectives for intervention. The short-term objective is change in the present. The target language goal is followed over time and the observed change or lack of change is recorded. It is the result of the current intervention at the current time. Long-term objectives are those that address the future status of the child. These objectives seek to answer the question, "Will current intervention influence the course of the child's future language skills by preventing or reducing the need for further intervention?" For some children with language impairment, dismissal from intervention with age-appropriate speech and language abilities is the long-term objective. For other children, the long-term objective may be a specified level of communication functioning. This type of long-term objective may change over time as the child learns more information and encounters new communication needs.

Dismissal from intervention, based on assessment, is one of the most difficult team decisions, particularly if there has been little progress. Fey (1988) proposes some helpful guidelines for determining when a child might be dismissed from intervention. He suggests that dismissal criteria should be determined *prior* to the initiation of therapy. The decision to dismiss a child from intervention can be viewed as a hypothesis about the current functioning of the child, which can be altered depending on the child's state. Three scenarios where dismissal is appropriate are:

1. when the child is no longer making gains (or has "plateaued"), despite efforts to modify intervention;
2. when the child has achieved all the goals set forth and is no longer at risk for academic or social consequences as a result of a speech and language impairment; and
3. when the child's progress is general, and not specific to intervention.

Fey has placed arbitrary time guidelines on this decision-making process. He suggests that the intervention program should be reevaluated when at least one subgoal (i.e., a step below a goal) is not reached in one month's time. Reevaluation includes possibly changing the goals, altering the type of intervention approach, or the interventionist. If changing the intervention approach, goals, or interventionist still does not result in positive change for the child within six months, then the team may consider discontinuing the intervention. This decision should be made with extreme caution, and without penalizing the child because the team has not successfully implemented appropriate communication goals. Should dismissal occur, the language interventionist should consider re-enrolling the child in intervention six months following dismissal. Importantly, it is recommended that the child be tracked following dismissal at three-month intervals. Tracking the child's progress on specific criteria without intervention allows for an objective view of the child's development.

Treatment efficacy and dismissal of a child from language intervention are topics that continue to be studied. For the time being, the best practice for a language interventionist is the careful monitoring of intervention to determine if intervention is responsible for positive change and a priori determination of the ultimate outcome for each child.

SUMMARY

Assessment is a series of events that provide professionals with a better understanding of a child's speech and language abilities. The information derived reflects the performance of that child on a given day and are subject to error from the test instrument, the child, and the examiner. Keeping these cautions in mind, professionals who undertake assessment with children should have a healthy respect for the complex task of describing a dynamic, interactional system such as speech and language. An accurate reflection of a child's current abilities in the context of the classroom and home with important providers and peers are key components in an accurate assessment.

Finally, it should be remembered that assessment is a continual process that repeats itself for each child, not only during specified periods of the year. As the child participates in intervention, the language interventionist needs to constantly assess changes in the child's communication, environment, and caregivers and modify interventions accordingly.

DISCUSSION QUESTIONS

1. A child has been referred to you by a kindergarten teacher who is concerned about her talking and listening skills. Discuss the types of things you will do to determine if this child has a language disorder.
2. In groups of three to four evaluate the reliability and validity of various screening tests or formal assessment tests using the psychometric criteria in Table 6.3.
3. Discuss how you will assess a child whose cultural background differs from mainstream Western culture. What are some guidelines to follow?
4. Break into groups and discuss how one ensures the representativeness of language sampling and how one might collect language samples within the classroom.
5. Discuss how you would go about documenting that a child's language disorder has an adverse effect on his or her education? What types of information could you gain from classroom observation. Be specific.
6. Discuss some of the pros and cons of cognitive referencing. How would you convince your district supervisor that cognitive referencing should not be used?

REFERENCES

Bloom, L., & Lahey, M. (1978). *Language development and language disorders*. New York: Wiley.

Brinton, B., & Fujiki, M. (1994). Ways to teach conversation. In J. Duchan, L. Hewitt, & R. Sonnenmeier (Eds.), *Pragmatics: From theory to practice* (pp.). Englewood Cliffs: Prentice Hall.

Brown, R. (1973). *A first language.* Cambridge, MA: Harvard University Press.

Casby, M. (1992). The cognitive hypothesis and its influence on speech-language services in schools. *Language, Speech, and Hearing Services in Schools, 23,* 198–202.

Chapman, R. S. (1981a). Computing mean length of utterance in morphemes. In J. F. Miller (Ed.), *Assessing language production in children* (pp. 111–138). Baltimore: University Park Press.

Chapman, R. S. (1981b). Exploring children's communicative intents. In J. F. Miller (Ed.), *Assessing language production in children* (pp. 22–25). Baltimore: University Park Press.

Cirrin, F. M. (1994). Assessing language in the classroom and the curriculum. In J. B. Tomblin, H. L. Morris, & D.C. Spriestersbach (Eds.), *Diagnosis in speech-language pathology* (pp. 135–164). San Diego: Singular.

Cole, K. N., Mills, P. E., & Kelley, D. (1994). Agreement of assessment profiles used in cognitive referencing. *Language, Speech, and Hearing Services in Schools, 25,* 25–31.

Coufal, K. L. (1993). Collaborative consultation for speech-language pathologists. *Topics in Language Disorders, 14,* 1–14.

Crystal, D. (1979). *Working with LARSP.* London: Edward Arnold.

Dale, P. S. (1991). The validity of a parent report measure of vocabulary and syntax at 24 months. *Journal of Speech and Hearing Research, 34,* 565–571.

Dodge, K. (1985). Facets of social interaction and the assessment of social competence in children. In B. Schneider, K. Rubin, & J. Ledingham (Eds.), *Children's peer relations: Issues in assessment and intervention.* New York: Springer-Verlag.

Dore, J. (1978). Requestive systems in nursery school conversations: Analysis of talk in its social context. In R. Campbell & P. Smith (Eds.), *Recent advances in the psychology of language: Language development and mother-child interaction.* New York: Plenum Press.

Fey, M. E. (1986). *Language intervention with young children.* Boston: College-Hill Press.

Fey, M. E. (1988). Dismissal criteria for the language-impaired child. In D. Yoder & R. Kent, (Eds.), *Decision making in speech-language pathology* (pp. 50–54). Burlington: B. C. Decker.

Fey, M. E., & Johnson, B. W.(1998). Research to practice (and back again) in speech-language intervention. *Topics in Language Disorders, 18,* 23–34.

Gallagher, T. (1991). Language and social skills: Implications for clinical assessment and intervention with school-age children. In T. Gallagher (Ed.), *Pragmatics of language,* San Diego: Singular.

Glascoe, F. P. (1991). Can clinical judgment detect children with speech-language problems? *Pediatrics, 87,* 317–322.

Goffman, L., & Leonard, J. (2000). Growth of language skills in preschool children with specific language impairment: Implications for assessment and intervention. *American Journal of Speech-Language Pathology, 9,* 151–161.

Goldstein, H. (1990). Assessing clinical significance. In L. Olswang, C. Thompson, S. Warren, & N. Minghetti (Eds.), *Treatment efficacy research in communication disorders* (pp. 91–98). Rockville: American Speech-Language-Hearing Foundation.

Guess, D., Sailor, W., & Baer, D. (1974). To teach language to retarded children. In R. Schiefelbusch & L. Lloyd (Eds.), *Language perspectives: Acquisition, retardation, and intervention.* Baltimore: University Park Press.

Guess, D., Sailor, W., & Baer, D. (1978). Children with limited languages. In R. Schiefelbusch & L. Lloyd (Eds.), *Language intervention strategies* (pp. 101-144). Baltimore: University Park Press.

Hadley, P., & Rice, M. (1991). Conversational responsiveness of speech- and language-impaired preschoolers. *Journal of Speech and Hearing Research, 34,* 1308–1317.

Huang, R., Hopkins, J., & Nippold, M. A. (1997). Satisfaction with standardized language testing: A survey of speech-language pathologists. *Language, Speech, and Hearing Services in the Schools, 28,* 12–23.

Hughes, D. L., Fey, M. E., & Long, S. H. (1992). Developmental sentence scoring: Still useful after all these years. *Topics in Language Disorders, 12,* 1–12.

Klee, T. (1992). Developmental and diagnostic characteristics of quantitative measures of children's language production. *Topics in Language Disorders, 12,* 28–41.

Klee, T., Carson, D., Hall, L., & Muskina, G. (1994). Screening language development in 24-month-old children. Poster presented at the 15th Symposium on Research in Child Language Disorders. University of Wisconsin-Madison, June.

Lee, L. (1974). *Developmental sentence analysis.* Evanston: Northwestern University Press.

Leonard, L. B. (1974). A preliminary view of generalization in language training. *Journal of Speech and Hearing Disorders, 39,* 429–434.

Liles, B. Z. (1985). Cohesion in the narratives of normal and language-disordered children. *Journal of Speech and Hearing Research, 28,* 123–133.

Linder, T. W. (1993). *Transdisciplinary play-based assessment.* Baltimore: Brookes.

Loeb, D., & Leonard, L. B. (1988). Specific language impairment and parameter theory. *Clinical Linguistics and Phonetics, 2,* 317–327.

Long, S. H., Fey, M. E., & Channel, R. (2000). Computerized Profiling, Version 9.2.7. [Computer Program, available as Freeware on the Internet at: [http://www.cwru.edu/artsci/cosi/faculty/long/research/cp.html] Department of Communication Sciences, Case Western Reserve University.

Margulies, C., Creaghead, N., & Rolph, T. (1980). Pragmatic checklist. Presented at the OSHA Convention, March.

McCabe, A., & Peterson, P. (1990). What makes a narrative memorable? *Applied Psycholinguistics, 8,* 73–82.

McCabe, A., & Rollins, P. (1994). Assessment of preschool narrative skills. *American Journal of Speech-Language Pathology: A Journal of Clinical Practice, 3,* 45–56.

McCauley, R., & Swisher, L. (1984a). Psychometric review of language and articulation tests for preschool children. *Journal of Speech and Hearing Disorders, 49,* 34–42.

McCauley, R., & Swisher, L. (1984b). Use and misuse of norm-referenced tests in clinical assessment: A hypothetical case. *Journal of Speech and Hearing Disorders, 49,* 338–348.

McGregor, K., & Appel, A. (1994). Nonstandard approaches to assessment of word-finding problems in preschoolers. Miniseminar presented at the American Speech-Language-Hearing Association, New Orleans.

Michaels, S. (1981). "Sharing time": Children's narrative styles and differential access to literacy. *Language in Society, 10,* 423–442.

Michaels, S., & Cazden, C. (1985). Teacher/child collaboration as oral preparation for literacy. In B. Schieffelin & P. Gilmore (Eds.), *The acquisition of literacy: Ethnographic perspectives.* Norwood, NJ: Ablex.

Miller, J. F. (1981). *Assessing language production in children.* Baltimore: University Park Press.

Miller, J. F., & Chapman, R. S. (1979). The relation between age and Mean Length of Utterance in morphemes. *Journal of Speech and Hearing Research, 24,* 154–161.

Miller, J. F., & Chapman, R. S. (2001). *Systematic Analysis of Language Transcripts (SALT).* Madison: Waisman Research Center.

Miller, J. F., Freiberg, C., Rolland, M., & Reeves, M. (1992). Implementing computerized language sample analysis in the public school. *Topics in Language Disorders, 12,* 69–82.

Miller, J. F., & Yoder, D. E. (1984). *Miller-Yoder Language Comprehension Test* (Clinical Edition. Baltimore: University Park Press.

Olswang, L. (1993). Developmental speech and language disorders. *American Speech, Language, and Hearing Association, 35,* 42–44.

Olswang, L., & Bain, B. (1991). When to recommend intervention. *Language, Speech, and Hearing Services in the Schools, 22,* 255–263.

Olswang, L., & Bain, B. (1994). Data collection: Monitoring children's treatment progress. *American Journal of Speech-Language Pathology, 3,* 55–66.

Paul, R., & Smith, R. L. (1993). Narrative skills in 4-year-olds with normal, impaired, and late- developing language. *Journal of Speech and Hearing Research, 36,* 592–598.

Peterson, C., & McCabe, A. (1983). *Developmental psycholinguistics: Three ways of looking at a child's narrative.* New York: Plenum.

Plante, E., & Vance, R. (1994). Selection of preschool language tests: A data-based approach. *Language, Speech, and Hearing Services in the Schools, 25,* 15–24.

Prutting, C., & Kirchner, D. (1987). A clinical appraisal of the pragmatic aspects of language. *Journal of Speech and Hearing Disorders, 52,* 105–119.

Renfrew, C. (1977). *The bus story language test: A test of continuous speech.* Oxford: Author.

Rescorla, L. (1989). The Language Development Survey: A screening tool for delayed language in toddlers. *Journal of Speech and Hearing Disorders, 54,* 587–599.

Rice, M. (1983). Contemporary accounts of the cognition/language relationships: Implications for speech-language clinicians. *Journal of Speech and Hearing Disorders, 48,* 347–359.

Rice, M., & Sell, M., & Hadley, P. (1990). The social interactive coding system (SICS): An on- line, clinically relevant descriptive tool. *Language, Speech, and Hearing Services in the Schools, 21,* 2–14.

Richard, N., & Schiefelbusch, R. (1991). Assessment. In L. McCormick, & R. Schiefelbusch (Eds.), *Early language intervention* (pp.109–142). Columbus, OH: Merrill.

Rosen, A., & Proctor, E. (1981). Distinctions between treatment outcomes and their implications for treatment evaluation. *Journal of Consulting and Clinical Psychology, 49,* 418–425.

Scarborough, H., & Dobrich, W. (1990). Development of children with early language delay. *Journal of Speech and Hearing Research, 33,* 70–83.

Schraeder, T., Quinn, M., Stockman, I. J., & Miller, J. (1999). Authentic assessment as an approach to preschool speech-language screening. *American Journal of Speech-Language Pathology, 8,* 195–200.

Shulman, B. (1985). Test of Pragmatic Skills (Re. Ed.). Tucson: Communication Skill Builders.

Sturner, R. A., Layton, T. L., Evans, A. W., Heller, J. H., Funk, S. G., & Machon, M. W. (1994). Preschool speech and language screening: A review of currently available tests. *American Journal of Speech-Language Pathology: A Journal of Clinical Practice, 3,* 25–36.

Templin, M. (1957). Certain language skills in children: Their development and interrelationships. Child Welfare Monog. No. 26. Minneapolis: University of Minnesota Press.

Tjossem, T. (1976). Early intervention: Issues and approaches. In T. Tjossem (Ed.), *Intervention strategies for high-risk and handicapped children.* Baltimore: University Park Press.

Watkins, R., Kelly, D., Harbers, H., & Hollis, W. (1994). Using form-class indices to measure children's lexical diversity. Poster Session presented at the Symposium on Research in Child Language Disorders. University of Wisconsin-Madison, June.

Watkins, R., Rice, M., & Moltz, C. (1993). Verb use by language-impaired and normally developing children. *First Language, 13,* 133–144.

Westby, C. E., & Vining, C. B. (in press). Living in harmony: Providing services to Native American children and families. In D. Battle (Ed). *Communication disorders in multicultural populations* (3rd Ed.) (pp. 135–178). Woburn, MA: Butterworth-Heinemann.

Wetherby, A., & Prizant, B. (1993). *Communication and Symbolic Behavioral Scales.* Chicago: Riverside.

Wiig, E. H. (1990). *Wiig Criterion Referenced Inventory of Language.* New York: The Psychological Corporation, Harcourt Brace Jovanovich.

Wolf, M. M. (1978). Social validity: The case for subjective measurement or how applied behavior analysis is finding its heart. *Journal of Applied Behavior Analysis, 11,* 203–214.

CHAPTER 7

Ecological Assessment and Planning

Linda McCormick

Recall from Chapter 6 that assessments occur at a number of different junctures and each has a specific purpose. Initial assessment in school settings determines whether the child has a disability, whether special education is required, and what types of special or related services are needed. That assessment is usually implemented with young children who are just entering the public school system and with school-age children with mild to moderate disabilities who have been referred (most often by a concerned teacher) because they do not appear to be benefiting from instruction. Because eligibility is typically not an issue for students with severe and/or multiple disabilities, initial assessment focuses on specifying what types of special or related services they need.

Data generated by the initial assessment process generally include developmental information (i.e., test scores, normative information), some information furnished by the family about behavior at home, and some information from past service delivery settings (e.g., early intervention program). These data will help to determine if the child is eligible for special education and related services. The next questions that will have to be answered are:

- What would be an appropriate educational program for this child?
- What special services does this child need?
- What is the least restrictive environment for this child?

As discussed in Chapter 5, these questions are discussed and answered as part of the IEP process.

This chapter describes an assessment process that yields plans for assessment and planning for instruction and intervention. This process, which is called Ecological Assessment and Planning, can help the team formulate age-appropriate instructional and intervention objectives for any student and facilitate planning for their implementation in inclusive settings. It identifies objectives in all ability domains.

While we will concentrate on generating objectives and planning for language/communication skills, it is important not to lose sight of the fact that development in the different areas—language and communication skills, motor skills, cognitive or academic skills, social-adaptive behaviors, and self-care—is interrelated. Development in one area cannot be understood apart from development in other areas. Similarly, difficulties in one developmental area cannot be understood and addressed without considering other areas. Delays and disorders are rarely confined to a single developmental domain: Difficulties in one area invariably affect and are affected by the child's abilities in other areas. Even children with the label specific language disability (SLI) experience problems in other areas, for example, academics and/or social–adaptive behavior (Fey, Catts, & Larrivee, 1995).

Meeting the many and varied needs of all students, particularly those with moderate and severe disabilities, requires close collaboration among professionals. Collaboration is expedited when professionals are able to put aside the notion of assigning the various intervention areas to different professional disciplines. Thinking of speech and language as *belonging* to speech-language pathology, motor skills as *belonging* to physical therapy, cognitive, social, and academic skills as *belonging* to regular or special education, and self-care skills as *belonging* to occupational therapy is counterproductive. It ignores developmental interrelationships and it gives the impression that the different disciplines have *totally* separate and distinct knowledge bases and practices. This is certainly not the case: There is enormous overlap in the research and practice traditions that disciplines working with individuals with disabilities bring to the intervention arena. Finally, it is a disservice to these professionals and to the disciplines to hold a single professional or discipline solely responsible for all assessment, planning, and instruction in a developmental/skills domain. Professional disciplines (including general education) must pool their resources and share accountability to meet the diverse needs of children with disabilities.

ECOBEHAVIORAL ASSESSMENT APPROACHES

Simeonsson and Rosenthal (2001) divide group assessment procedures into three broad categories: (1) psychometric assessment (as described in Chapter 6), (2) qualitative–developmental, and (3) ecobehavioral. Psychometric assessment is based on the assumption that development is continuous and cumulative. The primary goal is normative comparison of child performance and diagnostic classification but it can also provide descriptive information. Qualitative–developmental assessment (best represented by the early work of Piaget [1929; 1957]), is based on the assumption that cognitive growth is understood as a sequence of transitions that reflect qualitative rather than quantitative change. The primary goal is to determine and analyze the nature and stage of development. The value of qualitative assessment approaches is that they are applicable to any child, regardless of the nature or severity of impairment or disabilities.

Like qualitative–developmental assessment, ecobehavioral assessment is a nonnormative qualitative approach. The major difference from qualitative–development assessment is that the focus is on the individual child in relation to his unique environment rather than on theoretically defined cognitive structures. There are three branches of the ecobehavioral approach: They are *functional analysis of behavior, ethology,* and *ecological assessment* (Simeonsson & Boyles, 2001). All three branches recognize the significant influence of the environment on behavior and development.

Functional Analysis

The functional analysis of behavior focuses on understanding the function (purpose) of problem behavior with the goal of increasing the quality of life of the individual. It is much broader than traditional behavior management, which often focused almost exclusively on decreasing or eliminating problem behaviors. Functional analysis is successful with individuals of all ages, for problems ranging from relatively mild academic difficulties to severe tantrums and self-injurious behavior.

A basic tenet of functional analysis is the belief that there is a significant relationship between controlling the environment with communication and controlling the environment with problem behavior. All behavior is viewed as communicative (having message value), regardless of its topography. Interestingly, this is exactly what the pragmatic perspective of language would predict (Watzlawick, Beavin, & Jackson, 1967).

Intervention based on functional analysis (referred to as **communication-based intervention, CBI,** and/**or positive behavior support**) typically teaches communication forms as a replacement for problem behaviors *as well as* environmental modifications. The defining characteristic of this intervention is the emphasis on using positive procedures and promoting development of adaptive behavioral repertoires (Carr et al., 1994; Durand, 1990; Evans & Meyer, 1985). The basic assumptions of functional analysis are:

- problem behavior can serve specific, adaptive purposes or functions;
- successfully changing problem behavior depends on discovering the purpose or function of the behavior;
- the same problem behavior may serve many different purposes;
- achieving successful functioning depends on expanding limited response repertoires; and
- successful intervention involves changing social systems and lifestyles.

Assessment and intervention are inseparably linked processes in functional analysis. The function of the challenging behavior is first analyzed and defined, generating a set of predictions about when and where the problem behavior is likely to be exhibited. Subsequent definition or description of these variables then provides information about (1) the effects of various setting events, (2) immediate antecedents, and (3) consequences of the problem behavior. A behavior support plan is developed from this information. The behavior support plan describes (1) contextual variables (e.g., physical feature of the setting, social interaction patterns, the daily/weekly schedule), (2) physiological variables (e.g., sleep/eating cycles, allergies, medications), and (3) alternative communication responses that serve the same function as the problem behavior.

There is a substantial and growing literature drawing on this perspective to assist professionals concerned with addressing problem behaviors. Janney and Snell (2000) provide particularly good coverage of the methods of functional assessment.

Ethology

Ethology is the study of behavior in its natural context with a focus on discovering the ways in which members of the species are alike and develop in similar ways. Because ethology grew out of the work of zoologists, more has been done to apply this theory to the study of animals than to humans. Research by ethologists is particularly concerned with genetically influenced behavior that has adaptive significance.

Ethologists acknowledge that we are largely a product of our experiences, but they are also quick to remind us that we are inherently biological creatures with inborn characteristics that affect the kinds of learning experiences we are likely to have. Probably the most well-known application of ethological theory is Bowlby's (1973) research concerning the development of attachments between infants and their caregivers. The contribution of ethology is pointing up the value of studying human behavior in normal, everyday settings and of comparing human development to development in other species.

Ecological Assessment

The roots of ecological assessment can be traced to the ecological psychology tradition of Barker (1978) and Bronfenbrenner (1979). The central thesis of ecological theory is that an organism cannot be studied properly in isolation from its environment. Simply stated, *behavior cannot be understood without considering its context*. Ecological theory views the developing person as embedded in a series of environmental systems that interact with one another and with the individual to influence development.

There are four environmental systems or contexts: (1) **microsystem,** (2) **mesosystem,** (3) **exosystem,** and (4) **macrosystem.** The microsystem is the system closest to the individual—immediate environments. For example, the primary microsystem for a first-born is the family: infant, mother, and father interacting with one another. Next removed is the mesosystem system, the interrelationships or linkages between microsystems. For example, unpleasant experiences at the day-care program (one microsystem) could upset the infant and, in turn, could disturb relationships within the family (another microsystem), ultimately affecting the infant's development. The next system in the series is the exosystem. Included in this system are social settings that the child never experiences directly but that, nonetheless, still influence his development. For example, children can be affected by whether or not their parents enjoy supportive social relationships, as well as by whether their parents have satisfying or stressful work environments. Finally, there is the macrosystem, the larger culture or subcultural context in which the microsystem, mesosystem, and the exosystem are embedded. At this level are shared understandings such as views about (1) the nature of human beings at different points in the life span, (2) what children need to be taught to function in society, and (3) how one should lead one's life as an adult.

Rhodes (1967) was the first to apply the ecological perspective to developing intervention programs. Referring specifically to students labeled "emotionally disturbed," he made the cogent point that *viewing disturbance as something residing in the student leads to preoccupation with trying to "fix" the child's flaws.* Disturbance should not be viewed as residing in the child but, rather, in the tension between the child and the demands of the environment. Disability labels simply reflect that tension—the fact that there is a discrepancy between the child's skills and abilities and the demands or expectations of that child's environment.

In the late seventies, Brown and colleagues (Brown, Branston, Hamre-Nietupski, Pumpian, Certo, & Gruenewald, 1979) described procedures to generate functional goals and objectives for students with severe and multiple disabilities drawn from the tenets of ecological theory. They called this assessment the *ecological inventory process.* Since that time it has been widely used with children with disabilities of all types and severity and across many environments. The ecological inventory process developed by Brown and colleagues has five stages. Table 7.1 presents a brief description of these stages.

The ecological assessment process described in this chapter expands and modifies that of Brown and colleagues. We focus on application of the process in only one domain—the school domain—but the same procedures can be applied in the other domains (home, community, recreation/leisure, vocational). Also, there is a specific focus on assessment and planning for language and communication, but skills in other domains are also noted.

TABLE 7.1   Steps in the ecological assessment process as described by Brown and colleagues

Step	Procedure
1. Identify curriculum domains.	Identified four curriculum domains thought to represent the major life areas for most students: domestic, recreation/leisure, community, and vocational. (School was considered an environment in the community domain.) Because it is such a significant area in the lives of children, many now include school as a separate domain (York & Vandercook, 1991).
2. Identify and survey current and future natural environments.	Identified and described the environments in each domain in which student needs and wants to function. Also identified environments where the student would function in the future. For example, current environments in the community domain might include the grocery store, the beach, the park, the doctor's office, etc. Future environments: a fast-food restaurant.
3. Divide the relevant environment into subenvironments.	Identified locations in the environments with specific activities (that the student needs to participate in to be part of the environment) as subenvironments. For example, if it is decided that the student needs to be prepared to do grocery shopping, then subenvironments of the grocery store would be identified (e.g., the cart area, fruit/vegetable section, shelf displays, meat department, check-out).
4. Inventory the subenvironments to identify the relevant activities that are performed there.	Identified the activities and routines necessary for *basic* performance and participation in the subenvironments through observations and interviews at the subenvironment site. Extensive considerations given to how many times an activity is needed, the student's age and current skills, his interests, the priorities of the parents, and the physical characteristics of the setting that dictate the various behaviors.
5. Examine the activities to isolate the skills required for their performance.	Broke activities into teachable units or skills. Skills were then further task analyzed into precise performance sequences.

Relationship to Developmental Assessment

How does ecological assessment relates to traditional developmental assessment? In the past many assumed that teaching skills from the normal development sequence would effectively remediate language delays and deviations and prevent further delays and disorders. Consequently, the major source of information for goals and objectives was descriptive studies of stages of development of the various language dimensions, specifically, phonology, syntax, morphology, and semantics. The focus of intervention then was facilitating acquisition of knowledge and skills in the order in which they occur (or are thought to occur) in normal development. This is called the *developmental stage model.*

Application of the developmental stage model to development of goals and objectives was based on these assumptions: (1) that the development of children with disabilities is essentially the same as that of children without disabilities, and (2) that children with disabilities are simply functioning at an earlier stage of development. Unfortunately, there is not substantial data to support these assumptions. So, while developmental information is certainly useful for explaining learning barriers and designing some intervention *procedures,* it is usually not a good source for intervention goals and objectives (Goodman & Bond, 1993; Keogh & Sheehan, 1981; Leonard, 1987). With many children, there is much more involved than simply developmental delay: many children have pervasive mental and physical limitations that prevent them from attaining normal development milestones. Further, there is general acknowledgment that the skills demonstrated by normally developing children may not be necessarily sequential *or* indispensable.

Reliance on data concerning developmental milestones as the sole source for goals and objectives may have negative consequences (Guess and Noonan, 1982). The potential for negative consequences derives from the fact that professionals waste a great deal of valuable intervention time (the child's and their own) if they rely exclusively on developmental data; in fact, normal milestones are *not* appropriate goals and objectives for children with disabilities. Still another possible negative consequence of preoccupation with teaching skills from normal development sequences may be restricted social experiences. While they undoubtedly mean well, professionals may take up so much of the child's day trying to teach the skills observed in younger, normally developing children that they leave the child little time for social and communicative interactions with peers. Limiting opportunities for interactions with, and learning from, peers (whether by design or inadvertently) ignores the child's communication needs and the fact that, even when the child's language skills are at a younger developmental age, the child's communication needs are likely to be similar to those of same-age peers.

Developmental information is, however, useful for planning intervention. It can contribute to understanding the child's language and communication limitations, adapting activities and materials, and developing intervention procedures, but it must be used selectively. What is most important is not to rely on information about the child's developmental skills as the major source for generating goals and objectives. Table 7.2 highlights the differences between ecological assessment and traditional assessment, summarizing the points set forth in this section.

TABLE 7.2 Differences between ecological assessment and traditional assessment

	Ecological Assessment	**Traditional Assessment**
Reference	Compares child's performance to the demands and expectations of activities and tasks in the child's environments	Compares child's test performance with that of a sample of similar children who were administered the same test items
Focus	Child's ability to meet setting and task expectations and participate in activities and routines in natural settings	Language forms and structures described in the normal development research as representative of children at the child's age or stage of development
Procedures	Observes the child's behavior in daily activities and interviews with persons who know the child well	Elicits the child's responses to a set of standardized tasks thought to represent major skills/abilities in the area
Assessment Context	Natural settings: Assessment team includes parents and peers	Contrived settings: Independent assessments by discipline representatives
Best Use of Results	To generate individualized goals and objectives and plan special instruction	To determine child's status relative to same-age peers; for diagnosis and determination of eligibility for special education services

ECOLOGICAL ASSESSMENT PROCEDURES

Ecological assessment differs from traditional assessment in that it considers the child's behavior in relation to environmental demands and expectations (rather than in relation to the performance of a test's standardized population). Ecological assessment examines the environments in which the child is expected to function in order to determine what adaptations need to be made and what needs to be taught to ensure the child's success in these environments. Because we are particularly concerned with language and communication in inclusive environments, the major focus of assessment is on the adequacy of the child's language and communication skills in the natural contexts where she needs to know and use language in order to participate with peers. The purpose of the ecological assessment–planning process is

- to generate information about the social, education, and functional activities and routines in natural environments (the classroom and other school environments) where the child with disabilities wants and needs to be an active and successful participant;

- to determine what resources and support the child will need to participate in and receive maximum benefits from activities and routines in the classroom and other school environments; and
- to plan for provision of needed resources and supports.

Ideally the ecological assessment–planning process is implemented after the child has been in the inclusive classroom for a brief period. Where this is not realistically possible, it can be implemented at any time prior to or after placement.

The ecological assessment–planning process is applicable to all students. It is appropriate for

- young children who are just entering inclusive preschool classes;
- children who, though they have been identified as eligible for special education and related services, will remain in their general education classrooms;
- children who are being moved (or have just been moved) from segregated to inclusive classes;
- children with disabilities who have been in inclusive classes for some time but need revised or expanded goals and objectives.

The remainder of this chapter describes procedures for ecological assessment and planning. Assessment and planning for language and communication are highlighted in the context of ecological assessment and planning for overall functioning. Because language and communication skills permeate and are inextricably essential to success in all aspects of children's lives, completely removing this domain from the ongoing stream of daily functioning is counterproductive. Thus, there are references to skills in other domains throughout.

The planning/support team should include the regular and special education teachers, the language interventionist, other therapists (e.g., OT, PT), parents, siblings, peers (for older students), and the student. The team may begin the process during the first week the child is in the inclusive classroom or anytime thereafter. The required observations may be implemented prior to placement by having the student join peers for key activities and routines in the inclusive classroom.

Table 7.3 shows the 10 steps of the individualized ecological assessment–planning process and the expected outcomes at each step.

STEP 1: Person-Centered Planning: Getting to Know the Student.

The purpose of the first step is for team members (including the family) to begin to get to know the student and to get acquainted with one

TABLE 7.3 Overview: The ecological assessment–planning process

Steps	Outcome(s)
1. Person-centered planning: Getting to know the student.	A vision statement describing the student's strengths, capabilities, preferences, and needs as seen by the family, the team, and peers.
2. List activities/routines in a typical school day.	List of activities/routines for a typical school day for nondisabled peers.
3. Prioritize activities/routines and develop broad goal statements.	Broad goal statements for *at least* three first priority activities (e.g., _____ will participate in the arrival routine.
4. Observe/record the behavior of a nondisabled peer and/or conduct interviews to determine the key behavioral expectations for each priority activity/routine.	Description in the 1st column of the Discrepancy Analysis forms of the key behavioral expectations for each priority activity/routine.
5. Observe/record the behavior of the student from initiation to completion of each priority activity/routine.	Description in the 2nd column of the Discrepancy Analysis forms of the student's behavior for each priority activity/routine.
6. Compare student's behavior with behavioral expectations for each activity/routine. Note when the student does not meet expectation and behaviors/skills the student needs to learn.	Notation (+ or −) indicating student's skills relative to expectation (3rd column) of the Discrepancy Analysis forms. Description in the 4th column of the behaviors/skills the student needs to expand and/or learn for each priority activity/routine.
7. Highlight language/communication skills.	Indication of the language/communication skills that the student needs to learn.
8. Try to ascertain why key language/communication behaviors are not being demonstrated.	Description in the 5th column of the Discrepancy Analysis forms of variables impeding performance of desired language/communication behavior.
9. State language/communication objectives for each activity.	Language/communication objectives for each broad goal statement (Step 3).
10. Develop an Individualized Instructional Plan (including data collection procedures) for each objective.	An Individual Instructional Plan with adaptations, resources and supports, instructional procedures, and data collection for each language/communication objective.

another. Among the various titles for this process are *person-centered planning* (Mount, 1994), *group action planning* (Turnbull & Turnbull, 1992), and *McGill Action Planning System* (MAPS Forest & O'Brien, 1989). They all share two characteristics: (1) involvement of the student's family members and friends, and (2) a focus on developing a positive profile or vision for the student (what the student *can* do, instead of on his/her weaknesses).

The purpose of visioning in the ecological assessment process as described in this chapter is to

- identify the current and potential resources and natural supports in the student's home and school environments;
- insure that key people in the student's life are fully aware of the student's strengths; and
- develop a common vision for inclusion of the student in the general education classroom.

Key people in the student's life (family members, the student, professionals and paraprofessionals, two to five classmates when feasible, and anyone interested in the child's future) are assembled to share information and learn about one another. The visioning process provides practical information that will be useful in the development of the Individualized Instructional plans for identified objectives (Step 10).

The meeting typically lasts two or three hours (split into two sessions when a very young child is involved). Participants sit in a semicircle with a facilitator positioned at the open side of the circle. The facilitator's role is to introduce the participants and the process, solicit input, encourage and support interactions, ensure equal participation, and record responses to the questions that follow. Chart paper, an easel, and large markers should be available in order to record the participants' responses.

After introductions, the meeting begins with a brief summary of the student's strengths and positive attributes. The questions provided below can serve as a broad outline for the ensuing discussion.

The purpose of the first question is to give the team members an idea of what has happened in the student's life up to this time. Parents are asked to summarize the key milestones that have affected their child's life and her school experiences.

What Is _____ 's History?

Family members and peers should be encouraged to talk about milestones in the child's life.

> **Example: These were Jennie's family's responses
> to the question "What is Jennie's history?"**
> She and her twin are the youngest of four children.
> Dad is in the military.
> The twins were premature.
> Janie was able to come home from the hospital three weeks before we were able to bring Jennie home.
> She has a history of seizures, ear infections, and asthma.

> Where we lived last year, Jennie was in a special education kindergarten class.
>
> She walked at about 20 months and said her first word at about age 3.

The next question is intended to encourage the family to think about what they want for the student and what they think the student would want. The student, if capable of doing so, should be encouraged to contribute to this discussion. The goal is to project a vision that will give direction to planning. The parents are encouraged to talk about what they really want, not what they think is available, for their child. Parents of very young children often find it difficult to think about adulthood. They may be more comfortable focusing on the nearer future (e.g., five years from the present).

What Is Your Dream for _____ 's Future?

Example: These were Jennie's family's responses to the question "What is your dream for Jennie's future?"
She will participate in regular education classes all through school.
She will graduate from high school with her sister.
She will have friends like Janie.
She will someday be able to live independently in a place that she likes, with people she likes.
She will be able to carry on a conversation.
She will have an opportunity to do things that she likes and does well.

The next question is the most difficult to ask parents but it is extremely important. It makes explicit what is in the parents' hearts. The response tells the team what they must work to avoid.

What Is Your Nightmare?

Example: These were Jennie's parents' responses to the question "What is your nightmare?"
She will not progress developmentally.
She will have to be in a special education class.
She will not have friends.
She will have to live in a group home.
She will not be able to go places with the family.
She will be placed in an institution.

The next question is intended to begin a general brainstorming session that continues until no one can think of anything else to say. Because they know the student best (and in different contexts) it is especially important for family members and peers to describe the student. They should be encouraged to share descriptive statements and anecdotes about the student's life and unique and positive characteristics. At the end, each team member may be asked to circle three words they feel best describe the student.

Who Is _____?

Example: These were Jennie's family's and peers' responses to the question "Who is Jennie?"
She is a lovable, helpful, happy, and spunky little girl.
She is very motivated.
She is lively, curious, and full of energy.
She wants to learn—is inquisitive.
She is a twin, and her sister is her best friend.
She is excited about being in a "real" class like her sister.
Her favorite color is blue.
She is small and fragile looking.
She likes to be around people.
She has a good attention span.
She likes to go to birthday parties.
She likes to go to the beach.
She likes to be read to before bed.

The facilitator should ask team members to identify the student's strengths and unique gifts and abilities. The questions, "What can the student do?" "What does she like to do?" and "What does she do well?" are asked to get everyone, especially the parents, to focus on positives.

What Are _____'s Greatest Strengths (or Gifts)?

Example: This was the list that was generated in response to the question "What are Jennie's greatest strengths or gifts?"
People are drawn to her because she is so lovable and she is always happy.
She is almost able to dress herself.
Her motivation.
Her determination.
Her curiosity.
Her energy.
Her desire to learn.
Her sociability: She really likes people.
Her attention span.
She likes books.
She has Janie as a model for age-appropriate behaviors.
She's spunky and independent.

This question gives each team member an opportunity to identify the student's needs and challenges from his or her unique perspective.

What Are _____ *'s Greatest Needs and Challenges?*

> **Example: This was the list that was generated in response to the question "What are Jennie's greatest needs and challenges?"**
> She needs to be able to communicate well enough that people who are not familiar with her will know what she wants.
> She needs to be challenged to use language in more situations.
> She needs more independence with dressing (especially shoes).
> She needs more interactions with peers.
> She needs words.
> She needs consistent expectations.
> She needs to initiate communication.
> She needs to use the toilet without having to have a reminder.
> She needs her own friends.

Ideally, the student's school day will be the same or very similar to that of her peers. The issue is, what supports need to be in place to achieve this.

What Would _____ *'s Ideal School Day Be Like?*
And What Do We Need To Do To Make It Happen?

> **Example: These were the responses to the questions "What would Jennie's ideal school day be like?" and "What do we need to do to make it happen?"**
> The schedule for Jennie's ideal school day would be the same as that of her first-grade classmates.
> The team needs to (1) adapt first-grade curriculum activities (especially the academic activities that call for beginning reading and writing), and (2) identify alternative activities that have the same format for some time slots.

The outcome of the visioning process is a positive "picture" of the student and a shared vision for the student's participation in the inclusive classroom. The facilitator should summarize the participants' contributions with emphasis on the student's strengths, interests, and the available supports to facilitate successful inclusion. A written summary of the team's visions (copied from the chart paper) may be included in the student's records and also provided to the family.

STEP 2: List Activities/Routines in a Typical School Day.

The next step is to outline the activities and routines of a school day for a nondisabled student in the inclusive classroom. This can be accomplished through observation and/or by interviewing the teacher and one or more students in the class. Ask them to think step-by-step through the day and provide a detailed schedule of activities and/or routines on a typical day. Include settings (e.g., classroom, playground, cafeteria, gym). Begin with the student's arrival on the school campus and "talk through" the day until she leaves the school grounds in the afternoon.

STEP 3: Prioritize Activities/Routines and Develop a Broad Goal Statement.

The reason for prioritizing activities and/or routines is straightforward. Assessment, planning, and intervention should begin with a subset (at least three) of the daily activities/routines. Once the student is participating successfully in these activities/routines, the process is replicated with another subset of activities/routines.

Formulate a broad goal statement for each activity/routine in the set of prioritized activities/routines. The following are some examples of broad goal statements: Jennie will participate with peers at morning circle; Beau will eat lunch with peers in the cafeteria; Libby will participate in math activities.

STEP 4: Observe and Record the Behavior of a Nondisabled Peer and/or Conduct Interviews to Determine the Key Behavioral Expectations for Each Activity/Routine.

The information from completing this step and the next four steps is written on the Discrepancy Analysis form. You should construct a form with five columns similar to the one shown in Figure 7.1. Each activity will require *at least* one blank form.

The objective of this step is to determine and write in the key behavioral expectations for each of the activities/routines in the first column of the Discrepancy Analysis form. There are two ways to approach this: observe a student participating in the activity/routine and/or interview the teacher to determine the behavior expected of students. Enumerate the behaviors expected of students (what they are expected to do and say) from initiation until completion of the activity/routine.

Example: The activities at morning circle (one of the priority activities selected for Jennie) are:

1. Move to the morning circle area when the jingle is played
2. Sit on carpet square with eyes on teacher
3. Raise hand when the teacher asks "Is _____ here today?"
4. Respond to weather and calendar questions
5. Join in songs
6. Indicate desired free-play activity when asked
7. Take clothespin for selected area when offered
8. Move to free-play area when name is called

FIGURE 7.1   Discrepancy Analysis Form

Discrepancy Analysis

Student: _____ Date: _____ Activity/Routine: _____

Key behavioral expectations? What do peers do in the activity/routine?	Student's behavior in the activity?	Does student meet expectation?	Discrepancy? What does the student need to expand and/or learn to meet at least minimal expectations?	Possible explanation(s): • Strategy deficiency? • Skill deficiency? • Behavior problem? • Instructional problem? • Environmental problem?

Academic lessons in each curriculum domain (i.e., language arts, science, math, social studies), while they have different goals, materials, and tasks each day, have a similar format. Describe the typical sequence of behaviors, not the content or specific assignments. For example, for individual work the behavioral expectations might be to assemble materials, listen to directions, ask questions if the directions are not clear, begin the task, raise hand to have answers checked, and hand in completed work. (Note that the student with severe disabilities will undoubtedly be working on functional reading and math, but these key activity expectations for that student will be the same.)

STEP 5: Observe/Record the Behavior of the Student from Initiation to Completion of Each Priority Activity/Routine.

The goal here is to observe and record the student's behaviors in each of the priority activities. This information goes in the second column of the Discrepancy Analysis form. The focus is on recording precisely what the student does and says in the activity. As an illustration, refer to the example above for morning circle in Jennie's preschool class. Jennie was observed during morning circle for two days. She followed the other children to the circle area and sat on a carpet square. Jennie did not respond when the teacher asked, "Is Jennie here this morning?" nor did she respond to other teacher questions (the day of the week, what she had for breakfast, etc.). She made an effort to join in the songs and seems to be learning the accompanying gestures. At the end of circle, when asked which of the free-play areas she wanted to go to, she grabbed at the clothespins and threw them on the floor. When her name was called to move to a free-play area, she left the circle and started wandering around the room picking up objects at random. When observing the student, also take note of whether it takes the student longer than peers to respond and/or perform the behavior, what the student seems to be responding to, and which peers might be potential supports for the student. For example, Jennie seemed to be following the other children rather than responding to the jingle saying it was time to move to circle.

STEP 6: Compare the Student's Behavior with Behavioral Expectations for Each Activity/Routine. Note When the Student Does Not Meet Expectations and Behaviors/Skills the Student Needs to Learn.

Compare the student's behavior in each activity or routine with the behavioral expectations and note in the third column that the student performs the expected behavior (*yes* [+]) or does not perform the behavior as expected (*no* [–]). In the fourth column, indicate what the student needs to learn.

This example illustrates Step 6: Michael, a seven-year-old with Down syndrome, has been placed in an inclusive second-grade classroom. Data from observations of the morning arrival routine indicate that, when the bell rings, Michael moves with his peers into the classroom, finds his desk, sits down, and joins the class's choral response to the teacher's "Good morning class." (The teacher comments that he learned this by watching his peers during the first three days of school.) Unfortunately, Michael's participation in the morning routine ends at this point. During the next 8 to 10 minutes, the teacher takes lunch count, points to the date on a calendar, asks questions about the day's weather report that is written on the chalkboard, and outlines the day's special activities. Michael looks around the room, shuffles noisily through the contents of his desk, and turns to the side to look at (and occasionally touch) Britney who sits across the aisle. Michael does *not*

- raise his hand in response to the question, "Who is eating in the cafeteria today?" (he always buys his lunch in the cafeteria);

- attend to the teacher when she is talking about the weather or answer the question, "What kind of weather are we having today?" with one of the weather words (i.e., *rain, warm, cold, hot, sunny, cloudy*);
- look at peers when they answer the weather question;
- look at the teacher when she is describing and writing special activities for the day (on the chalkboard); or
- copy the words noting the special activities on his daily schedule (as the teacher instructs the class to do).

The team is working on several Discrepancy Analysis forms for Michael. The five behaviors above are listed on the fourth column of the Discrepancy Analysis form for the morning arrival routine.

STEP 7: Highlight Language and Communication Skills.

Highlight behaviors related to receptive as well as expressive language, and written as well as oral language. The team working on the Discrepancy Analysis forms for Michael discussed the fact that most of the behaviors he needs to learn involve cognitive, social, and language skills. All of the behaviors listed above were highlighted for Michael as they clearly involve language.

STEP 8: Try to Ascertain Why Key Language/Communication Behaviors Are Not Demonstrated.

The purpose of this step is for the team to explore possible reasons why the language /communication behaviors are not being demonstrated. It will be one *or some combination* of the following: a *strategy deficiency,* a *skill deficiency,* a *behavior problem,* an *instructional problem,* or an *environmental problem*.

- The student does not recognize what he is supposed to do or say. The behavior(s) is in his repertoire but he does not know that he is expected to perform it in those particular circumstances. He does it when prompted but not in response to natural cues. This is a *strategy deficiency*.
- The student's inability to perform the skill is related to his disability (i.e., motor limitation, sensory deficit). If the student's disability precludes performance of the skill in a manner similar to peers it will be necessary to consider a response that will accomplish the same purpose. This is a *skill deficiency*. (Selection and facilitation of functionally equivalent responses are discussed in Chapters 8 and 12.)
- The student is not motivated to perform the skill. This is a *behavior problem*.

- The student does not know how to perform the skill: he has never received instruction on it. The problem is *lack of instruction*.
- The way the physical or temporal environment is arranged impedes the performance of the skill. This is an *environmental problem*.

These possible explanations for the child's performance deficiencies are noted in the fifth column of the Discrepancy Analysis form. Recall the example of Michael above. In considering factors that may be contributing to his performance deficiencies in the arrival routine, the team discussed these questions:

1. Is he able to hear the teacher's questions and directions? Is his hearing in the normal range? Is his desk location optimal? Michael's hearing is in the normal range but there is often background noise during this activity (a possible environmental problem).
2. Does he understand what the teacher is asking? Does he understand that the appropriate response mode is to raise his hand (for the lunch count)? Michael may not understand the teacher's request for students to raise their hand if they are eating in the cafeteria (a possible strategy deficiency).
3. In other contexts, Michael has been able to answer questions about expected events and environmental conditions. However, Michael may not know the answers to the weather questions and he has not been taught to look at peers when they are answering the teacher's questions. Also, he may not know that the teacher expects every student to answer the questions (an instructional problem).
4. Has Michael ever been taught to copy from the chalkboard before? The consensus was that, while he copied information from sheets of paper into his notebook, he probably had not been asked to copy from the chalkboard (an instructional problem).

STEP 9: State Language/Communication Objectives for Each Activity.

The team should state an instructional objective for each of the language/communication behaviors when the student's performance does not meet expectations. These should be listed under the broad goal statements generated in Step 3. For example, under the broad goal, "Jennie will participate at morning circle in the classroom each morning," one of the objectives was *Jennie will raise her hand and nod or say "yes" when the teacher asks "Is Jennie here today?"*

STEP 10: Develop an Individualized Instructional Plan for Each Objective.

Construct an Individualized Instructional Plan form with four columns as shown in Figure 7.2. Discuss the explanations for the student's lack of required/expected skills (Step 8) and consider environmental manipulations and instructional strategies. The intervention will depend on whether the problem is a strategy deficiency, a skill deficiency, a behavior problem, an instructional problem, and/or a problem related to arrangement of the environment. Decide what environmental manipulations (supports and adaptations) will be required for the student to learn and perform the desired response. Then complete an Individualized Instructional Plan for each objective. This plan should show prompts, environmental modifications and supports, materials, and the people responsible for the manipulations and/or instruction.

List strategies to facilitate and support learning and performance of the targeted skills, and skill, material, or equipment adaptations that may eliminate the need to teach specific skills or make learning easier. Identify peers who might assist the student as special friends or as communication partners.

Data collection in inclusive classrooms may seem like a daunting task, but it is essential to determine whether the supports and instructions are effective. Planning for data collection means deciding what student responses will be recorded, when they will be recorded, and by whom. Assuming three objectives for each of three priority activities means collecting data on nine discrete responses over the school day.

Depending on the student's objectives, a repeated-trial assessment may be most appropriate for those skills requiring instruction. The observations already completed in Step 5 of the ecological assessment–planning process provide a baseline measure of how well the student performs the skill without prompting or instruction. Instruction requires provision of prompts in the context of the activity to help the student make the desired response. (This is done with care so as not embarrass or stigmatize the student.) Prompts may be *verbal* (e.g., a direction, the initial sound of a word or the first word in a sentence), *visual* (e.g., a gesture, a picture card or sequence of pictures or symbols on a chart, a manual sign), or *physical* (guiding the student's movement). Prompts, supports, and adaptations are described in Chapter 8.

In most cases, the best time to record data is after the activity. *Immediately* after the activity each day, record how many and what type of prompt(s) the student needed in order to respond. Decisions as to what type of prompts will be provided and how and when they will be provided are made prior to beginning instruction.

Data-collection forms are forms on which to record observations and instructional manipulations. Data-collection forms usually allow for data recording over some reasonable period of time, a week or a

FIGURE 7.2 Individualized Instructional Plan

Individualized Instructional Plan

Student: _____ Date: _____ Activity/Routine: _____

Objective: _____

Supports? Describe needed environmental, personnel, and/or peers supports.	**Adaptations?** Describe task modifications, prosthetics, or environmental adaptations.	**Instruction?** Describe instructional methods, including Prompts and consequences.	**Data Collection?** Describe how you will monitor instruction.

---

month or even longer. At a minimum, all data-collection forms should include three types of information:

- *situational information:* the student's name, the target response, the activity, the date and beginning and ending times of the observation or activity, and the observer or person doing the instruction
- *response information:* number and quality of responses, whether responses were prompted or independent (student initiated), type of prompts, and /or other supports required.
- *summary information:* total time of the activity/observation, totals for the responses recorded, and anecdotal comments to explain or describe the data.

It is possible to develop data-collection forms that can be used for many different responses. Typically there is a grid with space for noting the number of trials provided, the type of prompt(s) needed (or whether the response was independent), and the quality of the responses.

SUMMARY

This chapter has described an ecological assessment–planning process that plans for language and communication skills within a child's typical school day. Chapter 8 will describe important dimensions of the instruction/intervention process: (1) the focus of intervention; (2) methods and procedures; (3) the instructional environment; (4) relationships and responsibilities; (5) scheduling; and (6) measurement and evaluation.

DISCUSSION QUESTIONS

1. Some have noted that reliance on information about developmental milestones as the sole source for goals and objectives could have negative consequences. Discuss this issue and the alternatives.
2. Discuss the major assumptions of the ecological model and consider possible applications of this model (i.e., for service delivery, working with parents, etc.).
3. Compare ecological assessment and traditional assessment approaches.

ACTIVITY/PROJECT

Use the ecological assessment process guidelines for an assessment/planning project with a student with severe language disorders. Prior to beginning the project, get the permission of the school and the parents to assess and plan for the student. Follow the steps as outlined in Table 7.3 and described at length in the chapter. Use the forms (Figure 7.1 and 7.2) as provided or develop your own forms.

REFERENCES

Barker, R. G. (1978). *Habitats, environments and human behavior*. San Francisco: Jossey-Bass.

Bowlby, J. (1973). *Attachment and loss: Vol. 2: Separation*. New York: Basic.

Bronfenbrenner, U. (1979). *The ecology of human development: Experiments by nature and design*. Cambridge, MA: Harvard University Press.

Brown, L., Branston, M. B., Hamre-Nietupski, S., Pumpian, L., Certo, N., & Gruenewald, L. (1979). A strategy for developing chronological age-appropriate and functional curricular content for severely handicapped adolescents and young adults. *Journal of Special Education, 13,* 81–90.

Carr, E. G., Levin, L., McConnachie, G., Carlson, J. L., Kemp, D. C., & Smith, C. E. (1994). *Communication-based intervention for problem behavior.* Baltimore: Brookes.

Durand, V. M. (1990). *Severe behavior problems: A functional communication training approach.* New York: Guilford Press.

Evans, I. M., & Meyer, L. H. (1985). *An educative approach to behavior problems: A practical decision model for interventions with severely handicapped learners.* Baltimore: Brookes.

Fey, M. E., Catts, H. W., & Larrivee, L. S. (1995). Preparing preschoolers for the academic and social challenges of school. In M. E. Fey, J. Windsor, & S. F. Warren (Eds.), *Language intervention: Preschool through the elementary years.* pp. 3–38. Baltimore: Brookes.

Forest, M., & O'Brien, J. (1989). *Action for inclusion.* Toronto, Ontario: Center for Integrated Education, Frontier College.

Goodman, J. R., & Bond, L. (1993). The individualized education program: A retrospective critique. *Journal of Special Education, 26,* 408–422.

Guess, D., & Noonan, M. J. (1982). Curricula and instructional procedures for severely handicapped students. *Focus on Exceptional Children, 14,* 1–12.

Janney, R., & Snell, M. E. (2000). *Behavior support.* Baltimore: Brookes.

Keogh, B. K., & Sheehan, R. (1981). The use of developmental test data for documenting handicapped children's progress: Problems and recommendations. *Journal of the Division for Early Childhood, 3,* 42–47.

Leonard, L. B. (1987). Is specific language impairment a useful construct? In S. Rosenberg (Ed.), *Advances in applied psycholinguistics* (Vol. 1, pp. 1–39). New York: Cambridge University Press.

Mount, B. (1994). Benefits and limitations of personal futures planning. In V. J. Bradley, J. W. Ashbough, & B. C. Blaney (Eds.), *Creating individual supports for people with developmental disabilities* (pp. 97–108). Baltimore: Brookes.

Piaget, J. (1929). *The child's conception of the world.* New York: Harcourt, Brace.

Piaget, J. (1957). *The language and thought of the child.* New York: Meridian Books.

Rhodes, W. C. (1967). The disturbing child: A problem of ecological management. *Exceptional Children, 33,* 449–455.

Simeonsson, R. J., & Boyles, E. K. (2001). An ecobehavioral approach in clinical assessment. In R. J. Simeonsson & S. L. Rosenthal (Eds.), *Psychological and developmental assessment* (pp. 120–140). New York: Guilford Press.

Simeonsson, R. J., & Rosenthal, S. L. (2001). Clinical assessment of children: An overview. In R. J. Simeonsson & S. L. Rosenthal (Eds.), *Psychological and developmental assessment* (pp. 1–15). New York: Guilford Press.

Turnbull, A., & Turnbull, R. (1992, Fall-Winter). Group action planning. *Families and Disabilities Newsletter* (Beach Center on Families and Disability, Lawrence, KS).

Watzlawick, P., Beavin, J. H., & Jackson, D. D. (1967). *Pragmatics of human communication.* New York: W. W. Norton.

CHAPTER 8

Language Intervention and Support

Linda McCormick

Language and communication instruction/intervention should be guided by what we know about how and why language is learned: that it is learned in the context of interactions in daily activities and routines, as a tool for communicating meanings and controlling the environment. In inclusive schools, all students are provided appropriate educational opportunities and support to meet their individual needs (Stainback & Stainback, 1990). The resources, knowledge base, and personnel of special education (teachers, language interventionists, and therapists) combine with those of general education to facilitate and assist development and maintenance of challenging, supportive, and appropriate programs in all general education settings. In contrast, traditional schools tend to establish and maintain homogeneous environments where children with disabilities are served in separate classes and are the only students to benefit from the special resources provided by personnel in special education. Table 8.1 highlights the major differences between special education and speech-language intervention in traditional schools and special education and speech-language intervention in inclusive schools. This chapter is organized according to these differences, which range across six dimensions: (1) the focus of intervention; (2) methods and procedures for special instruction; (3) the instructional environment; (4) professional relationships and responsibilities; (5) scheduling; and (6) measurement and evaluation.

THE FOCUS OF INTERVENTION

The ecological assessment–planning process yields goals and specific intervention/instructional objectives for each goal. There are two basic issues with respect to intervention:

1. how to modify and adapt existing environmental conditions; and
2. what methods and procedures to use to help students achieve their individualized goals and objectives.

TABLE 8.1   Comparison of traditional and inclusive schools

| Dimensions | Traditional Schools | | Inclusive Schools |
	Special Education	Language Intervention	Special Education and Language Intervention
Focus of Intervention	Developmental skills Functional/adaptive skills	Linguistic concepts/rules Linguistic forms and structures	Teacher–Child interactions Curriculum adaptations
Methods and Procedures	Contrived instructional contexts Adult controlled Individual instruction Massed trials	Contrived therapy contexts Adult controlled Individual instruction Massed trials	Milieu language teaching Scaffolding Routines and script training Interactive modeling Situated pragmatics Systematic instruction Structured teaching Picture exchange communication system
Instructional Environment	Special education classroom Resource room Homogeneous groupings	Therapy room Special education classroom Homogeneous groupings	Regular classroom Other school settings Home/community environments
Professional Relationships and Responsibilities	Autonomous decision making Little opportunity for collegial interactions Periodic unidiscipline in-service training	Autonomous decision making Little opportunity for collegial interaction Periodic unidiscipline in-service training	Shared decision making Many opportunities for collegial interactions Continuous interdisciplinary training
Scheduling	Individual instruction Small-group instruction	Individual or small-group therapy weekly or biweekly	Block scheduling Regular consultation
Measurement and Evaluation	Formative and summative evaluation Quantitative data	Formative and summative evaluation Quantitative data	Formative and summative evaluation Authentic assessment Qualitative and quantitative data

Broad outcomes for children who are experiencing difficulties with language and communication (whether a delay, a disorder, or minimal or severe difficulties) will be to

- increase the number of functions accomplished with language,
- enhance and expand language and literacy competencies, and
- increase the number of social and physical contexts in which language is used spontaneously and effectively.

These outcomes will be achieved by facilitating and supporting effective teacher–student interactions, and maximizing opportunities for meaningful participation in activities in all school environments (and, to the extent possible, also in home and community environments).

Teacher–child interactions and the curriculum are the major environmental conditions that are available for manipulation. There are numerous possibilities for modifying these variables.

Teacher–Child Interactions

What children learn in the classroom (and how well they learn it) is largely dependent on teacher–child interactions. These interactions are likely to be most successful when the communicative competence that children bring to school matches that of their teacher. Miscommunications will be relatively infrequent and the children will be socialized effectively into the school environment. In many cases, however, the patterns of interaction that children encounter in their first classroom are completely new to them. They have not had experience with adults who are in positions of absolute authority, nor have they had experience with the type of communication patterns used by teachers (Garcia, 1992). Thus, miscommunications and unsuccessful exchanges far outnumber effective exchanges, and instruction and socialization efforts suffer.

Communication in the majority of American classrooms has been characterized as "rigid" (Saville-Troike, 1982). There are rules governing classroom interaction (e.g., you must raise your hand and not speak until called on), prescribed space arrangements (everyone in desks that are arranged in rows or sitting around tables), implicit control precepts (peer interactions are not supposed to occur except when the teacher permits them), and a great deal of question asking on the part of teachers. Even when the rules, arrangements, and precepts are stated explicitly (e.g., "Do not answer until you have been called on"), they are extremely difficult for children with language/learning difficulties.

In American classrooms, teachers use questions to elicit information from children in order to monitor and evaluate their comprehension of materials. Many children, at least when they enter school, are not accustomed to having an adult ask them questions for which the adult already knows the answer.

Typical classroom discourse patterns are also a problem. Children have difficulty with the turn-taking exchange pattern, known as the IRE exchange structure, which is repeated over and over again in most lessons. In the IRE structure, the teacher **I**nitiates a question, the student **R**esponds, and the teacher **E**valuates the student response (Blank & White, 1986; Cazden, 1988). Most children with language difficulties will not be successful in the general education classroom unless they are specifically taught and provided with practice with the IRE exchange pattern. Instruction on the IRE structure should focus on

- how and when to respond during a teacher-directed lesson;
- how to penetrate the structure if they want to say something that is outside the format or content of the lesson;
- how to get the teacher's attention;
- when it is appropriate to speak to the teacher in front of the group and when to speak to the teacher in private;
- the appropriate way to answer the teacher;
- with whom they can interact during the lesson (e.g., assigned partner).

The lesson presentation sequence is another aspect of teacher–child interactions. Many teachers use the lesson presentation steps recommended by Englert (1984) and Rosenshine (1983):

1. Review previous lessons with related information.
2. Tell students what they are expected to learn from the lesson.
3. Overview key points and planned activities to provide an anticipatory set.
4. Present salient information that is essential to acquisition of the targeted skills and concepts.
5. Maintain an appropriate pace of presentation and include active participation devices (e.g., games, self-assessment) to hold students' attention.
6. Provide examples and demonstrations before asking students to respond on their own.
7. Provide verbal and visual prompts and physical assistance to prevent incorrect responses.
8. Ask frequent and varied questions to maintain interest and test students' understanding.
9. Provide positive, clear, and immediate feedback for errors and provide an example or demonstration of the correct response.

Note that each step in the lesson presentation sequence relies on the oral presentation of information. Students with language difficulties understand what they *see* better than what they hear. They have problems

- focusing and maintaining attention;
- understanding and following through on verbal directions;

- dealing with changes in routines;
- organizing tasks; and
- receiving and using verbal information.

So, regardless of whether they are able to meet the academic demands of the lesson, they are not likely to be successful because they may not understand or be able to remember the review, the key points, the examples, and the directions.

The lesson presentation sequence is not an exception: In the typical general education classroom, because most information (e.g., homework assignments, quizzes, field trips, special projects) is given orally, children with language difficulties are decidedly at a disadvantage because of their difficulties understanding, using, and retaining verbal information. These problems can be prevented or at least attenuated by providing visual tools and supports. Many teachers provide some visual strategies but few exploit their worth.

Visual tools and supports can mediate and improve receptive *and* expressive language and communication processes for both verbal and nonverbal students. Visual supports can provide concrete, meaningful information in a logical and sequential form, thus reducing the need for repetition of directions and instructions. Visual aids can let students know what is expected of them, which allays the anxiety associated with transitions and change. In the lesson presentation sequence, for example, teachers can display pictures and/or icons depicting the review information, what is expected from the current lesson, key points and planned activities, salient new information, and samples of expected outcomes. Another example would be to provide pictures or icons illustrating the steps in the lesson and needed materials.

In summary, classroom observations by the language interventionist and/or the special education teacher should determine (1) how teacher communication expectations compare with the type of communicative competence that prevails in the child's cultural community, (2) specific reasons and possible remedies for teacher–child miscommunications, and (3) how visual aids and support can be used to supplement.the oral presentation of lessons.

The Curriculum

Some educators define curriculum to include virtually everything that happens in the child's school day, unplanned as well as planned experiences (e.g., Dittman, 1977). This view conceptualizes curriculum as a theoretical framework for experiences to promote the emotional, intellectual, and physical learning outcomes necessary for success in society. Others restrict the term to include what appears in the textbooks (or in the teacher's planbook) for a particular age or grade level (including goals and objectives, scope and sequence charts, teaching suggestions, environmental arrangements, materials and activities, evaluation procedures, etc.) (e.g., Johnson-Martin, Attermeier, & Hacker, 1990). We prefer to think of curriculum as *what* is to be learned.

In inclusive classrooms (or any classroom for that matter), all children do not need to be doing the same thing at the same time but, to the extent possible, they should be in the same curriculum. As Nelson (1994) points out, in most cases, the value of keeping students in the regular curriculum "far outweighs potential disadvantages associated with any particular curriculum" (p. 105). There is, however, a qualifier. The contention that all students should be in the same curriculum assumes (1) that the curriculum has a scope and sequence broad enough to accommodate students at a wide range of functioning levels, and (2) that the substance of what is taught and the instructional outcomes will not be affected by modifying the sequence of tasks and the way tasks are taught *or* by changing instructors.

Maintaining students with disabilities in the same curriculum as their peers without disabilities does not mean simply giving them more practice on certain skills or repetitions of lessons. Nor does it mean that language interventionists and special education teachers should abdicate total responsibility for language instruction and support to classroom teachers. The regular curriculum should be an important source for (1) determining communication intervention needs and goals, (2) designing intervention activities, (3) selecting and modifying materials, and (4) monitoring progress. This requires thoroughly and deliberately analyzing the language and communication expectations of the curriculum, determining where the student is having (or is likely to have) difficulties, and selecting or designing and implementing appropriate adaptations. This is done by the team—the general and special education teachers, the language interventionist, and other therapists as indicated—as part of the ecological assessment and planning process.

Functional life curricula (sometimes called community-based instruction, functional curriculum, or life skills instruction) are curricula for students with moderate and severe disabilities. Development of functional curriculum approaches arose from the need to teach skills that would have direct and immediate utility in students' lives in their communities and, equally pressing, the need to prepare students for a successful transition from school to adult living. Functional skills include personal care, communication, ambulation, and self-direction, which can be learned and practiced in a wide variety of settings.

The relationship between functional curricula and traditional academic curricula has been debated for well over a decade. Current trends emphasize the importance of melding the opportunities of the general education curriculum with appropriate and individualized functional outcome goals. Using strategies such as ecological assessment and cooperative learning, the team should plan to embed instruction of basic motor, personal care, communication, social interaction, and functional academic skills within the curriculum activities and daily routines of the general education environments (e.g., cafeteria, gymnasium, science lab). One way to do this is to develop a matrix that lists objectives for the child along one axis and the daily schedule (both academic lessons/classes and routines (e.g., homeroom, lunch) on the other. The team then decides which objectives can be taught logically and naturally during which activities and which objectives will require special scheduling because they cannot be taught naturally in the context of the day's activities. Chapter 12 discusses intervention for students with severe disabilities, including the use of a planning matrix.

Curriculum-based assessment (CBA) is a method of analyzing and assessing the curriculum and then sampling the child's performance on critical academic skills and concepts. There are a number of CBA approaches, but they all generally share these salient features: test items are drawn from children's curricula; repeated testings occur across time; and the assessment information is used to formulate instructional decisions. CBA is similar to the ecological assessment and planning process in that it is a general outcome measurement system, but it has a narrower focus. Whereas ecological assessment samples student performance in whatever activities are deemed important in the setting (academic or nonacademic), CBA is typically limited to sampling student performance on curriculum tasks and materials. It generally focuses specifically on performance in the areas of literacy and mathematics.

Both the curriculum-based language assessment approach and the ecological assessment–intervention approach emphasize adapting and individualizing instruction and the curriculum to reflect the interaction of the child's unique characteristics with curriculum expectations, teacher linguistic expectations, and peer interactions. In situations where there is clearly a need for a special instruction, it is still possible to use pieces of the regular curriculum.

Whether the team uses the CBA process and/or the ecological assessment and planning process (or both) to generate goals and objectives for children with language and communication difficulties, it is likely that lessons, activities, and materials will need to be adapted to make them accessible. Procedures for individualizing or adapting curriculum lessons and activities for students whose learning difficulties are primarily in the area of language and communication, and for those with more severe and/or pervasive language-learning disabilities, are on the same continuum. The range of possible adaptation for both groups is described in Table 8.2.

TABLE 8.2   Guidelines for adapting lessons/activities

No Difference: The student with disabilities participates in the same lesson/activity with the same objective(s) and using the same materials as peers without disabilities. Because objectives for the student with disabilities are the same as for peers without disabilities, there is no need for adaptations.

Physical Assistance: The student with disabilities participates in the same lesson/activity with the same objective(s) and using the same materials, but the student with disabilities is provided with physical assistance to enable participation. For example, a buddy may help a peer with physical disabilities by placing shapes on the felt board for him, helping him dip the brush into the paint jar, or taking notes for him.

Adapted or Different Materials: The student with disabilities participates in the same lesson/activity with the same objective(s), but the student with disabilities uses adapted or different materials. For example, a student with physical disabilities might use adapted scissors and adapted writing implements (pen or pencil) and need to have the writing paper taped in place on her desk. A child with visual impairment might use a laptop computer for writing, rather than pen or pencil.

Different Stimuli: The student with disabilities participates in the same lesson/activity with the same objective(s), but the student with disabilities is provided with more or different instructional stimuli. For example, some children may benefit from having multisensory stimuli when new concepts or complex instructions are being presented. The steps in a task may need to be presented one at a time and then left visible on the board or an overhead.

Different Response Level: The student with disabilities participates in the same lesson/activity, but the objectives—the response requirements—are at a different level. For example, a child with severe language difficulties is not expected to respond verbally to all of the questions about the story: He is required to answer only one question, "Was the story about a little boy or a little girl?" by pointing to a picture on his communication board.

Totally Different Objectives: The student with disabilities participates in the same lesson/activity with the same materials, but the objectives have a totally different focus because the student needs more functional goals with direct application to daily life. For example, when the focus of a science lesson for second graders is investigating how different kinds of liquids behave when poured (and recording their observations on a simple graph), the objectives for the student with disabilities may be (1) pouring without assistance, (2) making choices when presented with two options, and (3) following one-step directions.

Curriculum Adaptations for Children with Language-Learning Disorders

That the difficulties children with language disorders experience with oral language comprehension, auditory analysis, memory, and word finding and retrieval seem to translate to difficulties with reading, writing, and spelling skills is viewed as strong evidence for a relationship between oral language difficulties and literacy (Bashir, 1989; Sawyer, 1991; Wiig, 1990). As children move through the grades, what was initially an oral language disorder may be manifested as serious difficulties with written language, specifically difficulties in processing and comprehending what they read (Westby & Costlow, 1991). Scaffolding strategies are one way to facilitate language learning in written contexts. (These are described in the next section.)

Adapting materials for children with language-learning disorders is more than simplifying vocabulary, shortening sentences, or rewriting prose at a lower grade level. The information provided in daily lessons can be supplemented to make it more accessible. Some ways to supplement lessons are by

- providing advance organizers,
- highlighting important idea units,
- helping students identify different levels of importance of ideas, and
- teaching students to use task-appropriate cognitive strategies.

As discussed earlier in the chapter, visual aids such as pictures, charts, time lines, and outlines make information more accessible with a minimum of words. A series of pictures or a flowchart is many times more an effective way to convey a process than a paragraph or two filled with transitional adverbs and complex compound sentences. Flowcharts are especially useful for children who are having difficulty learning how to compare and contrast ideas. Time lines can be used to demonstrate and teach sequencing, and outlines are a good format to highlight specific points and reduce extraneous information. With an outline, comprehensible chunks of words and phrases can convey essential information in a concise manner.

The goal when adapting written material is to eliminate extraneous details by reducing the amount of text. Main ideas and the supporting facts are highlighted with bold typeface, underlining, and italics. (If, during the course of the lesson, students express an interest in details, they can be provided.) Once detail has been eliminated, the next consideration is the vocabulary and the grammar. New vocabulary should be clearly introduced and explained prior to reading; after reading, the new words can be reinforced with charts, pictures, and discussion. Because synonyms are often confusing to students who are trying to grasp the essence of a new concept, they should be minimized. Finally, it is important to use simple verb tenses in explanations and descriptions and to simplify word order in sentences by eliminating clauses and relying on a simple sentence (subject–verb–object) format. Written instructions can be simplified by using the active voice and limiting the use of pronouns and relative clauses.

Use concept analysis to teach new concepts. Concept analysis identifies critical or relevant attributes of the concept—those attributes that are present in all examples of the concept. These are the defining characteristics of the concept because they must be present for the concept to exist. Noncritical or irrelevant attributes may or may not be present in the concept. For example, concept analysis of the concept "square" yields these critical attributes: four sides, straight lines of equal length, four 90-degree angles, and enclosed space. Noncritical attributes include size, color, and orientation in space. To teach the concept, show examples of instances of the concept and also examples of noninstances (in this case, examples of squares and examples of figures that are not squares) and then comparing the two. Assess understanding by asking questions that verify that the student has the meaning and recognizes critical components of the definition.

Adaptations for Children with Severe and Multiple Disabilities
Adaptations for children with severe and multiple disabilities may involve modifications of the physical environment. The physical and/or occupational therapist will help the team understand the child's mobility skills (how she travels within the classroom and other school and community environments), appropriate positioning (so the child can participate as efficiently as possible in classroom activities), and possible adaptations that can support and/or substitute for fine and gross motor control. (These adaptations are especially important when selecting and teaching an augmentative communication system.) The language interventionist and the special education teacher can help others on the team understand the child's communication repertoire, specifically what symbols (e.g., words, signs, pictures) and what communication modes (e.g., speech, gestures, manual signing, a communication device) the child understands and uses spontaneously.

Goals and objectives for children with severe and/or multiple disabilities target specific skills and concepts necessary for participation in daily activities and routines. Many children with severe and multiple disabilities are able to participate in some activities/lessons (e.g., creative movement, library book selection, homeroom, listening to a story or tape) with no adaptations (or only very minor adaptations). Others require modified or different materials (larger paper, adapted scissors), modified or different instructions (pictorial instructions, instructions on audiotape), modified or different outcome expectations (e.g., fewer and/or less sophisticated responses, partial rather than full participation), and/or full or partial support and assistance (by a peer partner or an adult). These are discussed in Chapter 12.

Adaptations will necessitate developing different objectives for some students with moderate and severe disabilities. These alternative objectives may come from what is sometimes called the *implied curriculum* (Dittman, 1977). Examples of implied curriculum skills and concepts that are very important outcomes for children with severe and multiple disabilities include:

- sharing learning experiences and being part of a cooperative group;
- asking for (and giving) assistance;
- requesting materials;
- indicating activity and partner choices;
- following directions, and
- securing and organizing materials for an activity and returning them to their place when the activity has ended.

INTERVENTION METHODS AND PROCEDURES

Providing language instruction, facilitation, and support in the classroom and other school settings where children want and need to use language and communication has several major advantages:

- New skills and concepts are more likely to generalize because there are numerous opportunities to practice and use them in both social and academic interactions.
- Children receive more help because the teaching staff learns how to incorporate language instruction and practice into daily classroom activities and how to support carryover.
- Problems such as missed academic periods and increased isolation from peers that occur when students are regularly removed from their classrooms are avoided.

There is no one intervention method or set of instructional procedures that has been found to be superior for all children or all language goals (Yoder, Kaiser, & Alpert, 1991), nor is it possible to designate specific instructional procedures to use with particular objectives. The instructional procedures planned and implemented with a particular child depend on the child's objectives and his present functioning. Several procedures may be used to work on the same objective, and one procedure may be used to work on many objectives.

This section will describe procedures to teach functional communication skills in inclusive classrooms: milieu language teaching, scaffolding, routines and script training, interactive modeling, situated pragmatics, systematic instruction, structured teaching, and the picture exchange communication system. Several of these procedures were originally developed to be implemented in separate therapy settings. They have now been demonstrated to be effective when used in the context of either small- or large-group activities in natural settings.

Milieu Language Teaching

Milieu language teaching is an umbrella term covering a number of naturalistic language teaching procedures (Kaiser, Hendrickson, & Alpert, 1991): (1) child-cued modeling (Alpert & Kaiser, 1992), (2) mand-model teaching (Warren, McQuarter, & Rogers-Warren, 1984), (3) time delay (Halle, Marshall, & Spradlin, 1979), and (4) incidental teaching (Hart & Risley, 1968).

Milieu language teaching is based on observations of caregivers interacting with their normally developing children. Parents tend to

- talk about objects, events, and/or relations that have attracted the child's attention;
- model, imitate, and expand desired and actual child communication efforts;
- repeat and clarify words, statements, and requests that the child does not seem to understand; and
- use techniques such as higher speech frequencies and stress to call the child's attention to important sentence elements.

Although grounded in a behavioral approach to language intervention, milieu language teaching does not use a rigid direct instruction format. The topic of each teaching interaction and the reinforcement are defined by the child. Typical intervention targets include increasing the frequency of communicative behaviors, producing longer and more complex utterances, and expressing familiar functions with more advanced forms. The basic elements of milieu language teaching are (1) arranging the environment to create reasons for communication, (2) identifying communication or language targets, and (3) applying the teaching procedures.

Milieu teaching procedures (modeling, mand-modeling, time delay, and incidental teaching) require the immediate presence of an adult to mediate between the child and the desired or needed object or activity. The major difference in the milieu teaching model and most other naturalistic intervention models is that it uses explicit prompts. The child is prompted to use more advanced ways to communicate whatever message he has just tried to communicate. Detailed instructions for implementing milieu language teaching are provided in Chapter 10.

Scaffolding

Scaffolding is supporting children in such a way that they can understand and/or use language at a level that is more complex than could be grasped or produced independently. Scaffolding can be provided to assist children to understand and use any element of language, including specific vocabulary words, figurative language, syntactic structures, or elements of discourse structure. As children become more independent in the use of language, scaffolding is reduced and then gradually withdrawn. For example, when reading a story, scaffolding might take the form of explicit questioning about the elements of the story (e.g., Who was the story about? Where did it take place?). With older students, scaffolding questions could focus on more complex aspects of the plot, such as the characters' motivations. The challenge is (1) knowing when there is a mismatch between the communicative demands of the task or situation and a child's abilities, and (2) determining the nature of the mismatch so that scaffolding can be provided.

Conceptually, scaffolding draws from the same caregiver–child research as the milieu teaching model. The major difference between the two is precisely when modeling and expansion strategies are applied and the degree of structure. The concept of scaffolding was introduced by Vygotsky (1962, 1978) in his conceptualization of the dynamic regulation that goes on between the infant and caregivers in a nurturing environment. It was later used by Bruner (1975, 1986) to describe parents' use of language and gestures to segment ongoing experiences into meaningful elements appropriate to their child's level of understanding. In typical caregiver–child interactions, adults request only those behaviors (language and motor skills) that they know their child can produce. The difficulty of requests is gradually increased with just enough support that the child can be successful and, at the same time, challenged. Scaffolding provides a kind of "communication safety net," reducing the student's need to take risks when learning new skills.

Routines and Script Training

Routines are activities with a social or a maintenance purpose that are repeated frequently (usually on a daily basis) and always in almost the same way. They provide excellent opportunities to teach sequences of behavior, including language forms and functions. Social routines include games, rhymes, jokes, songs, storytelling, social amenities, and courtesies. Maintenance routines include classroom business activities (e.g., taking attendance, collecting lunch money), preparation activities (getting in line, preparing for a lesson, preparing for assembly, recess, lunch, or dismissal) and functional routines (cleaning up, distributing materials, toileting). Both social and maintenance routines may be viewed and taught as scripts.

Most classrooms (especially preschool and primary classrooms) have many routines that can be used as instructional contexts, or new routines can be developed to teach language. Once a new routine is well established, children anticipate what will happen next so they can be prompted to assume responsibility for whatever behavior should occur in the routine.

Some routines are more suitable contexts for promoting language and communication skills than others. When selecting a routine to use as an instructional context, consider (1) the type of materials involved, (2) time requirements, and (3) the number and repetitiveness of the component actions and subroutines. The following questions aid selection of routines to use for language facilitation and/or support (Halle, Alpert, & Anderson, 1984):

- Does the routine include a variety of attractive, interesting, and desirable objects and materials? Interesting objects and materials are more likely to stimulate language and communication.
- Can the routine be completed quickly? The faster a routine can be completed and another begun, the greater the number of new communication opportunities.
- Does the routine contain many actions? Each action in a routine is an opportunity for language, so the more actions, the more opportunities to prompt language.

Once a routine is selected and/or established, then it can be interrupted or varied. The unexpected departure from the anticipated sequence or anticipated action typically prompts a comment, protest, or request. The following are some ways to interrupt a routine:

- **Delay provision of an expected and desired material or event.** For example, consider the sequence of actions at snack time: one child distributes the napkins, another sets around the paper cups, the teacher pours juice or milk, and another child passes fruit or crackers. If, after the cups are set out, the teacher "forgets" to pour juice or milk, the children are likely to comment or protest the departure from routine (e.g., "No juice" or "I want juice" or "You forgot").
- **Provide an incomplete set of materials.** When a routine requires a prescribed set of materials, providing children with an incomplete set of materials (e.g., the toothpaste is missing from the tray with the other tooth-brushing materials) generally elicits a protest or request for the missing object(s). The adult simply waits until the children notice and comment on the missing object.
- **Make "silly" mistakes.** Children are quick to comment on or protest absurdities and inappropriate actions, such as holding a

book upside down. Intentionally violating expectations or calculated "silliness" has the additional advantage of helping children develop a sense of humor.

The first two strategies are especially effective in stimulating peer prompting. For example, when a child is "inadvertently" missed while pouring juice, a peer might say something like: "Tell Miss Kim that you didn't get juice" or "Ask for some juice." The use of routines with preschoolers is discussed at more length in Chapter 10.

Scripts are generalized representations of familiar events or routines that show the established order of the elements (Nelson & Gruendel, 1986). All people have scripts that they use when they describe routine events and when they want to predict what might happen in unfamiliar circumstances. Even very young children form scripted representations of routines and familiar events (e.g., a birthday party). Similarly to older children and adults, they use their scripts, which are either temporally ordered (one event always follows another in time) or causally ordered (one event must occur before another can occur), to structure their verbal accounts of experience and to aid their recall. When events do not proceed as a child anticipates, adults generally help the child make comparisons and understand that there can be different versions of the same event (e.g., "I realize this isn't what you expected but, at some birthday parties, the gifts are opened before the cake and ice cream").

Although the line between them is often blurred, using naturally occurring routines and script training are somewhat different. Using routines involves identifying (and sometimes teaching) naturally occurring routines that can be used as contexts to encourage and teach language and communication, whereas script training typically involves actually writing and teaching something like a play script. The goal in script training is to create interactive, systematic repetitions of events in which each "actor" plays her predictable role so that children can (1) practice social roles, (2) observe and model the language skills of others, and (3) learn to solve interpersonal conflicts. In the course of practicing the social roles in various events (e.g., going shopping, going to a restaurant, getting a haircut, a field trip to the zoo) the participants learn the expectations and the linguistic demands of the roles.

Script training is an effective strategy for teaching children the sequence, requirements, and roles for familiar events and routines when there is evidence that they have not developed generalized event representations on their own or lack the language ability to express their scripts. To maximize the effectiveness of script training, there needs to be a preparatory session when the children are given background, introduction, and priming for the "play." Roles are introduced, the use of props is demonstrated, and the basic goals of the play are discussed. As children practice their roles and exchange essential props, the familiar, repetitive structure of the scripts enhances the likelihood of successful interactions.

When a child seems to know what will happen next in a routine, whether that knowledge is verbalized or not, it is evidence of some kind of generalized representation for the routine. For example, when a child knows what to do when the 8:20 bell rings and when he enters the cafeteria this indicates that he has a script for these routines (whether he can tell us about them or not). There are numerous classroom activities which, because they require a child to recall elements of a script, teach scripting. They begin with "show and tell" in the preschool years, through literacy activities (e.g., "what I did on my summer vacation") in the elementary grades, to expository discourse in middle school and high school.

Interactive Modeling

The basic premise underlying **interactive modeling,** which is also called *recasting* (Nelson & Gruendel 1986), interactive language instruction (Cole & Dale, 1986), or focused stimulation (Leonard, Schwartz, Chapman, Rowan, Prelock, Terrell, Weiss, & Merrick, 1982), is that increasing the frequency of exposure to targeted language features enhances their saliency (and, thus, the probability that they will be learned). Interactive modeling gives children with language difficulties more deliberate and focused practice, more time, more repetitions, and heightened focus on new words and concepts. With interactive modeling, students are presented with multiple exemplars of target forms or operations in contexts where the form is semantically and pragmatically appropriate. For example, target language forms or operations might be embedded in play activities (e.g., "Simon says"), routines (e.g., making snacks), and/or curriculum activities. The child is neither requested nor required to respond.

These are the steps in implementing interactive modeling (Fey, Cleave, Long, & Hughes, 1993):

1. Identify the student's specific language targets.
2. Determine activities that provide semantically and pragmatically appropriate conditions for the student to hear the language target(s).
3. Model the language target(s) frequently during the identified activities.
4. Recast the student's attempts to produce the target(s) through simple expansions or by changing the sentence modality (e.g., recast a declarative sentence as a yes-no question to highlight auxiliary form).

5. Use false assertions to encourage the child to produce sentences that use the target(s) (e.g., "That's not your book," said to evoke "Yes, it is") and contingent queries to elicit semantic details omitted from an original message (e.g., "Which one did he take?").

6. Ask forced-alternative questions that provide a model of the correct use of the target(s) (e.g., "You do want it or you don't want it?" to evoke "I don't want it") or ask questions about a story to give the student practice in producing the targeted features. Interactive modeling is described at more length in Chapter 10.

Situated Pragmatics

Situated pragmatics is instruction that provides contextual support to increase the inclusion of children with language and communication disorders in the social and cultural mainstream (Duchan, 1995). The basic goal is to help the child make sense of what is going on and to provide an emotionally safe environment so that the child participates willingly and meaningfully.

Possible support contexts are (1) the social context, (2) the emotional context, (3) the functional context, (4) the physical context, (5) the event context, and (6) the discourse context. Supports in the various contexts are tailored to fit the child's difficulties or to build on strengths. The specific methods depend on what is going on in the situation, who the interactants are, the child's needs in that context, and the supporter's goals for the child. Table 8.3 provides examples of support and possible techniques in the six situated pragmatics contexts.

Situated pragmatics can be used to (1) develop vocabulary, (2) teach expression of targeted speech acts, and (3) facilitate understanding and use of targeted grammatical structures. When developing vocabulary, the focus is on teaching words as tools to express ideas about objects and events of interest to the child. Vocabulary goals should be words that are functional for the child. They should be taught as a related set in the context of an everyday event. Children with a limited vocabulary are encouraged to use words to express their communicative intents or their favorite objects and ideas in order to participate in daily events. To teach expression of particular intents, such as requests, the targeted functions are elicited and modeled in a variety of contexts with the goal of supporting the child's efforts to use language to get what he or she wants. A situated pragmatics approach to improve understanding and use of language structure first considers the pragmatic impact of the targeted structure, then functional communicative contexts that highlight the importance of the structure are identified or developed.

TABLE 8.3 Examples of support and possible techniques in the six situated pragmatics contexts

---

Examples of support for language learning in the **social context** *include:*
- helping the child identify and understand his or her role in the setting;
- helping the child understand his or her role in relation to the others in an interaction.

Possible technique(s)—enact scripts involving family roles, teacher–child roles, etc.

Examples of support for language learning in the **emotional context** *include:*
- helping the child and family members attune to the affect or emotional tone of one another;
- creating contexts in which the child can take a valued and important role, leading to positive self-esteem.

Possible technique(s)—use events in stories to develop understanding of emotions; provide emotional support when the child experiences frustration or difficulty.

Examples of support for language learning in the **functional context** *include:*
- helping the child associate intent with communicative acts, either nonverbal (e.g., pointing to request) or verbal (e.g., using a word, phrase, or sentence to make a request);
- helping the child detect the motivations behind the behavior and language of her communication partners.

Possible technique(s)—design events the child is excited about and ways the child can request the events and items within the event; use stories to interpret the motivations of others to the child.

Examples of support for language learning in the **physical context** *include:*
- offering interesting, manipulable objects and pictures as props for learning about the world;
- creating interesting and suggestive spaces (e.g., accessible theme areas) in the room.

Possible technique(s)—create alternative spaces in the classroom that the child can manipulate; provide communicative support at afterschool programs where children are able to socialize informally.

Examples of support for language learning in the **event context** *include:*
- allowing the child to watch and then act as an apprentice in an event until he is comfortable engaging directly in the event;
- helping the child expand familiar routines by inserting new elements into various slots in the routine.

Possible technique(s)—develop joint interaction routines between the child and different adults; create scripts with the child to help him understand and participate in complex or rule-based events.

Examples of support for language learning in the **discourse context** *include:*
- arranging space and allocating sufficient time for discourse;
- providing props that support initiations and enactments of discourse-based activities.

Possible technique(s)—create opportunities for the child to tell about an emotional event in the past; scaffold answers to questions about past events using a notebook that goes between home and school.

Based on Duchan (1995).

Systematic Instruction

Systematic instruction is teacher-guided instruction using procedures based on applied behavior analysis (ABA) (Skinner, 1957). These procedures can be used for instruction of virtually any language and communication targets in any environments (contrived *or* natural). Linguistic and naturalistic approaches also use many of the behavioral methods associated with ABA but systematic instruction applies them in a more rigorous and structured manner. Systematic instruction is most commonly used with students with severe disabilities (including autism). The children who seem to benefit most from ABA are those who are nonverbal and noncompliant. Children with milder problems may benefit from the use of systematic instruction in combination with some of the other procedures described in this chapter (Dawson & Osterling, 1995).

The techniques that are "packaged" into the treatment approach called **Discrete Trial Training** (DTT) and identified with the work of Lovaas (1987) also fall under the broad umbrella of ABA. They are, in fact, systematic instruction procedures. There is nothing new about these procedures. They have been used very effectively by professionals for over three decades. Discrete trial training, however, has some specific intervention requirements that make it more rigorous and demanding than systematic instruction (e.g., the requirement for thirty to forty hours a week of one-to-one training by highly trained therapists).

The major goals of DTT are reducing behavioral excesses such as tantrums and acting-out behaviors and improving communication skills. Training begins with simple tasks and imitation activities and then builds to more complex activities that require greater use of language. Based on the premise that the reason children with autism are not learning is that they have not learned to focus their attention on learning tasks and cooperate with the teacher's instructions, DTT focuses on eliciting attention and reinforcing any attempts at compliance. Over time, after innumerable repetitions, the child develops an initial repertoire of communication skills and some basic life and academic skills.

The time requirements and some of the other very rigid conditions (e.g., one-to-one training, the high level of training required by all of the trainers) associated with DTT are difficult, if not impossible, for many schools and families to manage. Critics argue that the same improvement possible with DTT could be achieved with fewer hours of discrete trial training. This would leave children time to also learn how to play, socialize, and generally function in groups.

Systematic instruction typically involves some drill and practice with trials on specific forms and/or structures. The behavioral term for repeated drill and practice on a single skill is *massed trial instruction*.

Most linguistic approaches also provide some drill and practice (particularly in the initial acquisition phase of instruction) (Cole & Dale, 1986). In linguistic approaches the targets for drill and practice may include forms or structures exemplifying particular inflectional morphemes and specific syntactic rules. In a behavioral approach the targets for massed trial instruction are more likely to be request forms (e.g., "more," "want _") that can be used across a range of naturalistic contexts.

Drill and practice procedures need not involve removing the learner from the natural environment to a distraction-free setting. It is usually possible to provide practice trials in the context of ongoing activities (i.e., situated pragmatics contexts). In fact, there are some activities and routines in which repetitions of a single response occur naturally (e.g., turn-taking in a social routine, saying "goodbye" to peers who are leaving a setting one at a time).

Systematic and intensive instruction is best used in small groups in the context of ongoing classroom activities. This avoids the stigma of singling out a student for "special" instruction. Systematic instruction uses the following procedures: modeling, task analysis, shaping, prompting, and reinforcement.

Modeling

Modeling is "showing how," a teaching strategy that provides a demonstration in order to prompt the desired motor or verbal behavior. Imitation is just the opposite. Imitation is a learning strategy. Imitation is performance of a response that matches, or at least approximates, a model. When modeling is used as a teaching strategy, the model or demonstration is usually preceded by a verbal direction (e.g., "do it like this," or "say _"). An instance (or, at the very least, a picture) of the concept being labeled should be present and should be the focus of the child's attention when modeling a word or manual sign. When modeling, placing stress on critical aspects of the stimulus increases the likelihood of imitation. For example, when teaching names of shapes, the format would be (1) display the circle shape, and (2) say "This is a circle. Say . . . circle" (with a pause between the words *say* and *circle* and the word *circle* emphasized).

Task Analysis

Task analysis is breaking down a skill into small steps to make it easier to teach. Once the target skill has been identified and stated as an instructional objective, these task analysis steps are implemented:

1. Either perform the skill (or watch someone else perform the skill) and record the behaviors required to execute the skill successfully.
2. Eliminate unnecessary or redundant steps.
3. Sequence the steps in the order in which they are performed or in terms of difficulty.

4. Prompt the student through the task and make any modifications in step size that is necessary (based on the student's performance).

Task analysis must be individualized for students because the size of the steps depends on a child's ability level. There should be just enough steps to allow efficient instruction. One student might need a ten-step task analysis to acquire a particular skill while another might need to have the same behavior broken down into a twenty-step process. Each step in the task analysis should be clearly stated in measurable terms.

Shaping

Shaping is a procedure for teaching the steps in the task analysis. Shaping begins with reinforcement of the closest approximation of the first step and systematically builds on slight changes in that behavior (called *reinforcement of successive approximations*). Each step or approximation is reinforced until it is learned, and then the next behavior (the next closer approximation) is taught until eventually the complex target behavior is produced. Shaping can be used with prompts to further encourage the development of new skills when reinforcement of successive approximations alone does not have the desired results.

Prompting

Prompting can be thought of as "priming" a desired response. Prompts are assists or supports that are provided to increase the likelihood that the learner will respond correctly. Prompts are introduced during the acquisition phase of instruction and faded as soon as the desired behavior is occurring with predictable frequency. There are response prompts and stimulus prompts. Response prompts include verbal directions, modeling, and physical guidance. Stimulus prompts are cues that are used in conjunction with the task materials to ensure a correct response. Examples include movement cues (e.g., the teacher points to the correct picture), position cues (e.g., the correct picture is placed closest to the student's right hand), and redundancy or exaggeration cues (the stimulus is altered by exaggeration, repetition, or adding a dimensional cue such as color, size, or shape). The two criteria for judging the effectiveness of instructional prompts are (1) whether they elicit the desired response, and (2) whether they can be faded.

A student is prompt-dependent if she waits for a prompt rather than attempting a response on her own. This is a major concern when using prompts. The following steps will help to avoid students becoming prompt-dependent:

- develop and use a written plan for when and how prompts will be delivered and what correction procedures will be used;
- select prompts that minimize errors but do not interfere with the instructional sequence;

- have the student's attention before delivering the prompt;
- pair natural prompts with instructional prompts and fade the instructional prompts as soon as possible; and
- use prompts that focus the student's attention on the most relevant characteristics of the stimulus.

Fading

Fading is the gradual removal of an instructional prompt so that the desired behavior is performed independently or only with naturally occurring supports. Fading is accomplished by shifting from partial prompts, or by reducing the amount of assistance. The type of fading strategy used depends on the type of prompt: The sound intensity of auditory prompts can be faded; the size of spatial and movement prompts can be decreased; the color intensity of visual prompts can be faded. The primary concern when using fading is maintaining the student's correct responding when prompts are removed. If, as prompts are being faded, the student begins to perform the behavior incorrectly, or stops performing the behavior at all, this means that the prompts were faded too fast. When fading procedures are properly executed, whatever level of responding that was evident *with* the prompts is maintained when they are removed.

Reinforcement

Reinforcement is *any* event that immediately follows a response that has the effect of increasing the probability that the response will be repeated. Reinforcement and reinforcers are often misunderstood and misrepresented as simply providing a treat (e.g., candy, raisins, trinkets) or praise after an appropriate behavior. The only way to determine whether an object or event is reinforcing is by reference to its effects on the response that it follows. An event is not reinforcement *unless* it increases (qualitatively and/or quantitatively) the behavior it follows. For some individuals treats and praise are *not* reinforcers in that they do not increase the probability that the response they follow will be repeated.

Another misconception is that use of reinforcement is limited to behaviorists and behavioral programs. *Everyone* provides reinforcement of one type or another. The major difference between behaviorists and others is the way the event is described and how systematically the reinforcement is provided.

Availability of a reinforcer in the learner's natural environment is an important consideration in selecting reinforcers for a particular child. Contrived and artificial reinforcement conditions should be avoided in favor of naturally occurring events. If contrived reinforcement must be used, it should be replaced or faded as quickly as possible toward natural consequences. In normal learning circumstances, a child's efforts to communicate are reinforced, not the form of the communication. Even primitive communication efforts are typically responded to with attention, if not the receipt of a requested object or event. The more meaningful and appropriate the child's communication efforts, the greater the likelihood that the intent of the message will be correctly interpreted and responded to.

Structured Teaching

Structured teaching superimposes a high level of organization in the child's environments as a way to develop skills and minimize behavioral difficulties (Mesibov, Schopler, & Hearsey, 1994). The structured teaching approach is most commonly associated with Division TEACCH (Treatment and Education of Autistic and related Communication-handicapped Children) at the University of North Carolina, where it is used specifically with children with autism. The Division TEACCH procedures are similar in some ways to milieu teaching strategies, but there is considerably more emphasis on receptive language and substantially more attention to structuring the environment. Structured teaching also uses some instructional techniques from systematic instruction, for example, directions, prompts, and reinforcements. The unique aspect of this approach is using physical organization, individual work systems, visual structure, and routines to help children organize themselves and respond appropriately to their environments.

Physical Organization

One of the basic premises of the structured teaching approach is that children with autism have difficulty differentiating between dissimilar events and seeing how distinct activities are related to one another (Mesibov, Schopler, & Hearsey, 1994). Structured teaching describes ways to arrange the physical environment so that the child has consistent, visually clear areas and boundaries for different activities, for example, designating a specific location in the classroom for individual work so that the child knows what to expect when she is in that location. Children are helped to focus on the relevant aspects of their tasks by blocking out as many extraneous sights and sounds as possible. This is done by using dividers (bookshelves, window shades) or distributing work areas around the classroom. Some boundaries that can be used to separate specific activity areas include rugs, bookshelves, partitions, tape on the floor, and the arrangement of furniture.

Schedules

Visual schedules are supports for children with receptive language difficulties and attention and memory problems. They help students remember what is planned, predict daily and weekly events, and organize their time accordingly. Structured teaching recommends providing two types of schedules: a general classroom schedule and individual students' schedules. Individual schedules help students remember what to do during the activities listed on the general schedule.

Individual Work Systems

Students' work systems tell them (at a level they can understand) what they should do while in their independent work areas. They communicate four types of information: (1) expected tasks, (2) how *much* work is expected, (3) how the student will know when she is finished with the work, and (4) what happens when the work is completed.

Visual Structure

Visual structure is achieved by using visual clarity, visual organization, and visual instructions. Visually clear tasks and materials have distinctive shapes, patterns, or color, for example, the students' individual materials, their work areas, and their chairs might be color-coded. Materials are organized into containers to make them easier for students to manage and work with. Visual instructions are simply visual representations of how a task is to be carried out. They may depict the task requirements, sequence of steps, relevant concepts, and other implementation details.

Routines

The routines that are part of structured teaching are different from the routines described in the section on routines and script training. The routines in structured teaching are not established with a view to interrupting them to elicit language. Based on the premise that children with autism develop stereotypical and unproductive ways of approaching certain tasks, structured teaching attempts to redirect this tendency toward productive routines. The first routine taught to children in the structured teaching approach is "first work and then play" (Mesibov, Schopler, & Hearsey, 1994). This routine can then be used throughout the day and across many activities. Checking their schedules and following the directions from their work system are other examples of routines that, once established, are extremely productive for the student.

Picture Exchange Communication System

The **Picture Exchange Communication System** (PECS) is an augmentative system for teaching functional communication skills (Bondy & Frost, 1994; Frost & Bondy, 1996) to young children with autism and other severe disabilities (Schwartz, Garfinkle, & Bauer, 1998). The PECS training does not require any prerequisite behaviors and it is relatively easy and inexpensive to use. Like milieu language teaching, it is based on child initiation and generalization strategies are embedded in the teaching protocol. Children are taught to request multiple items with many communication partners in different settings.

PECS training begins with reinforcer assessment—providing children with arrays of materials to determine their reinforcement preferences. Initial training then requires two adults, one who serves as the communicative partner, and another to be the instructor and provide prompts while seated behind the child. The second adult is faded as soon as possible, based on how well the child grasps the idea that she is to provide the picture in exchange for the desired object. Using a combination of forward and backward prompting techniques, children learn to scan an array of 2 × 2 inch line drawings/symbols, select the symbols for what they desire, place the symbols on a strip of laminated poster board next to a symbol meaning "I want," and hand the strip with the affixed symbols to an appropriate adult. All training takes place in the classroom and other natural environments (e.g., playground, cafeteria) in the context of ongoing activities. A unique aspect of this training is the focus on teaching children to be persistent.

THE INSTRUCTIONAL ENVIRONMENT

Where instruction is provided is a major difference between traditional and inclusive schools. In traditional schools, special instruction was usually provided in a special education class, a resource room, or a therapy room. In inclusive schools, special instruction for language and communication and other skills occurs in heterogeneous groups in the regular classroom and other school settings (i.e., the playground, cafeteria, halls, gymnasium). Students with disabilities spend the school day alongside peers who are not disabled. This sends the message to peers, families, school personnel, and others in the community (and, most importantly, to the students themselves) that they belong.

Functional living and vocational skills are taught in nonschool environments (e.g., home, vocational, and other community settings), the contexts in which they naturally occur. Children are encouraged and supported in such contexts by appropriate special education and vocational rehabilitation staff, but the actual instruction should be provided by the people who are responsible in those settings (e.g., parents, employers).

The defining characteristic of the inclusive classroom is children and adults who look for and find ways to support and nurture each other's learning so that everyone succeeds. Some ways to create inclusive environments are:

- **Eliminate competitions.** Emphasize that everyone does his or her "personal best." Create bulletin boards and other displays that feature the work of all children, not just the work of the high performers.

- **Plan activities that encourage feelings of "togetherness."** Some activities that encourage this attitude and draw the class together are plays, choral singing, and other performances. Students work together to write a play script, produce the scenery, paint advertising posters, make popcorn for the production, and so on. For music performances, students can take turns teaching and leading songs.

- **Use "we" language.** Using *we* rather than singling out individual students or small groups within the class (e.g., "the first reading group") encourages and supports group achievement and solidarity. When there is an issue with a particular child or a small group, engage the whole class in problem solving. Inclusive language helps students.

- **Encourage sharing of information, instruction, and support.** Arrange the class into cooperative support groups and set this rule: If one person in the group has a problem of any sort, she consults first with her group before coming to the teacher for help.

- **Encourage students to recognize each other's accomplishments.** Many times, students are more attentive to the misdeeds of their classmates (as evidenced by tattling and recriminations) than to their accomplishments. Turn this around by focusing attention on positive acts and achievements, making it clear that there is no competition, that everyone can succeed and everyone can be happy for others' accomplishments.

- **Discuss cooperation and/or conflict resolution.** Reading books with cooperation themes is one way to initiate discussions about personal and classroom applications of cooperation and conflict resolution. Another idea is for students to write their own book about cooperation in which they record the things they have accomplished as a class that would not have been possible without cooperation and collaboration.

PROFESSIONAL RELATIONSHIPS AND RESPONSIBILITIES

As noted earlier in this chapter, the organization of traditional schools had the effect of isolating special and regular education teachers from one another and isolating therapists from each other and from teachers. Regular education teachers were primarily concerned with their children and their rooms; special education teachers were concerned with their children and their rooms. Therapists worked independently to facilitate development of specific skills for specific children (children assigned to their caseloads). Because people were never in the same place at the same time, it was all but impossible to form any type of professional (or personal) relationships. They did not have the opportunities or support for getting to know one another and learning to work together in a meaningful way. Working together in a meaningful way depends on overcoming physical, attitudinal, and logistical barriers.

The hallmark of inclusive schools is togetherness and positive interdependence, which has both professional and personal benefits for teachers and therapists. There is recognition that no one person can effectively address the diverse educational, social, and psychological needs of all children and focus on maximizing each person's contributions and performance through modeling, feedback, and mutual support. Everyone acknowledges and is comfortable with the fact that special education and related services personnel and general education teachers bring unique but complementary skills to the special instruction process. Teachers learn about language instruction, and language interventionists learn about curriculum and classroom management skills.

The team structure provides a supportive collegial atmosphere that enables professionals to practice creative thinking and problem solving. In addition to assuming new roles, adults learn new professional skills (as well as interpersonal skills). They learn to accept, trust, and help one another, to communicate accurately and unambiguously, and to resolve conflicts constructively. In the process of developing meaningful, reciprocal, and interdependent relationships they create a rich learning environment for all students.

SCHEDULING

Staffing arrangements in inclusive schools are different than traditional schools, where grouping of students with disabilities is based on what is judged to be the intensity of their needs. In traditional schools, staffing patterns are based on the staff-to-student ratio and the percentage of the day the student receives services. A special education teacher, called a Resource Teacher, may serve as many as twenty-five children with mild to moderate disabilities. Because they are considered to have minimal needs, these children receive special instruction weekly for varying periods of time. Teachers with separate classes (usually called Self-Contained Classroom Teachers) serve children regarded as having more intensive needs. They may serve children with mild to moderate disabilities in classes with twelve to fifteen children or children with severe and multiple disabilities in classes with six to eight children. In traditional schools, language interventionists usually try to schedule at least a half hour of therapy every week or every other week for each child in their caseload. In inclusive schools, rather than serving children with the same "intensity of needs" in homogeneous groups, special education teachers are assigned to a grade level. The number of children for whom they are responsible depends on the students' instructional needs. Language interventionists in inclusive schools also function differently. In addition to providing direct support and team-teaching, they participate in team decision making focused on planning, coordinating, and monitoring language intervention efforts for the children in their caseload.

An example will illustrate how one inclusive elementary school has chosen to organize services. In the planning process, based on data indicating that the percentage of children eligible for special education services in the primary grades in the district is generally 15 to 16 percent, the Dalton School Primary Inclusion (DSPI) team predicted that there would be ten to fifteen children with disabilities at each primary grade level (K–3). (This is based on three classrooms at each level with an average enrollment of twenty-eight students.) When school started, the actual count of children eligible for special education services was ten, twelve, fourteen, and fifteen for kindergarten, first, second, and third grades, respectively. It was decided to distribute children with disabilities evenly among the classes and to assign a special education teacher and a teaching assistant to each grade level (the classroom-based special instruction arrangement described below). A language interventionist was assigned to serve all four levels and a physical therapist was assigned to serve children in grades K–6.

Staffing arrangements in inclusive schools generally fall into two broad categories: direct contact/service arrangements and consultation arrangements. Each arrangement, of course, requires different scheduling.

Direct contact/service arrangements include:
  1. **Co-teaching.** The language interventionist and the special education teacher share responsibility for instruction for the entire class with the general education teacher. In addition to sharing teaching responsibilities, the classroom team equally shares instructional problem solving and decision making for all children (with and without disabilities). As this arrangement usually includes some children with severe disabilities, the team may also include an occupational and/or physical therapist and parents. The language interventionist might lead the class in brainstorming a list of guidelines (on a large piece of poster paper) before providing opportunities to practice some class presentations. The guidelines one class developed looked like this: (1) use a loud enough voice so that everyone can hear and look at the

audience (most of the time); (2) begin by giving the name of whatever you are showing or naming the experience you are going to describe (e.g., "my first fishing trip"); (3) tell two or three things that you think are interesting about the object or the experience; and (4) ask if anyone in the class has questions or comments and wait long enough for people to think of a question or comment. Each child (including the children in the class with language disorders) copies the list of guidelines in her notebook and the large chart is posted in the classroom. The learning of the children with language disorders is further facilitated by several demonstrations (provided by students without disabilities) that highlight each of the guidelines.

2. **Classroom-based special instruction.** In the classroom-based direct services model, the language interventionist modifies and presents existing curriculum activities for individual children and/or groups of children with similar goals and objectives or expectations (ASHA, 1993). The special education teacher develops and provides modified activities and curricula in the regular classroom for individual children and/or a group of children with behavioral and/or academic difficulties in the regular classroom. Both the language interventionist and the special education teacher base their instruction on and draw from the classroom curriculum and routine activities. Decisions are also made as a team, but because the language interventionist and the special education teacher are not in the classroom at all times, they may be less involved in problem solving and decision making for children without disabilities. This model differs from co-teaching in that most of the instruction provided by the support professionals (the language interventionist and the special education teacher) is for the children in the class who have special instructional needs. This special instruction and support may be provided individually or as part of a small group that includes both children with and without disabilities. In this model the support professionals serve a number of classrooms.

Consultation arrangements include:

1. **Collaborative support.** The language interventionist and the special education teacher participate as team members in decision making for children with special instructional needs. The support team, which includes the classroom instructional staff, family members, the special education teacher, the language interventionist, and other related services professionals, collaborate for continuous assessment, develop goals, plan programs, identify and arrange curriculum adaptations, and monitor program implementation and program effectiveness. The language interventionist and/or the special education teacher and the

regular education teacher may provide some direct classroom-based services as a team. In this model, the support professionals consult and provide technical assistance and formal and informal training for many classrooms.

2. **Expert support.** After assessing the child, the support professional meets with the team (made up of the teaching staff, the special education teacher, and the parents) to provide intervention suggestions and recommendations. The expert consultant may also provide technical assistance and in-service training for those who will deliver the services.

All of these models have several things in common: All call for collaboration and communication among administrative personnel, support personnel, teaching staff, and parents, and all present major scheduling challenges.

In co-teaching, particularly if there are a number of children with severe disabilities, the language interventionist and/or the special education teacher may be in the general education classroom full-time. The success of co-teaching depends on total parity, recognition of each other's strengths, and commitment to common goals for the students. With classroom-based special instruction, the language interventionist and the special education teacher schedule regular blocks of time for their special instruction activities and also time for planning with the teaching staff how they can meet individual student language and communication objectives in the context of the classroom curriculum, daily routines, and interpersonal exchanges. When language interventionists and special education teachers serve as collaborative consultants to the classroom teacher, they must allocate large time blocks for team meetings and blocks of time for classroom observations (to learn about the curriculum and the strengths and needs of the children as they relate to social and academic functioning and to monitor the effectiveness of intervention strategies and children's progress). Collaborative consultation models may also include some direct classroom-based language intervention services, which are provided jointly by the language interventionists and/or the special education teacher and the classroom teacher.

MEASUREMENT AND EVALUATION STRATEGIES

Measurement and evaluation are different procedures with different purposes. Measurement is systematic data collection in order to evaluate student progress and make programming decisions. The basic steps in the measurement process are (1) determining what is to be measured, (2) defining the target behavior or event in observable terms, and (3) selecting an appropriate data-recording system for observing, quantifying, and summarizing the behavior. Evaluation is analysis of the data collected in the measurement process for the purpose of decision-making. Evaluation may be summative or formative.

Summative Evaluation and Formative Evaluation

Summative and formative evaluation differ in purpose, time, and level of generalization. **Summative evaluation** takes place after an intervention has been implemented (typically the annual review called for by the IDEA). The purpose is to document that the promised services have been provided and that goals and objectives have been achieved. **Formative evaluation** is undertaken before and during instruction to find out whether the planned intervention efforts are being provided and whether they are proving to be effective. Formative evaluation is primarily to assist identification of strengths and weaknesses in the intervention/teaching process.

In most cases it is possible and desirable to use both qualitative and quantitative evaluation methods. Quantitative research and evaluation methods report results in numbers in an effort to describe, explain, and predict relationships. Qualitative methods are also concerned with description (and understanding what is occurring), but they use words, rather than numbers. Qualitative methods are concerned with process rather than simply outcomes or products. The goal is to construct a picture of what is occurring. The assumption behind the use of qualitative data is that the meaning of behaviors cannot be separated from the context. Intervention is evaluated according to whether it results in socially valid (i.e., important and meaningful) changes in children's lives and whether it uses strategies that are socially valid (i.e., acceptable and sustainable) in the classroom and other natural settings.

Used in the broadest sense, qualitative methods include investigative methodologies and data collection procedures described as ethnographic, naturalistic, anthropological, or participant-observer. Qualitative methods are a way to examine the processes of teaching and learning, the intended and unintended consequences of the intervention procedures, the relationships among children and with adults, and the sociocultural contexts within which teaching and learning occur most effectively.

The term for assessment that provides both qualitative and quantitative information about the child's performance of skills in actual rather than contrived tasks is **authentic assessment** (Wiggins, 1989). Authentic assessment is not a single method. It is any measure that provides information about the child's behaviors in daily activities. Some methods for authentic assessment include observations, interviews, checklists, photographs, anecdotal records, and diaries. Checklists, anecdotal records, and observations are described below.

Checklists make it possible to obtain a great deal of information in a relatively short time. They can provide both specific and general information about children's understanding and use of different language forms, structures, and functions. An advantage of checklists is the potential to obtain information to address several different questions at once. Checklists can be used to document (typically with a checkmark) whether the student performed the targeted behavior when performance was appropriate and whether it was performed correctly or incorrectly.

Anecdotal records are a type of narrative recording. They may be written or recorded on audio- or videotapes. Notes about a student's use of language in specific contexts and activities and the appropriateness of an activity or certain materials in eliciting language are particularly useful. They may be recorded when the events occur or sometime thereafter. Some professionals write notes with reminders and questions such as these:

1. "3/14 (10:30): Susannah said 'Can I play?' twice (without being prompted) to Brandon and Kyle. They were playing the Fishing Game during free play. She seems to be developing a special friendship with Brandon."
2. "4/16: Need to remember to discuss with the team how to get Cory to respond to choice situations. Also, need to ask Donna for some ideas as to what to do to get Nicole to use words for feelings."

Anecdotal records provide an objective description of a specific behavior at a specific time in a specific situation. Every anecdotal recording should include the student's name, the date and time, a description of the behavior that occurred, where it occurred, and both the stimulus for and the response to the behavior. It should include everything that the student said and did in the situation (and to/with whom) as well as what is said and done to/with the student. Facts should be clearly separated from interpretations.

Interpreting written narrative data is simplified by providing an indication of the time and organizing the descriptions into three columns. Events that occur before the communicative utterance are recorded in the first column: the student's specific language or communication behaviors (verbal and nonverbal) are recorded in the second column, and the effect or response to the student's language/communication behavior is recorded in the third column.

Observations are essentially a series of "snapshots" depicting different sequences of behaviors and events as they occur in their natural contexts. Selection of the most appropriate lens for the snapshots depends on the questions being asked, practical considerations (e.g., time available for data collection), and what dimension of the behavior is of concern (e.g., rate, duration). The methods for collecting observation data are (1) event or frequency recording, (2) duration and latency recording, and (3) interval recording.

Event or frequency recording involves counting the number of times the target behavior occurs during a specified time period. This method is appropriate for recording discrete behaviors of short duration with easily discernible beginnings and endings. Sentences, phrases, words, syllables, and phonemes are examples of discrete behavior units that, if not delivered at an extremely high rate, can be tallied. Frequency recording is realistic for classroom data collection because it can be incorporated easily into daily routines. The only data collection devices required are a pencil or pen and paper or a counter (handheld or worn on the wrist). When recording frequency of occurrences, it is critical also to record the number of trials (opportunities for the response) when performance is based on opportunity. For example, it is meaningless to record the number of "appropriate requests for assistance in the cafeteria" without a record of the number of times such requests were indicated.

Duration recording is used when the length of time a behavior occurs is of interest. The number of seconds or minutes from initiation to termination of the target behavior is recorded. Duration recording is most appropriate for behaviors that (1) occur at rates too high to make tallying a possibility; (2) occur for extended time periods; and (3) are variable in length (e.g., conversation, dramatic play). One way of recording duration data is the time accumulation method. The stopwatch is started as the behavior begins, stopped when the target behavior ends, then restarted when the target behavior is begun again, and so on for the length of the observation period. Over time, if the stopwatch is not returned to zero, this produces a record of the accumulated time of instances of the behavior. Latency is the time between a stimulus, or prompt, and the student's response. **Latency** is a concern when it affects the functionality of a skill (for example, if the student takes so long to respond to a request for a toy that the peer starts playing with something else).

Interval recording permits fairly sensitive measurement of both duration and frequency simultaneously. The observation period is divided into equal time intervals (usually from 5 to 50 seconds) depending on the average frequency and duration of the behavior. Regardless of the number of times the target behavior occurs during an interval, the interval is checked only once. When more than one behavior is being observed or recorded, or when more than one child is to be observed and recorded, there may be separate rows of interval cells for each behavior or each child, or a single row of cells where a symbol is recorded (for the behavior or child). When using an interval recording system it is important to specify in advance the proportion of the interval in which the behavior must occur in order to be scored. For example, does the interaction have to occur for the entire interval to be scored? Or will it be scored if it occurs during part of the interval? If it needs to occur for only part of the interval, how long must it occur?

Summary

This chapter has considered six dimensions of programming in inclusive schools: (1) the focus of intervention; (2) methods and procedures for intervention; (3) the instructional environment; (4) professional relationships and responsibilities; (5) scheduling; and (6) measurement and evaluation. For teachers and language interventionists, as well as for families and administrators, inclusion is a new way of thinking and a new way of acting. This chapter has discussed ways that team members can collaborate to modify classrooms and other school environments to accommodate the needs of children with language and communication difficulties.

The approach to data collection and evaluation of behavior change described in this chapter encourages teachers and language interventionists to think broadly and to commit to documenting important, relevant, and functional outcomes.

Discussion Questions

1. Contrast present-day special education and language intervention services with past special education and language intervention services. Specifically, focus on the six dimensions discussed in the chapter: intervention focus, methods and procedures, instructional environment, professional relationships and responsibilities, scheduling, and measurement and evaluation.
2. Discuss the IRE pattern and how it can be modified for students with severe language disorders.
3. Describe a typical general education curriculum for reading for a particular grade level and discuss possible adaptations for a student with severe language disorders.
4. Discuss implied curriculum skills and concepts. What is the value of these skills and concepts for students with severe and multiple disabilities?
5. Describe systematic instruction procedures and discuss when and how these procedures should be used with a child with severe language disorders.

References

Alpert, C. L., & Kaiser, A. P. (1992). Training parents to do milieu language teaching with their language-impaired preschool children. *Journal of Early Intervention, 16,* 31–52.

American Speech-Language-Hearing Association. (1993). Guidelines for caseload size and speech-language service delivery in the schools. *ASHA, 35* (Suppl. 10), 33–39.

Bashir, A. S. (1989). Language intervention and the curriculum. *Seminars in Speech and Language, 10,* 181–191.

Blank, M., & White, S. (1986). Questions: A powerful but misused form of classroom exchange. *Topics in Language Disorders, 6,* 1–12.

Bondy, A., & Frost, L. (1994). The picture exchange communication system. *Focus on Autistic Behavior, 9,* 1–19.

Bruner, J. S. (1975). The ontogenesis of speech acts. *Journal of Child Language, 2,* 1–19.

Bruner, J. (1986). *Actual minds, possible worlds.* Cambridge, MA: Harvard University Press.

Cazden, C. B. (1988). *Classroom discourse: The language of teaching and learning.* Portsmouth, NH: Heinemann.

Cole, K. N., & Dale, P. (1986). Direct language instruction and interactive language instruction with language-delayed preschool children: A comparison study. *Journal of Speech and Hearing Research, 29,* 206–217.

Dawson, G., & Osterling, J. (1995). Early intervention in autism: Effectiveness and common elements of current approaches. In M. J. Guralnick (Ed.), *The effectiveness of early intervention: Second generation research.* Baltimore: Brookes.

Dittman, L. L. (1977). *Curriculum is what happens: Planning is the key.* Washington, DC: National Association for the Education of Young Children.

Donahue, M., & Bryan, T. (1984). Communicative skills and peer relations of learning disabled adolescents. *Topics in Language Disorders, 4,* 10–21.

Duchan, J. F. (1995). *Supporting language learning in everyday life.* San Diego: Singular.

Englert, C. (1984). Measuring teacher effectiveness from the teacher's point of view. *Focus on Exceptional Children, 17,* 1–16.

Fey, M., Cleave, P. L., Long, S. H., & Hughes, D. L. (1993). Two approaches to the facilitation of grammar in children with language impairment: An experimental evaluation. *Journal of Speech and Hearing Research, 36,* 141–157.

Frost, L., & Bondy, A. (1996). *The picture exchange communication system training manual.* Cherry Hill, NJ: Pyramid Educational Consultants.

Garcia, G. E. (1992). Ethnography and classroom communication: Taking an "emic" perspective. *Topics in Language Disorders, 143,* 45–66.

Halle, J. W., Alpert, C., & Anderson, S. (1984). Natural environment language assessment and intervention with severely impaired preschoolers. *Journal of the Association for the Severely Handicapped, 4,* 1–14.

Halle, J. W., Marshall, A., & Spradlin, J. (1979). Time delay: A technique to increase language use and facilitate generalization in retarded children. *Journal of Applied Behavior Analysis, 12,* 431–439.

Hart, B., & Risley, T. (1968). Establishing the use of descriptive adjectives in the spontaneous speech of disadvantaged preschool children. *Journal of Applied Behavior Analysis, 1,* 109–120.

Johnson-Martin, N. M., Attermeier, S. M., & Hacker, B. (1990). *The Carolina curriculum for preschoolers with special needs.* Baltimore: Brookes.

Kaiser, A. P., Hendrickson, J., & Alpert, C. L. (1991). Milieu language teaching: A second look. In R. G. Gable (Ed.), *Advances in mental retardation and developmental disabilities* (Vol. 4, pp. 63–92) London: Jessica Kingsley.

Leonard, L. B., Schwartz, R., Chapman, K., Rowan, L., Prelock, P., Terrell, B., Weiss, A., & Merrick, C. (1982). Early lexical acquisition in children with specific language impairments. *Journal of Speech and Hearing Research, 25,* 554–559.

Lovaas, O. I. (1987). Behavioral treatment and normal educational and intellectual functioning in young autistic children. *Journal of Consulting and Clinical Psychology, 55,* 3–9.

Mesibov, G. B., Schopler, E., & Hearsey, K. A. (1994). Structured teaching. In E. Schopler & G. B. Mesibov (Eds.), *Behavioral issues in autism* (pp. 195–207). New York: Plenum.

Nelson, K., & Gruendel, J. (1986). Children's scripts. In K. Nelson (Ed.), *Event knowledge: Structure and function in development* (pp. 399–429). Hillsdale, NJ: Lawrence Erlbaum.

Nelson, N. W. (1994). Curriculum-based language assessment and intervention across the grades. In G. P. Wallach & K. G. Butler (Eds.), *Language learning disabilities in school-age children and adolescents* (pp. 104–113). New York: Merrill-Macmillan.

Rosenshine, B. (1983). Teaching functions in instructional programs. *Elementary School Journal, 85,* 335–339.

Saville-Troike, M. (1982). *The ethnography of communication: An introduction* (1st ed.). Baltimore: University Park Press.

Sawyer, D. J. (1991). Whole language in context: Insights into the current great debate. *Topics in Language Disorders, 11,* 1–13.

Schwartz, I. S., Garfinkle, A. N., & Bauer, A. (1998). The Picture Exchange Communication System: Communication outcomes for young children with disabilities. *Topics in Early Childhood Special Education, 18,* 144–159.

Skinner, B. F. (1957). *Verbal behavior.* New York: Appleton-Century-Crafts.

Stainback, W., & Stainback, S. (1990). *Support networks for inclusive schooling.* Baltimore: Brookes.

Vygotsky, L. (1962). *Thought and language.* Cambridge, MA: MIT Press.

Vygotsky, L. (1978). *Mind in society: The development of higher psychological processes.* Cambridge, MA: Harvard University Press.

Warren, S. G., McQuarter, R. J., & Rogers-Warren, A. K. (1984). The effects of teacher mands and models on the speech of unresponsive language-delayed children. *Journal of Speech and Hearing Research, 49,* 43–52.

Westby, C. E., & Costlow, L. (1991). Implementing a whole language program in a special education class. *Topics in Language Disorders, 11,* 69–84.

Wiggins, G. (1989). A true test: Toward more authentic assessment. *Phi Delta Kappan, 70,* 703–713.

Wiig, E. H. (1990). Language disabilities in school-age children and youth. In G. J. Shames & E. J. Wiig (Eds.), *Human communication disorders: An introduction* (3rd ed., pp. 193–220). New York: Merrill/Macmillan.

Yoder, P. J., Kaiser, A. P., & Alpert, C. L. (1991). An exploratory study of the interaction between language teaching methods and child characteristics. *Journal of Speech and Hearing Research, 34,* 155–167.

CHAPTER 9

Language Intervention with Infants and Toddlers

Ken M. Bleile and Becky S. Trenary

$\mathbf{T}$his chapter describes the major principles and procedures that govern language intervention with infants and toddlers. Special attention is given to providing language intervention to children with medical problems because of the challenges such children raise in care provision. The section that follows provides background information on three children whose case studies are used heuristically at various points in the chapter. Major topics addressed include the philosophical and research foundations of early language intervention, the organization and settings of care, safety precautions, assessment, and treatment.

CLINICAL CASES

The following three case studies are composites of several real clients and serve to emphasize that language disorders in infants and toddlers often occur as part of larger developmental and medical problems as well as underscore that, in most cases, the medical and developmental problems that give rise to language disabilities are unexpected: an eagerly awaited child is born with a genetic disorder that causes mental retardation; a mother and father are expecting one child, discover they are having twins, and the twins are born prematurely. Families differ enormously in how they cope with such unexpected difficulties surrounding what should have been one of the most joyous of times. Discussion of how professional caregivers can support and provide assistance to families of children with language disorders is provided in Chapter 4.

Thomas

Thomas was born with Down syndrome, a genetic abnormality caused by an additional chromosome added to the twenty-first pair (Batshaw, 1991). Shortly after Thomas's birth, it was explained to his mother that Down syndrome is the most common cause of mental retardation, affecting approximately 1 in 700 births. She was also told that most children with Down syndrome are moderately retarded, and that these children often suffer from heart conditions, weak muscle tone, and respiratory problems.

The first months at home Thomas developed slowly but steadily, although he was a difficult child to feed. Thomas underwent heart surgery at six months to correct a faulty valve, and during that time in the hospital he appeared to regress in some of his earlier developmental gains. At one year Thomas still was not babbling. A language assessment undertaken at that time estimated his developmental level to approximate that of a child 6 months old. At two years, Thomas was just beginning to use single words to express his thoughts and needs. A language assessment indicated that Thomas's language development approximated that of a one-year-old toddler.

Jean and Jennifer

Mr. and Mrs. Smith were thrilled when they realized they were going to have a baby, and they were doubly thrilled—and shocked!—when a sonogram taken early in pregnancy revealed the presence of twin girls. The pregnancy proceeded normally until the twenty-second week, when Mrs. Smith began to experience cramping. The babies, named Jean and Jennifer, were born in the twenty-forth week, fully three months premature.

The tiny infants were placed in incubators where they received around-the-clock medical attention in a neonatal intensive care unit (NICU). It was explained to their parents that the children were experiencing difficulty in breathing on their own because their lungs lacked surfactant, a secretion normally formed in the last month of pregnancy that helps the lungs to breath (Metz, 1993). It was also explained that both children were at-risk for future developmental problems due to possible damage to their immature neurological systems (Bernbaum & Hoffman-Williamson, 1991).

Despite the potential medical problems, Jennifer grew steadily stronger and in three months was discharged from the hospital, small but healthy, a few weeks after the expected full-term due date. Jean's medical course was more complicated. Jean's neurological system was too immature to regulate her body, and her lungs were unable to supply the breaths needed to sustain life. At two months, Jean was placed on mechanical ventilation, which kept her alive by breathing for her, even while the life-saving breaths administered by the machine damaged Jean's fragile, immature lungs, resulting in Broncho Pulmonary Dysplasia (BPD). Jean survived these early medical crises to be raised in a hospital until she was one year old.

Near her first birthday, Jean was discharged from the hospital to her home, where she continued to receive mechanical ventilation for two more months. At fourteen months, Jean was weaned from mechanical ventilation, although she continued to breath through a tracheostomy tube placed in her throat for an additional three months. At twenty-four months, a developmental assessment indicated that Jean's language skills approximated those of a child fourteen to sixteen months old; her sister Jennifer's language was assessed and found to approximate that of a child near eighteen months.

PHILOSOPHICAL AND RESEARCH FOUNDATIONS

Early intervention seeks to be proactive, so that language disorders can be eliminated or reduced before they can adversely affect a child's social and educational development. The consequences of uncorrected language disorders are often severe. Adults with language disorders generally are less well educated and have lower incomes than their peers, while persons with even mild impairments in language sounds are judged by their peers to be immature, tense, nervous, and afraid (Aram, Ekelman, & Nation, 1984; Crowe Hall, 1991; Hall & Tomblin, 1978; Silverman & Paulus, 1989). For children such as Thomas, who experience intellectual or cognitive impairments, the ability to use language effectively may mean the difference between living and working in a restricted or unrestricted environment.

Support for early intervention comes from research in neurology, language development, and psychology. The first two years of life are the most rapid period of neurological development in a person's life. During this period the brain grows to approximately 70 percent of its adult size, myelinization occurs throughout the central nervous system, and such critical areas for language as the cortex and hippocampus largely develop (Damasio, 1990; Ojemann, 1991). During this period the brain also has more connections between cells than it will during any subsequent time, perhaps reflecting a greater potential for learning (Bach-y-Rita, 1990).

Language development is intimately connected to the growth and development of the human brain. Not surprisingly, then, the first two years of life are the most rapid period of language development.

During this period the child first learns to control his or her speech mechanism, acquires and refines basic turn-taking skills, learns to understand hundreds of different words, and has begun to acquire the fundamental patterns of syntax (for detailed reviews, see Paul, 1995).

The first two years of life also provide the foundation on which later social development is based (Yarrow, Rubenstein, & Pedersen, 1975). Family bonds establish a level of support and security that is needed for the child to learn and grow socially. Language disorders may interfere with bonding between parent and child, especially if the child also experiences concomitant medical or cognitive deficits (Hock-Long, Trachtenberg, & Vorters, 1993). For example, as with many other parents of children with Down syndrome, Thomas's parents needed to be encouraged to believe that their son could benefit and learn from parent–child interactions. Jean's parents also required counseling about how to interact with their daughter during her early months of life when the tracheostomy precluded her from vocalizing.

The efficacy of both early intervention in general and early language intervention in particular has been demonstrated in multiple studies (Bricker, Bailey, & Bruder, 1984; Infant Health and Development Program, 1990; Mantovani & Powers, 1991; Ramey & Campbell, 1984; Warren & Bambara, 1989; Warren & Kaiser, 1988; White, Mastrapierl, & Casto, 1984; Wilcox, Kouri, & Caswell, 1991; Yoder, Warren, Kim, & Gazdag, 1994). The largest study to date investigated the effects of early intervention on intelligence in infants born prematurely at eight different clinical settings (Infant Health and Development Program, 1990). Results of the study indicated that children who received early intervention had intelligence quotients from 6.6 to 13.2 points higher at three years of age compared to those children in the study who received only routine follow-up. The lowest gains in intelligence were obtained by children with the lowest birthweights, perhaps reflecting reduced potential for learning. A striking finding of the study was that children who did not receive early intervention were 2.7 times more likely to have IQ scores in the mentally retarded range at three years than those who did receive early intervention (Bleile, 1995).

ORGANIZATION OF CARE

Early intervention teams function under different models of service in the assessment and treatment of children with language disorders. The model of service selected depends on the setting of treatment and who comprises the early intervention team. In a multidisciplinary approach, each professional works primarily independently from the rest of the team. Assessments and treatment plans are specific to the discipline and child-focused rather than emphasizing family involvement in goal planning and the facilitation of intervention. This team model lacks in meeting the current requirements in early intervention services designed to incorporate all disciplines cooperatively along with the family in the decision-making process of the child's treatment.

A more cooperative team model is the interdisciplinary approach that suggests conducting individual assessments by each discipline, then collectively deciding on treatment goals for the child based on the recommendations provided by each professional. The child's caregivers contribute additional input on selecting treatment targets, which are then facilitated by each member of the early intervention team.

The third model of team approaches for providing early intervention services is the transdisciplinary approach. This approach has become more prevalent as the view of providing early intervention has evolved. The family and early intervention professionals collaborate equally to provide the most effective services for the child. Assessment is family-centered and more naturalistic in obtaining information about the child. Findings of the assessment are freely exchanged between team members and integrated into a global representation of the child's abilities. In this approach, one professional is selected as the primary provider of treatment services while consulting with other team members. Family participation during intervention is a key component of the transdisciplinary approach.

Settings of Care

The classroom is the setting for inclusion with most school-age children with language disorders. The early intervention classroom is only one of several important settings in which an infant or toddler may receive language intervention. Other settings in which language intervention is provided include acute care and rehabilitation hospitals and the child's home. In all these settings the persons responsible for language intervention are the child's early intervention team, which includes the child's parents and at least one professional whose educational training lies in language development and its disorders.

Acute Care

Acute care hospitals are designed to serve persons whose medical condition requires intensive medical attention. The location of language intervention in an acute care hospital most often is bedside and the immediate area around the bed. Some acute care facilities also provide areas for small groups of less medically involved children. Language intervention is typically based on quiet play and activities of daily living.

(Re)habilitation

As the child's medical condition stabilizes, he or she is moved to a unit or hospital for less medically acute patients. The location of language intervention in a rehabilitation facility is likely to be bedside, the area around the bed, and a room or room area set aside for early intervention activities. Language intervention is built around play and activities of daily living. For long-term hospital patients such as Jean, the clinician's efforts are directed to providing the child the best possible environment for development. For more short-term patients (such as Jennifer and Thomas, the latter of whom was hospitalized for heart surgery at six months), the clinician's efforts are devoted to trying to prevent the child's loss of developmental skills.

The Community

While hospitals are excellent places to overcome medical problems, even the best medical facility is a poor setting in which to raise a child (Fridy & Lemanek, 1993). In recognition of this, hospitals attempt to discharge children as soon as possible. As a result, community-based clinicians increasingly provide care to children with significant, even life-threatening medical needs, including those with seizure disorders, pervasive developmental delay, mental retardation, HIV, Fetal Alcohol Syndrome, environmental neglect, and in-place tracheostomies.

The home is the community location for language intervention for children with severe illnesses or those attached to relatively cumbersome medical equipment (as Jean was when she received mechanical ventilation). The locations of home intervention typically are areas that the child frequents, such as the bedroom, kitchen, and living room. Language intervention is likely to be built on quiet play and activities of daily living, possibly including those involving medical equipment. To illustrate, Jean was taught simple names for parts of her tracheostomy.

Care for less severely affected and more mobile children is provided in community early intervention classrooms and playgrounds. Language intervention is typically undertaken in those places that the child frequents, such as play areas, meal areas, and changing stations. The activities on which intervention is based are those of functional importance in the child's daily life.

SAFETY PRECAUTIONS

Prior to providing any language intervention services to infants and toddlers, clinicians must be knowledgeable of basic safety procedures, including cardiopulmonary resuscitation (CPR) for children. The appendix of this chapter lists common sense guidelines to follow for infection control. Additionally, clinicians working with children with medical needs must be well versed in the safety procedures for the populations with which they are in contact. At first, persons new to working with children with medical needs may find that medical issues impose a barrier between establishing a relaxed, natural rapport with the child. After some time to adjust, however, clinicians usually report that the child's medical needs cease to dominate their attention, and that they are able to interact with the child confident that they are providing care safely.

Children with medical conditions such as those listed in Table 9.1 may sometimes experience sudden, even life-threatening changes in their medical status (Bernbaum & Hoffman-Williamson, 1991). Whether the setting is an acute care hospital unit or a community early intervention center, clinicians who work with children with medical needs must be able to recognize and respond appropriately to emergency situations, if need arises. The most common physiological warning signs (or red flags) associated with mechanical ventilation, tracheostomy assistance, cardiac conditions, gastrointestinal conditions, shunts, and seizures are discussed below. If physiologic warning signs are observed, the clinician should immediately contact a member of the medical or nursing staff.

Mechanical Ventilation

Mechanical ventilation is provided through a machine that breaths in and out for the patient. Jean, one of the children described at the

TABLE 9.1 Medical conditions that can involve life-threatening changes in medical status.

Conditions	Definition
Mechanical ventilator	A machine that breathes in and out for patients with airway disorders whose lungs are unable to breath without assistance
Tracheostomy	A surgical opening below the larynx on the anterior neck that acts as an artificial airway for breathing
Seizure	A relatively common type of abnormal electrical discharge in the brain that causes from mild to severe changes in behavior and cognition
Shunt	A device that diverts excess cerebrospinal fluid from a ventricle to another part of the body where the fluid is then safely absorbed
Gastrointestinal conditions	Problems in one or more of three conditions areas: controlled movement of food through the body, digestion of food, and absorption of nutrients
Cardiac conditions	Medical problems affecting the heart that may occur either as isolated medical problems or in conjunction with other disabilities

beginning of this chapter, received ventilator assistance through a tracheostomy tube for the first year of her life secondary to Broncho Pulmonary Dysplasia, which is the primary indicator for mechanical ventilation in young children (Metz, 1993). The most commonly encountered physiological warning signs in children receiving mechanical ventilation include changes in skin color, exaggerated breathing, coughing, alteration in heart or respiratory rate, and lethargy or irritability.

Tracheostomy

Tracheostomy is a surgical opening below the larynx on the anterior neck (Handler, 1993). Persons receiving tracheostomy assistance breathe through a hole (stoma) placed in the anterior neck. Approximately 30 percent of children who receive tracheostomies also are ventilator-assisted (Bleile, 1993). The most common daily hazards associated with tracheostomy care involve blockages that make breathing difficult or impossible. The physiological warning signs of blockage include a blue tint around the lips or nailbeds, flared nostrils, fast breathing, a rattling noise during breathing, mucus bubbles around the tracheostomy site, coughing or gagging, clammy skin, restlessness, and lethargy or irritability.

Seizures

A seizure is a type of abnormal electrical discharge from the neurons in the cortex. Seizure disorders are prevalent among many populations of children with developmental disabilities, occurring in approximately 16 percent of children with mental retardation, and 25 percent of children with cerebral palsy, spina bifida, and hydrocephalus (Wallace, 1990). Thomas, anther child described at the beginning of this chapter, is at-risk for a seizure disorder because he is mentally retarded. The physiological warning signs associated with seizures include pallor, irritability, staring, nystagmus, changes in muscle tone, and vomiting.

Shunt

A shunt is a device that diverts cerebrospinal fluid from a brain ventricle to another part of the body, where the fluid is then absorbed. Shunts are used with children with hydrocephalus, a condition in which the fluid-filled ventricles in the brain become enlarged. Approximately 60 to 95 percent of children with neural tube defects also experience hydrocephalus (Charney, 1992). Physiological warning signs suggesting a shunt malfunction include headaches, vomiting, lethargy, and a bulging fontanel (soft spots on the heads of infants).

Gastrointestinal Conditions

Gastrointestinal conditions involve problems in one or more of three areas: controlled movement of food through the body, digestion of food, and absorption of nutrients. If a child cannot receive enough nourishment by mouth (per oral) to sustain life and continued growth, the youngster is fed via a gastrostomy or jejunal tube placed into the stomach or small intestine. Jean experienced feeding difficulties but did not require tube feeding. Physiological warning signs of problems with a gastrostomy or jejunal tube include the presence of formula leaking from the tube at either the clamp or skin site, in and out movement of the tube, increased irritability, and emesis.

Cardiac Conditions

Cardiac conditions are medical problems affecting the heart, and may occur as isolated medical problems or in conjunction with other disabilities. Cardiac conditions are relatively common among children with Down syndrome. Thomas had a cardiac condition requiring surgical intervention at six months. Physiological warning signs associated with cardiac conditions include changes in skin color, increased heart and/or respiratory rate, chest retractions, nasal flaring, and lethargy or irritability.

ASSESSMENT

Federal law as well as clinical sense mandates that a language assessment be undertaken prior to treatment. Topics pertinent to children of all ages were discussed in Part Two of this book. Topics in assessment that are particular to infants and toddlers are discussed in this chapter. As elsewhere in this chapter, this section describes clinical options rather than a particular early intervention approach or program.

Overview

The primary purpose of most assessments is to determine if intervention is warranted (see Table 9.2). The first type of information used to make a decision is the parent interview (or a medical chart review), which reveals the child's background, the nature of the family's concerns, and the presence of any risk factors that might affect the prognosis for future development. The second type of information used to decide if treatment is warranted are nonstandardized and standardized assessments, which provide insights into the child's current communication abilities. Nonstandardized assessments are

TABLE 9.2   Major purposes of three aspects of language assessment of infants and toddlers.

Aspect of Assessment	General Purpose
Parent interview	To understand better the family's perspective To identify areas in the child's history that might affect the child's language development
Nonstandard assessment	To provide a first estimate of which language milestones the child has attained To serve at times as the sole means of assessment, especially with children who are otherwise untestable
Standardized assessment	To allow the clinician to determine if a child is acquiring language at the same rate as other children

particularly useful with otherwise untestable children and they often provide insights into developmental areas not described in standardized test instruments. Standardized assessment instruments provide important means to compare a child's performance to a peer group.

Inclusion

The language assessment typically includes a variety of persons in a range of different locations, allowing the clinician to better understand how and when the child communicates in daily situations. For example, the assessment of Jean while she was in the rehabilitation hospital revealed that she was communicative with a favorite nurse during diaper changing, but grew increasingly withdrawn and quiet in situations where other children were present. If the child has a medical condition (as was the case with Jean), a nurse or other qualified staff member knowledgeable about the child's medical status should be consulted prior to the assessment to rule out the existence of medical complications that would either interfere with the assessment or exacerbate the child's medical problems (Bleile & Miller, 1994).

An inclusive setting is not ideal for all aspects of the assessment. Many standardized test instruments, for example, are designed to assess a child's language abilities in settings that are free from possible distractions. To use the normative information on such instruments requires the clinician to assess children in similar environments. Many aspects of phonology are also difficult to assess in inclusive settings because of the effect of noise and other distractions on the clinician's transcription of the child's speech.

Standardized assessments and phonological test should be performed in quiet and clean locations when the child appears calm and alert. Either the parent or clinician may elicit language from the child; in many cases, a parent is better at this task because of his or her greater familiarity with the child. The child and the caregiver (or clinician) should be positioned in such a manner that eye contact between the two is easily achieved and maintained. If a child has physical limitations or special motoric needs, positioning should be undertaken with guidance from an occupational or a physical therapist (Bleile & Miller, 1994).

Parent Interview

Most clinicians typically begin the assessment with a parent interview or, if the parents are unavailable, with a review of the child's medical chart or educational records, if either exist. In addition to helping the clinician understand the family's perspective on the child's communication behavior, the parent interview is used to identify areas in the child's background that might impact the child's present ability or prognosis for future language development. Parent interviews can last from ten to thirty minutes, depending on the nature of the child's language difficulties, the ability of the parents to serve as reliable informants, and the clinician's style of interaction.

Parent Concerns

Early in the parent interview the clinician inquires into the family's concerns about the child's language development. Types of questions that elicit this information include, "What brings you to the clinic?" "What are your major concerns?" or "Can you tell me why you brought your child for a language assessment today?" followed by more direct questions about the nature of the family's concerns, should such concerns exist.

Background Information

One important interview goal is to explore those aspects of the child's background that may affect present or future language development. Because a child's physical well-being has an important influence on the rate of language development, a medical history should be conducted for all children. Another area that can influence language development is the child's exposure to language both in and outside the home. Lastly, the family's perception of when the child reached major language acquisition milestones reflects their perception of the child's current language development and potential for future development. Examples of questions typically asked about these topics are listed in Table 9.3.

TABLE 9.3   Types of questions used to elicit background information.

Questions

1. Medical History

   Did the mother or child experience pre- or perinatal medical complications?

   Does the child possess any diagnosed syndromes or conditions?

   Has the child ever been hospitalized?

   Does the child experience ear infections? If so, how frequently do (or did) they occur presently or in the past?

   What is the child's current health status?

2. Educational and Social Background

   How many siblings and parents reside in the child's household?

   Does the child have contact with any children outside the home?

   Is the child presently or has the child in the past been involved in any educational programs?

3. Language Milestones

   At what age did the child begin to babble?

   At what age did the child say his or her first word?

   At what age did the child begin to put words together into sentences?

   How does the child typically express his or her wants and needs?

Prognosis

An important purpose of the parent interview (or medical chart review) is to identify medical and nonmedical factors that may place the child at-risk for future language disorders. Clinicians typically explore the following issues:

- Does the child possess any medical conditions that may result in future language disorders (i.e., medical risk factors)?
- Is the child living in an environment that is likely to adversely influence language development (i.e., environmental risk factors)?
- Is there a history of language disorders in the child's immediate family (i.e., genetic risk factors)?

Current Language Abilities

After the parent interview is completed, most clinicians assess the child's current language development. This assessment, which typically requires from one half to one hour to complete, is undertaken to determine if the child is delayed in language development relative to the child's other developmental abilities and to the child's chronological peers. The assessment typically consists of two parts: nonstandard assessments and standardized assessments.

Nonstandardized Assessment

Nonstandardized assessments use observational techniques to determine which language milestones the child has attained. Some clinicians use the nonstandardized assessment to provide a first approximation of the child's language development, while for others the nonstandardized assessment serves as the sole assessment of the child's current language development abilities, especially with children who are otherwise untestable. Of the three children discussed at the beginning of this chapter, Thomas was unable to complete standardized assessment instruments, and his language development was assessed using only nonstandardized assessment techniques.

Topics typically included in a nonstandardized assessment are described below. Included in each topic are a sample of relatively well-researched and easily observed or elicited language milestones. See Chapter 1 for additional milestones and definitions of language use, content, and form.

Language Use

The two most typically encountered assessment topics for language use are turn-taking skills and the use of sound during interactions.

1A. TURN-TAKING SKILLS.   Many investigators believe that infants first acquire the "my turn–your turn" aspect of language use through interacting with caregivers during daily routines such as mealtime, diaper changing, and dressing, and while playing such interaction games as "peek-a-boo" and rolling a ball back and forth (Bruner, 1983; Snow & Goldfield, 1983). Additionally, turn-taking activities afford children excellent opportunities to acquire the meaning and phonological shape of words. Jean, for example, was taught the meaning of *ball* while she and her clinician rolled a bright red ball back and forth, because Jean appeared more attentive and motivated to learn the meaning of *ball* while playing this game than in other, more distracting situations.

1B. REPRESENTATIVE MILESTONES.   Most children can be encouraged to play sound-gesture games such as "peek-a-boo" by nine months (Capute, Palmer, Shapiro, Wachtel, Schmidt, & Ross, 1986), and by the end of the first year of life an infant can cover his or her own eyes in peek-a-boo and will initiate this and other sound-gesture games.

2A. SOUND DURING INTERACTIONS.   The child's gradual ability to use sounds to interact with others is one of the most significant accomplishments of the first two years of life. At first, sounds are little more than an activity that accompanies interactions with caregivers, similar to eye gaze and arm waving. Gradually, however, sound replaces eye gaze and pointing as the child's primary means of communication, allowing the child to express the increasingly complex thoughts and needs permitted by the youngster's rapidly evolving neurological system. Thomas, the child with Down syndrome, experienced significant difficulties in learning to use vocal sounds instead of pointing and grunting to express his needs and wants.

2B. REPRESENTATIVE MILESTONES. By three to four months an infant may coo, grunt, or squeal when spoken to, and by seven months may vocalize on seeing a bottle. The clinician can expect an infant near ten months old to use a ritualized intentional gesture in conjunction with a short sound to obtain a desired object from a caregiver, and can expect a toddler in the first months of the second year of life to communicate using a combination of facial expressions, gestures, single words, and vocalizations. A toddler around 16 to 18 months of age can use words to express wants and needs, and by twenty months children can use words to relate experiences (Hedrick, Prather, & Tobin, 1984).

Language Content

The most common areas of language assessed are receptive and expressive vocabulary.

1A. RECEPTIVE VOCABULARY. Perhaps the most profound linguistic insight achieved by the infant is that sound can signify meaning. An infant learns, for example, that a certain group of sounds (*daddy*) means one caregiver, that *mommy* means another caregiver, and that *kitty* means a strange little creature with soft fur. Typically, a child's receptive vocabulary (i.e., the words a child understands) is larger than the child's expressive vocabulary (i.e., the words the child speaks). All three children discussed in the beginning of this chapter experienced problems in word comprehension.

1B. REPRESENTATIVE MILESTONES. An infant four to six months old may respond to hearing his or her name, and by six months responds to "no" with inflection, although the child does not understand "no" if a different inflection is used (Hedrick, Prather, & Tobin, 1984). An infant six to seven months old understands "bye-bye" and turns to look when a family member is named ("Where's daddy?"). An infant eight to nine months old responds to "no" if the clinician says it in a "flat" voice. The infant also knows the name of a few common objects. A toddler twelve to thirteen months old responds to a few simple commands without gestures, such as "sit down," "come here," "clap hands," and "stand up." A toddler sixteen months old may be encouraged to point to such body parts as the ears, eyes, hair, mouth, and nose, and a toddler seventeen to eighteen months old lifts a foot or points to a shoe when asked, "Where are your shoes?" Lastly, a toddler twenty months old puts a block "in the box" when given that command.

2A. EXPRESSIVE VOCABULARY. Acquisition of expressive vocabulary (words actually used for communication, rather than words the child understands) has a central role in language acquisition during the first two years of life. Researchers hypothesize that children first acquire words as isolated "items," somewhat analogously to how a person in a foreign country, for example, might learn a word for *dinner,* another word for *taxi,* and another word for *museum* (Ferguson & Farwell, 1975). In no sense, however, is such a traveler "acquiring the country's language." Instead, the traveler is learning isolated words that are useful for meeting simple daily needs. The same may hold for the toddler in the early stages of word acquisition: the child learns a word for a favorite food, another to call a parent, and another to signal distress. Only later, after the child's vocabulary has grown to approximately fifty words, do most children begin to show evidence that they realize that certain words can be classified as nouns, that others can be classified as verbs, or that certain classes of words begin with the same sound (and, therefore, can be pronounced similarly), while other words all begin with another sound (and so can be pronounced differently than other words) (Bleile & Fey, 1993).

2B. REPRESENTATIVE MILESTONES. Many parents are able to accurately report the number of words a child regularly uses. Children typically are reported to acquire their first word by 11 months, speak two to three words by 12 to 13 months, speak four to six words by 14 to 15 months, speak seven to twenty words by 16 to 17 months, and possess a single-word vocabulary of fifty words or more by 20 to 21 months (Capute, Palmer, Shapiro, Wachtel, Schmidt, & Ross, 1986). Words can be elicited by asking parents to say which words their child speaks. To avoid the parent listing only the words the child "says well" (which happened with the mother of Jennifer and Jean), it should be explained that the clinician is interested in the number of child words, not how well the child pronounces the words. Many times, parents begin by listing a few words, but remember more words as the assessment session continues.

Language Form

The nonstandardized assessment of language form typically focuses on three aspects of phonology (prespeech vocalizations, use of sounds and syllables in words, and correct productions of consonants) and one area of syntax (combining words). Morphology (see definitions in Chapter 1) is typically not assessed because its developmental course has scarcely begun by children two years old or younger.

1A. PHONOLOGY (PRESPEECH).   Prespeech vocalizations produced during the first year of life are thought to provide "practice" for later speech development (Bleile, Stark, Silverman McGowan, 1993; Jusczyk, 1992; Locke, 1983; Locke & Pearson, 1992; Vihman & Miller, 1988). Through babbling, for example, the infant learns how to synchronize the velum, tongue, lips, and larynx for the purposes of producing sound.

1B. REPRESENTATIVE MILESTONES.   Around 3 to 4 months of age many infants may be observed or encouraged to produce cooing sounds, consonantlike noises made at the back of the mouth. Squeals, growls, raspberries, and trills are often heard when the infant nears 4 months. Reduplicated babbling (repetitions of the identical syllable, such as ba-ba-ba) begin to appear near 6 months and become well-established near 7 to 8 months of age. Around 10 months most infants produce nonreduplicated babbling (repetitions of different syllables, such as ba-di-du).

2A. PHONOLOGY (SOUNDS AND SYLLABLES IN WORDS).   Phonological units (sounds and syllables) constitute the building blocks of words. Some investigators hypothesize that the phonological problems of a toddler may "grow into" an expressive language problem by the time the child is a preschooler because the phonological problems place limitations on the child's ability to develop an expressive vocabulary (Paul, 1991).

2B. REPRESENTATIVE MILESTONES.   A child near 16 months old may produce around six different consonants at the beginning of words and may produce one or no consonants at the ends of words; these consonants need not be "correct" relative to the adult language. Commonly produced word-initial consonants during this period are *b, d, m, n, h,* and *w,* and the most common word-final consonant is *t.* The most common syllable shapes of words are CV (consonant-vowel), CVCV, and, less frequently, VC and CVC. If the child is 24 months old, the child's speech should contain nine to ten consonants at the beginning of words, and five to six consonants at the end of words. The most common word-initial consonants are *b, d, g, t, k, m, n, f, s, w,* and *h,* and the most common word-final consonants are *p, t, k, n, s,* and *r.* Approximately 70 percent of the consonants produced by a child near 24 months old may be correct relative to the adult language. The following consonants should be produced correctly in two out of three positions (initial, medial, final): *m, n, h, w, p, b, t, k, d,* and *g.*

3A. SYNTAX.   Syntactic development represents an important expansion in the ability of the toddler to express ideas and needs. A child, for example, who says the single word *dog* must depend on the listener's understanding of the nonverbal context to know if the child is saying, "I want my dog," "The dog is panting," or "The dog is barking." A child who says, "Want dog," is more likely to have his or her needs met, because more of the request is included in the linguistic message. Jennifer, for example, received intervention to facilitate use of syntax.

3B. REPRESENTATIVE MILESTONES.   Sometime between 20 and 24 months a child can be observed to begin to combine words, and by 24 months many children speak regularly in two- and three-word sentences. When assessing a child's syntactic abilities, the clinician should remember that what seems like a sentence to an adult may be a single word for a child. Jennifer, for example, learned "got to go" as a single word, without having analyzed the phrase into separable units. Many times, children's "word phrases" are clichés used by adults in specific situations, such as "off we go" (while daddy picks up the child), or "bye-bye now" (while mother hangs up the telephone). Because the child always hears these words together, the youngster hypothesizes that the sounds are all one word. To avoid attributing to the child more knowledge of syntax than is possessed, a word should occur in combination with at least three other words before concluding the child is making a sentence rather than a word phrase. For example, "off we go" would not be considered a word phrase, unless one of the words occurred in at least two other utterances, such as "daddy go" and "go home."

Standardized Assessment

A standardized assessment allows the clinician to determine if a child is acquiring language at the same rate as its peers, and may also provide information on the child's relative communication strengths and weaknesses, which can be useful in identifying possible treatment goals. The standardized assessment instruments listed below represent a range of options for assessing communication development with infants and toddlers. The list is divided into two parts: screening instruments and complete language evaluations.

1. SCREENING TESTS.   The following screening instruments are briefly summarized: *The Clinical Linguistic and Auditory Milestone Scale, The Rossetti Infant-Toddler Language Scale, The Early Language*

Milestone Scale-2, The Receptive-Expressive Emergent Language Scale-2, and *The Infant Scales of Communicative Intent.*

1a. Clinical Linguistic and Auditory Milestone Scale (CLAMS).

The *CLAMS* (Capute & Accardo, 1978) was developed by two well-respected developmental pediatricians to screen for language disorders in children from 0 to 2 years of age. Information on the *CLAMS* is obtained using parental report supplemented by direct observation. The test assesses twenty-five language milestones. The normative sample on which the *CLAMS* is based are 448 children, 69 percent of whom were Caucasian and 30 percent of whom were non-Caucasian (Capute, Palmer, Shapiro, Wachtel, Schmidt, & Ross, 1986). Approximately twenty minutes is required to complete the *CLAMS.*

1b. Rossetti Infant-Toddler Language Scale (Rossetti).

The *Rossetti* is a relatively new clinical instrument intended for use with children 0–3 years. Information on the *Rossetti* is elicited using incidental observation and parental report. Items were chosen for inclusion in the *Rossetti* based on "author observation, descriptions from developmental hierarchies, and behaviors recognized and used by leading authorities in the field of infant and toddler assessment" (p. 10). A normative sample was not obtained in the development of the *Rossetti.*

1c. Early Language Milestone Scale-2 (ELM-2).

The *ELM-2* (Coplan, 1993) is a screening instrument for use with children from 0 to 36 months old, and also assesses intelligibility in children 18 to 48 months old. Information on the *ELM-2* is obtained using parental report in conjunction with limited elicitation. The elicitation stimuli are real objects. The normative sample on which the *ELM-2* is based are 191 children aged from birth to 36 months. Approximately 1 to 10 minutes is required to complete the *ELM-2.*

1d. Receptive-Expressive Emergent Language Scale-2 (REEL-2).

The *REEL-2* (Bzoch & League, 1991) is a screening instrument for use with children 0 to 3 years old. The *REEL-2* is a new edition of an older instrument and the theory on which it is based is now somewhat out-of-date. Information on the *REEL-2* is elicited using parental report. The normative sample on which the *REEL-2* is based are "language-advantaged Caucasian infants" (p. 7). The number of children composing the normative sample is not provided, nor is information available on how long the clinician should allow for test administration.

1e. Infant Scales of Communicative Intent (Infant Scales).

The *Infant Scales* (Saint Christopher's Hospital for Children,

1982) is a screening instrument for children from birth to 18 months old that relies on direct clinical observation of behaviors. The *Infant Scales* has been largely superseded by more recently developed screening instruments although it is still used in some clinical settings in which obtaining parent reports is not feasible. No normative information on the *Infant Scales* is available, nor is there published information on how long the clinician should allow for test administration.

2. COMPLETE ASSESSMENT INSTRUMENTS. The following complete assessment instruments are briefly summarized: *The Sequenced Inventory of Communicative Development, The MacArthur Communicative Development Inventories,* and *The Preschool Language Scale-3.*

2a. Sequenced Inventory of Communicative Development (SICD). The *SICD* (Hedrick, Prather, & Tobin, 1984) is a well-respected in-depth language assessment instrument for use with children between 4 months and 4 years old. The *SICD* assesses both language reception and expression using a combination of direct elicitation techniques and parental reports. The elicitation stimuli for infants and toddlers are real objects. The normative sample for the *SICD* were 252 children aged from 4 to 48 months. The *SICD* requires from between 30 minutes for infants to 75 minutes for children 24 months or older. Both English and Spanish versions of the test are available.

2b. MacArthur Communicative Development Inventories (CDI). The *CDI* is a new, highly regarded language assessment instrument for use with children 8 months to 2 years 6 months (Fenson, Dale, Reznick, Thal, Bates, Hartung, Pethick, & Reilly, 1993). The *CDI* uses one form for infants 8 to 16 months (Words and Gestures) and another for toddlers 16 months to 30 months (Words and Sentences). Information is elicited using parent questionnaires. The normative sample for the *CDI* were 1789 children aged 8 through 30 months. Parents are typically able to complete the *CDI* in twenty to forty minutes, and speech-language clinicians require approximately ten minutes to score the results. Currently, only an English version of the *CDI* is available, although translations into several other languages (including Spanish) are underway.

2c. Preschool Language Scale-3 (PLS-3). The *PLS-3* (Zimmerman, Steiner, & Pond, 1992) is an in-depth assessment instrument for use with children from birth through 6 years, 11 months. The *PLS-3* assesses both language reception and expression using real objects and pictures. Earlier editions of the *PLS* tended to overestimate children's language development, perhaps because the normative sample on which the test was based was not completely representative of the

U.S. population. The normative sample on which the *PLS-3* is based are approximately 1900 children balanced for geographical region and racial and ethnic origin. The *PLS-3* requires less than one hour to administer and score.

Intervention

Language acquisition depends crucially on the child's neurological readiness to learn in conjunction with the availability of experiences afforded by the environment. The general educational strategy of early intervention is to manipulate the environment to maximize a child's opportunities to acquire language. In recognition that language acquisition depends on both the environment and the child's developmental readiness to learn, language treatment is said to "facilitate" or "stimulate" rather than "teach" language.

This section provides an overview of language treatment for infants and toddlers. The discussion focuses on underlying principles and procedures held in common by most clinicians and researchers rather than on enumerating the tenets of a particular language intervention approach (Greenspan, 1985, 1992; MacDonald, 1989; MacDonald & Carroll, 1992; Wilcox, 1989). The topics considered include inclusion, the role of parents, treatment goals, and facilitative techniques. Issues are raised for consideration at the conclusion of each subsection.

Inclusion

Inclusion brings language intervention out of the treatment room and into the child's natural setting, a goal supported by the vast majority of clinicians who provide language treatment to infants and toddlers (Greenspan, 1985; MacDonald, 1989; Wilcox, 1989). Perhaps one reason clinicians support the general idea of inclusion is its implicit recognition that language acquisition is different from other types of skill learning. To illustrate, language acquisition differs from a specialized motor skill such as tennis, which involves acquiring certain specific motor skills best learned through direct instruction from a tennis instructor. Instead, language is acquired indirectly as a child performs activities and interacts with other people. Within an inclusion model, restricting language treatment to a single person in a single discipline is unnatural and, in effect, is attempting to train language a few hours each week, as if acquiring one's language were a type of motor skill.

Inclusion also recognizes the facilitation of language as being the province of everyone with whom the child comes in contact. This view is in accordance with research that indicates language acquisition in its earliest stages is almost impossible to divorce from the contexts in which it occurs. As discussed in the assessment section, children first acquire words as items that accompany certain actions and activities. For example, a particular child may first acquire *bye* as the word that accompanies hand waving as a parent goes off to work in the morning. The same context specificity affects other areas of language acquisition. For example, the sentence "Throw ball" might be acquired as the words that accompany throwing a ball to a parent in a park, and the sound *b* might be acquired as the sound in a specific word, such as *balloon*.

An important hypothesis made by inclusion is that, because intervention occurs across a variety of settings and people, children should more readily generalize the results of treatment compared to children whose language treatment is confined to a therapy room. This hypothesis is supported by Wilcox, Kouri, and Caswell (1991), who studied vocabulary acquisition in twenty children aged 20 to 47 months. Half the children were randomly assigned to receive individual therapy and the other half received treatment in a classroom-based early intervention program. Results of the investigation indicated that the two groups were equivalent in vocabulary acquisition, but that generalization of learning to the home setting was superior in those children who received treatment in a classroom setting.

Issues

Some clinicians provide all language intervention within a classroom or other inclusive setting. The philosophical rationale for a total inclusion model is that this form of treatment better facilitates the acquisition and generalization of language than does working in a therapy room isolated from the child's daily activities. Inclusion also may be less expensive to provide than other types of language intervention because a clinician in an inclusive setting typically provides treatment to multiple children within the same treatment session.

A nearly opposite view is held by clinicians who provide all or nearly all language intervention within a therapy room setting. This view is founded on the belief that success in language intervention is best achieved in a quiet setting free from distractions through the efforts of an expert with extensive treating in language and its disorders. The efficacy of this model with children of all ages has been demonstrated in numerous studies (for extensive reviews see Fey [1986] and Warren & Kaiser [1988]). As long noted, however, a major limitation of the model is that generalization of treatment success to other people and places may be difficult to obtain (Wilcox, Kouri, & Caswell 1991). This problem can be partially offset through a strong parent and staff training program, as the critique that the therapy room model is too expensive can also be partially offset by holding group therapy sessions in the therapy room.

Some early intervention teams chose to provide language intervention using elements of both inclusion and a therapy room model. Within such approaches, intervention is typically undertaken inclusive settings, while treatment in a therapy room is reserved for special purposes. To illustrate, language intervention for Thomas typically occurred in an early intervention classroom. However, Thomas often appeared distractible when other children were present, so his clinician sometimes introduced new language goals in individual therapy sessions.

The Role of Parents

Parents have a special role on the early intervention team because they are ultimately responsible for all treatment decisions affecting their child (Trout & Foley, 1989). Importantly, this special status is derived from parents' legal guardianship of their child rather than from such extraneous factors as the parents' sexual orientation, marital status, and whether the child is a biological offspring or adopted.

The clinician's role is to serve as a resource to parents and to help them make the most informed decisions possible. This may involve providing written information about the nature of language development and a child's language disorder. Most clinicians also hold frequent meetings with parents to answer questions as they arise. Demonstrations of treatment techniques often are excellent means to help parents understand treatment issues.

It must be recognized that parents differ in their ability to participate as members of the early intervention team. Thomas's father, for example, frequently appeared angry and frustrated during meetings of the early intervention team, oftentimes expressing his unhappiness with Thomas's relative slowness in reaching developmental milestones. Other parents may lack the cognitive skills to grasp the questions asked of them by team members, while still others may only participate with the other members of the early intervention team erratically, if at all.

The early intervention team has legal obligations to contact law enforcement agencies if they believe that the parents' actions constitute child abuse. However, unless a court revokes legal guardianship, the parents continue to be the final arbitrators of all treatment decisions. If tensions between parents and other members of the team cannot be resolved informally, a consultation with a social worker or a clinical psychologist may be needed.

Issues

Occasionally, parents retain legal guardianship of their child, but refuse to become involved in the child's care, leaving all such matters to members of the early intervention team (Bleile, 1993). In an extreme case, parents of a hospitalized child may not visit or communicate with their child for years. In effect, in such situations the parents are asking the early intervention team to assume parental responsibilities.

The dual role of the early intervention team as both intervention provider and parent is fraught with legal and ethical perils as the parental role conflicts with the needs of other children. To illustrate, the team in its parental role may make "its" child their highest clinical priority, even while recognizing that other children they might serve have greater needs for language treatment. Some early intervention teams assume parental responsibilities for one or more children. Other teams, rather than allowing themselves to be caught in such a painful and unresolvable conflict, appoint a person (often a member of the clergy) whose sole function is to act as an advocate for the child. This person meets with the early intervention team, serving in the role of surrogate parent.

Treatment Goals

Language is a tool for communication. The clear lesson of research on language development is that a child acquires those aspects of language for which he or she has use (see discussion in the assessment section). Language intervention goals provide the child with a verbal tool through which the child expresses his or her states, thoughts, and needs. To illustrate, Thomas loved to interact with people around him; early language goals for Thomas included facilitating babbling and participation in peek-a-boo games as ways to interact with his caregivers. Similarly, during one period in development Jean appeared increasingly frustrated when adults could not understand what she wanted them to do; a language goal during this period focused on facilitating Jean's ability to name objects she wanted.

TABLE 9.4 Treatment goals for language intervention with infants and toddlers.

Language Domains	Treatment Goals
Language use	Turn-taking skills
	Vocalizations or speech during interactions
Language content and form	Receptive vocabulary
	Expressive vocabulary
	Prespeech vocalizations
	Sounds and syllables in words
	Combining words

As with adults, children have different needs and thoughts, and what seems important and functional to one may be of little or no importance to another. For this reason, functionality is determined on an individual basis. For example, a language intervention goal for a particular child may include facilitating the use of words such as *hi* and *bye,* while a vocabulary intervention goal for a child of the same age and developmental level might focus on facilitating the acquisition of words for various foods.

Individual differences in functionality are particularly striking when comparing children with medical needs to their nonmedically involved peers. Jean, for example, learned words for the mechanical ventilation and care of her tracheostomy far more quickly and with greater apparent interest than she did words for such things as trees, grass, and flowers. This is because Jean was surrounded by medical equipment, while she only knew trees, grass, and flowers from pictures in books. Stated differently, the names of parts of medical equipment were highly functional and interesting to Jean (as they are to many children with medical needs), while the names of objects outside the home represented abstract, vague concepts that she seldom directly experienced.

Representative Examples

Language intervention goals for infants and toddlers must be appropriate for children in the earliest stages of language acquisition, and include facilitating the child's awareness of basic rules of conversation (language use), the knowledge of word meanings (language content), and ability to vocalize and speak and to combine words into sentences (language form). The following are representative examples of language intervention goals for children at various levels of language development.

1. LANGUAGE USE.   Treatment to facilitate language use can begin as early as the first months of life when the child begins to awaken more frequently and for more extended periods of time. An early language use goal for Thomas, for example, included increasing attention and mutual eye gaze. In addition to increased vocalizations, early signs of the infant's involvement in interactions include eye widening, body movement, and smiling. For children between birth to 6 months, rattles and handheld toys are useful in facilitating interactions between the child and the speech-language clinician. Similarly, busy boxes excite the child and provide an activity that requires the joint attention of the child and caregivers.

For children 6 months or older, noise-making objects such as toy cars and drums are useful because they afford the child the opportunity to engage in reciprocal play. Jean and her caregivers, for example, took turns patting a toy drum. Participation in sound–gesture games and daily activity routines such as diaper changing, bathing, and eating also provide excellent opportunities to facilitate the development of language use.

Toddlers benefit from such turn-taking routines as rolling a ball, putting together big-piece puzzles with an adult, and pointing and identifying pictures in books. Toddlers also can be encouraged to vocalize in interactions through simple manipulations that "violate social norms." Jennifer's caregivers, for example, "took Jennifer's turn" in peek-a-boo and tried to feed a shoe to a doll. Alternately, the adult might hide or withhold objects, forcing the child to vocalize in order to obtain a desired toy.

2. CONTENT AND FORM.   Language content and form (both reception and expression) are often facilitated concurrently in naturally occurring contexts such as turn-taking routines or while playing. For example, changing the child's clothes provides opportunities to facilitate acquisition of the sounds, words, and syntax used with body parts, while mealtime offers chances to acquire aspects of language content and form associated with foods and actions such as opening, closing, chewing, and swallowing.

Issues

An important difference among clinicians concerns whether they treat language goals simultaneously or in sequence (Fey, 1986). The simultaneous treatment of language goals is sometimes called a horizontal approach and is depicted as a series of bidirectional arrows between language goals (a↔b↔c↔d↔e). The sequential treatment of language goals is sometimes called a vertical approach and is depicted as a series of unidirectional arrows between language goals (a → b → c → d → e).

A horizontal approach presents language "all at once" rather than focusing on only one or several language areas. To illustrate, within a horizontal approach the language goals for content, form, and use are presented simultaneously. Proponents of a horizontal approach observe that simultaneous learning is more typical than sequential learning in language acquisition. For example, when a parent says "please" he or she is simultaneous modeling form (the sounds in *please*), content (the meaning of *please*), and use (the social functions of *please*).

An argument against a horizontal approach is that it replicates an environment from which children with language disabilities have been unable to learn. Stated differently, a reason for language delay is that some children find it difficult to learn from an environment that presents content, form, and use simultaneously. A vertical approach provides more intensive, focused facilitation on selected language goals than does its horizontal counterpart.

An extreme version of a vertical approach would focus on a single language goal at a time. To continue with the example of *please,* a clinician using an extreme vertical approach might first facilitate use (the social purpose of *please*), then content (the meaning of *please*), and then form (the pronunciation of *please*). A difficulty with such an extreme version of a vertical approach is that content, form, and use are often closely bound together, making it difficult to facilitate them separately. For example, the content of *please* is difficult to facilitate without also facilitating its form.

Although either an extreme horizontal or vertical approach is possible, clinicians often adopt a position midway between the two. Such clinicians facilitate all aspects of language as they occur during a treatment activity (a horizontal approach), but also have additional language goals for specific aspects of language (a vertical approach). For example, while clinicians for both Thomas and Jean attempted to stimulate all aspects of language in every treatment session, they also devoted additional clinical attention to facilitating specific areas of content, form, and use.

Facilitative Techniques

Early language treatment relies on naturalistic techniques that model aspects of language use, content, and form (Hart, 1985; Nelson, 1989). These techniques constitute in large measure the child's "language learning lesson." The techniques that follow can be adapted to facilitate many different aspects of language, depending on the child's developmental needs. The techniques described are presented separately for the sake of simplicity; in clinical practice, they typically are used in conjunction with each other.

TABLE 9.5   Summary of rationales for treatment goals.

Language Domain	Rationale for Treatment Goal
Language Use	The fundamental rules of discourse and pragmatics are acquired in the course of interacting with caregivers in daily routines and simple games.
	An important development in discourse and pragmatics is the use of vocalizations and speech in interactions.
Language Content	The first steps in semantic development are undertaken as the child learns the names of familiar objects and people in the environment.
Language Form	The principles of phonology are acquired as the child first babbles and then uses sounds to say words.
	The ability to combine words into simple sentences represents a significant development in the acquisition of syntax.

1. Vocal Stimulation

Vocal stimulation encourages the child's use of sound in play (Bleile, 1995). The following sequence was used to stimulate vocal development with Thomas.

1. The clinician spoke with Thomas's caregivers to discover times of day during which he was most likely to engage in vocal play. When Thomas was 6 months old in development, it was found that sometimes he could be induced to vocalize by setting a mobile in motion, which appeared to have a soothing effect and induced him to coo. When Thomas was over 7 months in development, play with mirrors permitted Thomas to look at his own facial expressions and vocalize his apparent excitement.

2. The clinician waited until Thomas began vocalizing, and then imitated the sounds produced by Thomas. For example, Thomas said a raspberry and then the clinician responded with a raspberry.

3. After a few "turns" imitating Thomas's babble, the clinician began introducing syllables that the assessment indicated Thomas was able to produce. In most cases, Thomas was often "coaxed" into imitating the clinician. The clinician, for example, said "ba-ba-ba" and Thomas responded by saying "ba-ba."

4. Lastly, the clinician produced syllables slightly in advance of Thomas's developmental level. In many cases, Thomas attempted to imitate these new syllables. For example, the clinician babbled "da-da-da" when Thomas's babble was primarily composed of *b*.

2. Parallel Talk

Parallel talk provides linguistic labels that describe the child's activities or those aspects of the environment to which the youngster is attending. The rationale for engaging in parallel talk is that the child is more likely to acquire those aspects of language that refer to things and actions that it finds interesting. The following parallel talk sequence, for example, was used with Jean to facilitate acquisition of *ball* and *book*.

> *Jean picks up a ball.*
> Clinician: "Ball."
> Jean rolls the ball.
> Clinician: "Go, ball."
> Jean picks up a book.
> Clinician: "It's a book."

3. Expansions and Recasts.

Expansions and recasts "fill in the missing parts" in the child's utterances while retaining the child's meaning. Recasts are a specialized form of expansion, involving a change in mood or voice. Expansions and recasts are often used to facilitate a toddler's syntactic development, but are also valuable techniques to facilitate aspects of meaning and phonology. The following is an example of an expansion used with Jennifer to facilitate acquisition of two-word sentences.

> *Jennifer opens a book.*
> Jennifer: "Book."
> Clinician: "Book open." (expansion)
> Jennifer points to a ball.
> Jennifer: "Ball."
> Clinician: "It's a ball." (expansion)
> Jennifer picks up the book and opens it.
> Jennifer: "Book."
> Clinician: "Is the book open?" (recast)
> Jennifer: "Yes."

4. Expatiations

Expatiations are similar to expansions, except that new information is added. The following is an example of an expatiation used with Thomas to facilitate acquisition of /b/ in the beginning of words.

> *Thomas points to a picture of a bee.*
> Thomas: "ee."
> Clinician: "Bee is buzzing."
> Thomas: "ee."
> Clinician: "Bees like honey."
> Thomas: "Bee."

5. Buildups and Breakdowns

Buildups and breakdowns expand and reduce sentences to their parts. The following is an example of a buildup and breakdown sequence that was used with Thomas to facilitate acquisition of the form and content for the word *ball*.

> *Thomas rolls a ball.*
> Thomas: "Ball."
> Clinician: "The ball is rolling." (expansion)
> Thomas smiles.
> Clinician. "Ball. Rolling." (breakdown)
> Thomas laughs.
> Clinician: "Ball is rolling." (expansion)

6. Vertical Structuring

Vertical structuring is designed to facilitate the acquisition of multi-word utterances. Within vertical structuring, the child says a word, which is followed by a contingent question by the clinician (Scollon,

1976). The result is that the child and adult create a multiword sentence over several turns in conversation. The following is an example of vertical structuring that was used with Jennifer to facilitate the two-word sentence "Bike out."

> *Jennifer rides a tricycle to the door and then looks at the*
> *clinician.*
> Jennifer: "Bike."
> Clinician: "Where?" (contingent question)
> Jennifer: "Out."
> Clinician: "Bike out." (expansion)
> Jennifer: "Out."
> Clinician: "Bike out."
> Jennifer: "Bike out."

Issues

An important issue in early language intervention concerns who should be the agents of language change. Some clinicians believe their major role on the early intervention team is to train parents and other team members to implement language intervention techniques. For example, a clinician might explain to a parent about recasts and then model this technique with the parent's child.

The philosophical underpinnings of an advisory approach to language intervention are similar to those for inclusion. Primarily, training a variety of people to perform treatment techniques better reflects the nature of language acquisition, which typically occurs across a range of settings and persons. More practically, people on the early intervention team (especially parents) may have more opportunities to interact with the child than the clinician. Training such people to perform simple intervention techniques often greatly extends the number of treatment opportunities that the child receives.

Financial reasons may also motivate a clinician to assume an advisory role on an early intervention team. As the number of children requesting language services swells, early intervention teams are increasingly forced to become ever more efficient and cost-sensitive. The use of parents and other early intervention team members (including aides) often represents an important way to "stretch" early intervention budgets.

The primary philosophical argument against an advisory conception of the clinician's role is that other team members are not always well qualified to carry out treatment techniques. This argument may not present itself within a horizontal approach in which the goal is to stimulate all areas of language acquisition simultaneously. However, vertical approaches require whoever is performing intervention techniques to identify those aspects of content, form, and use being facilitated. Not all parents, aides, and other members of the early intervention team are sufficiently interested in and possess the abilities to carry out such treatments.

Use of other early intervention team members may also not be feasible in certain clinical settings. For example, early intervention teams in hospital settings may be more concerned with medical than developmental issues, and may be either unable or unwilling to spend the time required to learn language intervention techniques. Lack of parent involvement in any care setting may also hinder the clinician's best training efforts. Lastly, although training parents and other team members is cost-effective, clinicians in some settings have too many children on their caseloads to find time to establish training programs.

Most clinicians seek a middle ground between that of an advisory role and that of sole agent of language change. Clinicians typically do not think of language as "their territory," and so view the training of parents and others in treatment techniques as an important component of inclusion. For example, language intervention for Thomas, Jean, and Jennifer included training any willing parent and other team members in treatment techniques. Training typically was achieved using a combination of written materials, in-services, and modeling. Additionally, the clinicians also provided direct language intervention to the children.

Summary

Infants and toddlers may experience language disorders that place them at risk for future educational and social failure. The goal of early language intervention is to act proactively before negative consequences of a child's language problem have an opportunity to occur. A growing number of studies support the potential effectiveness of early intervention in general and language intervention in particular.

Early language intervention is provided by a team that includes the child's parents and at least one professional whose educational training is in the study of language and its disorders. Locations where language intervention may occur include acute care and rehabilitation hospitals, the child's home, and early intervention classrooms in community centers. Clinicians who work with infants and toddlers in any setting need to be knowledgeable about medical issues and safety precautions as well as having expertise in speech and language development, because children who receive early intervention are increasingly likely to have concomitant medical and genetic disorders.

The primary purpose of the language assessment is to determine if future treatment is warranted. Typically, the assessment consists of three parts: a parent interview (or medical chart review), nonstandardized testing, and standardized testing. An important goal of the assessment is to determine how the child uses language in his or her natural environment; this aspect of the assessment should be undertaken in an inclusive setting. However, the quiet of a therapy room or other removed setting may be needed to perform the transcription needed for the phonological aspect of the assessment. A similarly removed setting may be needed for standardized testing in order to match the conditions under which the normative language sample was obtained.

Language acquisition depends on neurological readiness in conjunction with experiences from the environment. The general purpose of language intervention is to maximize a child's opportunities to learn from his or her environment. This purpose is achieved through providing treatment in as natural a setting as possible, maintaining the parents' involvement in all clinical decisions affecting a child, developing language goals that guide treatment, and implementing facilitative techniques that maximize the child's language learning environment. Current issues that arise in early intervention include: How and to what extent should inclusion be undertaken? How should early intervention teams respond when parents are not involved? Should treatment goals be undertaken simultaneously or sequentially? Who should be the agents of language change?

QUESTIONS FOR DISCUSSION

1. What is the rationale for early intervention?
2. What is the difference between interdisciplinary and transciplinary models?
3. What are the relative advantages and disadvantages of standardized and nonstandardized testing?
4. What is the general educational strategy of early intervention?
5. What are the relative advantages and disadvantages of inclusion compared to individual therapy provided outside the child care or home enviornment?

REFERENCES

Administration on Developmental Disabilities. (1988). *Mapping the future for children with special needs: P.L. 99-457.* Iowa City, IA: University of Iowa Press.

Aram, D., Ekelman, B., & Nation, J. (1984). Preschoolers with language disorders: Ten years later. *Journal of Speech and Hearing Research, 27,* 232–244.

Bach-y-Rita, P. (1990). Brain plasticity as a basis for recovery of function in humans. *Neuropsychologica, 28,* 547–554.

Bailey, D., & Simonsson, R. (1985). *Family needs survey.* Chapel Hill: University of North Carolina.

Batshaw, M. (1991). *Your child has a disability: A complete sourcebook of daily and medical care.* Boston: Little, Brown.

Bernbaum, J., & Hoffman-Williamson, M. (1991). *Primary care of the preterm infant.* Philadelphia, PA: Mosby Year Book.

Bleile, K. (1993). Children with long-term tracheostomies. In K. Bleile (Ed.), *The care of children with long-term tracheostomies* (pp. 3–19). San Diego: Singular.

Bleile, K. (1995). *Manual of articulation and phonological disorders.* San Diego: Singular.

Bleile, K., & Fey, M. (1993). Issues and methods in the care of infants and toddlers. Annual convention of the American Speech-language-hearing Association. Anaheim, CA, November.

Bleile, K., & Miller, S. (1994). Toddlers with medical needs. In J. Bernthal & N. Bankson (Eds.), *Child phonology: Characteristics, assessment, and intervention with special populations* (pp. 81–109). New York: Thieme.

Bleile K., Stark R., & Silverman McGowan, J. (1993). Evidence for the relationship between babbling and later speech development. *Clinical Linguistics and Phonetics, 7,* 319–337.

Bricker, P., Bailey, E., & Bruder, M. (1984). The efficacy of early intervention and the handicapped infant: A wise or wasted resource? In M. Wolraich & D. Routh (Eds.), *Advances in developmental and behavioral pediatrics* (pp. 373–423). Greenwich, NY: JAI Press.

Bruner, J. (1983). *Child's talk: Learning to use language.* New York: Norton.

Bzoch, K. & League, R. (1991). *Receptive-expressive emergent language test* (2nd ed.). Austin, TX: PRO-ED.

Capute, A., & Accardo, P. (1978). Linguistic and auditory milestones during the first two years of life: A language inventory for the practitioner. *Clinical Pediatrics, 17,* 847–853.

Capute, A., Palmer, F., Shapiro, B., Wachtel, R., Schmidt, S., & Ross, A. (1986). Clinical Linguistic and Auditory Milestone Scale: Prediction of cognition in infancy. *Developmental Medicine and Child Neurology, 28,* 762–771.

Charney, E. (1992). Neural tube defects: Spina bifida and myelomeningocele. In M. Batshaw & Y. Perret (Eds.), *Children with disabilities: A medical primer* (pp. 471–488). Baltimore: Brookes,

Coplan, J. (1993). *Early language milestone scale.* Austin, TX: PRO-ED.

Crowe Hall, B. (1991). Attitudes of fourth and sixth graders toward peers with mild articulation disorders. *Language, Speech, and Hearing Services in Schools, 22,* 334–349.

Damasio, A. (1990). Category-related recognition defects as a clue to neural substrates of knowledge. *Trends in Neuroscience, 13,* 95–98.

Dunst, C., Trivette, C., & Deal, A. (1988). *Enabling and empowering families: Principles and guidelines for practice.* Cambridge, MA: Brookline Books.

Fenson, L., Dale, P., Reznick, J., Thal, D., Bates, E., Hartung, J., Pethick, S., Reilly, J. (1993). *MacArthur communicative development inventories*. San Diego: Singular.

Ferguson, C., & Farwell, C. (1975). Words and sounds in early language acquisition: English initial consonants in the first fifty words. *Language, 51,* 419–439.

Fey, M. (1986). *Language intervention with young children*. San Diego: College Hill.

Fridy, J., & Lemanek, K. (1993). Developmental and behavioral issues. In K. Bleile (Ed.), *The care of children with long-term tracheostomies* (pp. 141–166). San Diego: Singular.

Greenspan, S. (1985). First feelings: Milestones in the emotional development of your child from birth to age 4. New York: Viking.

Greenspan, S. (1992). *Infancy and early childhood: The practice of clinical assessment and intervention with emotional and developmental challenges*. Madison, CT: International Universities Press.

Hall, P., & Tomblin, B. (1978). A follow-up study of children with articulation and language disorders. *Journal of Speech and Hearing Disorders, 43,* 227–241.

Handler, S. (1993). Surgical intervention of the tracheostomy. In K. Bleile (Ed.), *The care of children with long-term tracheostomies* (pp. 23–40). San Diego: Singular.

Hart, B. (1985). Naturalistic language training techniques. In S. Warren & A. Rogers-Warren (Eds.), *Training functional language* (pp. 63–88). Baltimore, MD: University Park Press.

Hedrick, D., Prather, E., & Tobin, A. (1984). *Sequenced Inventory of Communication Development*. Seattle: University of Washington Press.

Hock-Long, L., Trachtenberg, S., & Vorters, D. (1993). The social worker's role with the family. In K. Bleile (Ed.), *The care of children with long-term tracheostomies* (pp. 203–222). San Diego, CA: Singular.

Infant Health and Development Program. (1990). A multisite, randomized trial. *Journal of the American Medical Association, 263,* 3035–3042.

Jusczyk, P. (1992). Developing phonological categories from the speech signal. In C. Ferguson, L. Menn, & C. Stoel-Gammon (Eds.), *Phonological development: Models, research, implications* (pp. 17–64). Timonium, MD: York Press.

Locke, J., (1983). *Phonological acquisition and change*. New York: Academic Press.

Locke, J. (1988). The sound shape of early lexical representations. In M. Smith and J. Locke (Eds.), *The emergent lexicon: The child's development of a linguistic vocabulary* (pp. 3–22). New York: Academic Press.

Locke, J., & Pearson, D. (1992). Vocal learning and the emergence of phonological capacity: A neurobiological approach. In C. Ferguson, L. Menn, & C. Stoel-Gammon (Eds.), *Phonological development: Models, research, implications* (pp. 91–130). Timonium, MD: York Press.

MacDonald, J. (1989). *Becoming partners with children: From play to conversation*. San Antonio: Special Press.

MacDonald, J., & Carroll, J. (1992). A social partnership model for assessing early communication development: An intervention model for preconversational children. *Language, Speech, and Hearing Services in Schools, 23,* 113–124.

Mantovani, J., & Powers, J. (1991). Brain injury in premature infants: Patterns on cranial ultrasound, their relationship to outcome, and the role of developmental intervention in the NICU. *Infants and Young Children, 4,* 20–32.

Metz, S. (1993). Medical management of the ventilator. In K. Bleile (Ed.), *The care of children with long-term tracheostomies* (pp. 41–55). San Diego: Singular.

McGongigel, M., Kaufmann, R., & Johnson, B. (Eds.). (1991). *National Early Childhood Technical Assistance System (NEC-TAS): Guidelines and recommended practices for the individualized family service plan* (2nd ed.). Chapel Hill, NC: National Early Childhood Technical Assistance System.

Nelson, K. E. (1989). Strategies for first language teaching. In M. Rice & R. Schiefelbusch (Eds.), *The teachability of language* (pp. 263–310). Baltimore, MD: Brookes.

Ojemann, J. (1991). Cortical organization of language. *Journal of Neuroscience, 11,* 2281–2287.

Paul, R. (1991). Profiles of toddlers with slow expressive language. *Topics in Language Disorders, 11,* 1–13.

Paul, R. (1995). *Language disorders from infancy through adolescence: Assessment and intervention.* Philadelphia, PA: Mosby Year Book.

Ramey, C., & Campbell, F. (1984). Preventive education for high-risk children: Cognitive consequences of the Caroline Abecedarian Project. *American Journal of Mental Deficiency, 88,* 515.

Saint Christopher's Hospital for Children. (1982). An assessment tool: The infant scales of communicative intent. *Update Pediatrics, 7,* 1–5.

Scollon, R. (1976). *Conversations with a one year old: A case study of the developmental foundation of syntax.* Honolulu: University Press of Hawaii.

Silverman, F., & Paulus, P. (1989). Peer relations to teenagers who substitute /w/ for /r/. *Language, Speech, and Hearing Services in Schools, 20,* 219–221.

Snow, C., & Goldfield, B. (1983). Turn the page please: Situation-specific language acquisition. *Journal of Child Language, 10,* 551–569.

Trout, M., & Foley, G. (1989). Working with families of handicapped infants and toddlers. *Topics in Language Disorders, 10,* 57–67.

Vihman, M., & Miller, R. (1988). Words and babble at the threshold of language acquisition. In M. Smith and J. Locke (Eds.), *The emergent lexicon: The child's development of a linguistic vocabulary* (pp. 151–184). New York: Academic Press.

Wallace, S. (1990). Rise of seizures (Annotation). *Developmental Medicine and Child Neurology, 32,* 645–649.

Warren, S., & Bambara, L. (1989). An experimental analysis of milieu language intervention: Teaching the action-object form. *Journal of Speech and Hearing Disorders, 54,* 448–461.

Warren, S., & Kaiser, A. (1988). Research in early language intervention. In S. Odom & M. Karnes (Eds.), *Early intervention for infants and children with handicaps. An empirical base* (pp. 89–108). Baltimore, MD: Brookes.

White, K., Mastrapierl, M., & Casto, G. (1984). An analysis of special education early childhood projects approved by the joint dissemination review panel. *Journal of the Division of Early Childhood, 9,* 11.

Wilcox, M. (1989). Delivering communication-based services to infants, mothers, and their families: Approaches and models. *Topics in Language Disorders, 10,* 68–79.

Wilcox, M., Kouri, T., & Caswell, S. (1991). Early language intervention: A comparison of classroom and individual treatment. *American Journal of Speech-Language Pathology, 1,* 49–62.

Yarrow, L., Rubenstein, J., & Pedersen, F. (1975). *Infant and environment: Early cognitive and motivational development.* Washington, DC: Hemisphere.

Yoder, P., Warren, S., Kim, K., & Gazdag, G. (1994). Facilitating prelinguistic communication skills in young children with developmental delay II: Systematic replication and extension. *Journal of Speech and Hearing Research, 37,* 841–851.

Zimmerman, I., Steiner, V., & Pond, R. (1992). *Preschool Language Scale-3.* San Antonio, TX: Psychological Corporation.

Appendix

Infection Control Guidelines

Although the topic of colds and hand washing may seem mundane, young children have relatively weak immunological systems, and diseases carried by staff members are a primary source of infection to children receiving early intervention services. The clinician should remain at home during illnesses such as colds and flues. Regardless of the number of sick days available, staff shortages, or other seemingly good reasons, the staff member who comes to work with an infection does children a great disservice. It is far better for a child with medical needs to miss a few treatment sessions because a clinician is ill than to be exposed to infection.

Staff members without infections can still spread infection from a sick child to the other children with whom the clinician comes in contact. The following basic infection control guidelines greatly reduce the chance that the clinician will carry disease from child to child:

HAND WASHING

Most infections in early intervention centers and hospitals are carried from child to child by staff members. The most effective means to reduce spread of infection is through careful washing after intervening with each child. Other times when washing should be performed are when coming on or off duty, when the hands are dirty, after toilet use, after blowing or wiping one's nose, after handling soiled child secretions, and on completion of duty. To wash, the speech-language clinician wets the hands and forearms, applies soap, and washes all areas of the hands and forearms for one to two minutes, being careful to wash nailbeds and between fingers. Afterwards, the soap is rinsed from the hands and forearms thoroughly. An unused paper towel is used to turn off the water faucet, and then the paper towel is discarded.

TOY WASHING

Toys are another source of infection because young children often place toys in their mouth, or may place a finger in their mouth or nose after playing with an infected toy. Gloves are worn to clean possibly infected toys. Each toy is wiped down with warm, soapy water and then rinsed. Next, the clinician sprays or wipes each toy with a disinfectant such as 1:10 solution of household bleach. The toy is then rinsed well and air-dried for ten minutes.

CHAPTER 10

Language Intervention in the Inclusive Preschool

Linda McCormick

Separate services for young children with disabilities were premised on these assumptions: (1) that the disabilities of preschoolers are such that they need different, intensive, and specialized, services that can only be provided in separate settings, and (2) that they are unlikely to benefit from the kind of experiences provided to their nondisabled peers. There is no empirical support for these assumptions: There is, in fact, a substantial research base suggesting just the opposite (e.g., Lipsky & Gartner, 1997; Peck, Odom, & Bricker, 1993). When provided with the supports they need (i.e., integrated special services, environmental and curricular adaptations, individualized methods and materials), young children with disabilities thrive in inclusive settings.

Daily interactions with peer models and exposure to the rich variety of experiences in inclusive settings provide them with continuous opportunities to observe, learn, and practice age-appropriate social, communication, and cognitive skills. Considering that the majority of activities in early childhood programs are designed to encourage language, social, cognitive, and motor-skill development, it is not surprising that developmental outcomes for children with disabilities in inclusive programs often surpass those of peers in separate special education classes (Strain, 1990). They demonstrate higher levels of social play and more appropriate social interactions. Additionally, they are more likely to initiate interactions with peers, and they have decidedly more advanced play skills (Demchak & Drinkwater, 1992; Fewell & Oelwein, 1990; Lamorey & Bricker, 1993).

Montgomery's (1995) observations over a period of time in an inclusive preschool with fourteen 2- to 4-year-olds highlight these benefits. Half of the children in the class she observed had diagnosed moderate-to-severe disabilities (autism, pervasive developmental delay, cerebral palsy, unknown neurological dysfunction, mental retardation). Related services (speech and language therapy, physical and occupational therapy) for these children were integrated into the daily routines. After only four months in the inclusive setting, the children with disabilities had learned

- where to hang their coats;
- to identify their own storage "bucket" for materials they would take home;
- to fingerpaint;
- where the painting shirts were kept and that they needed to put them on before painting;
- to play with peers in the playhouse (often imitating what they saw their peers doing);
- to play at the water table, the bean table, and the flour table;
- to "write" messages to peers and deliver them to the proper mailboxes;

Four of the children with disabilities learned to climb the fence in the backyard, two learned to "pump" in the swings, six learned to sit on the rug square with their own name on it, and four imitated unusual and fun words heard in the stories read in class. Montgomery notes that this is only a sampling of the outcomes she observed.

In addition to the social, linguistic, and cognitive benefits of inclusion, the increased probability for inclusion as the child gets older is another important benefit of the decision to place a child in an inclusive program (Miller, Strain, McKinley, Heckathorn, & Miller, 1993). Children of matched demographics and developmental levels who were placed in inclusive preschool programs were significantly more likely to be in inclusive elementary classes than were their peers who started off in segregated preschool programs.

Whether inclusion is successful has little to do with either the severity or the pervasiveness of the child's disability and everything to do with available resources and supports. The one qualifier attached to the assertion that inclusion seems to benefit all young children is that *there must be planning, staff training, and, most importantly, adequate supports.*

It is important to emphasize that inclusive programs do not penalize children without disabilities. Children without disabilities in inclusive programs achieve positive developmental outcomes comparable to those attained in programs that do not include children with disabilities (Odom & McEvoy, 1988; Strain, 1990). Particularly gratifying is the finding that they demonstrate greater understanding of and sensitivity to individual differences—more patience, compassion, and acceptance of others.

This chapter will describe intervention and instructional strategies for young children with language and communication impairments in inclusive early education settings. These strategies are compatible with best practices in both early childhood special education (ECSE) and general early childhood education (ECE). We are concerned with language and communication difficulties that are the child's primary disability or secondary to another disability, for example, learning disabilities, attention disorders, orthopedic impairments, multiple disabilities, hearing impairments, visual impairments, serious emotional disturbance, autism, mental retardation, or traumatic brain injury.

STRATEGIES TO ENCOURAGE LANGUAGE AND COMMUNICATION

Young children with disabilities have much in common with their nondisabled peers. Like their nondisabled peers, they learn from repeated and sustained interactions with objects, events, and people in their environment. Young children with disabilities have significant learning potential (as Montgomery's observations above so aptly illustrate), but learning is less likely to occur incidentally and acquisition of new skills and concepts may require more prompts, more repetition, and at least some systematic instruction. Young children with disabilities sometimes

1. fail to generalize,
2. are less goal-oriented,
3. have a shorter attention span,
4. show less persistence,
5. cannot express themselves, and
6. lack social competence.

Young children attend to, learn, and talk about what interests *them* (not what interests the adults in their environment). Thus, the challenge—if we hope to increase and enhance language and positive social interaction—is to provide an environment replete with people, objects, and activities that interest children. The single most essential element of language intervention in inclusive preschool programs is arranging the environment. **Environmental arrangement** entails selection and use of materials, arrangement of the physical space, and the provision of structure to activities. Unfortunately, many do not use environmental arrangement to promote language. Quite the opposite: Some environments are arranged in such a way that they discourage the use of language. Materials, toys, activities, drinking water, and foods (the things children want and need) are *too* available. Children can easily "help themselves" to whatever they want or simply wait for it to be provided by adults.

Arranging the Environment

Hierarchical intervention models stratify interventions by level of intensity, beginning with the least intense approach, which is developmentally appropriate practice (Bredekamp & Rosegrant, 1992; DEC recommended practices, 1993). Each successive level in the hierarchy is more intrusive because there is more structure and the need for more resources and more elaborate planning. The least intensive and intrusive intervention is first preference because the strategies are very similar to naturally occurring learning experiences: they "blend in" so well in the classroom that they are virtually indistinguishable from ongoing activities (Schwartz, 1998).

Environmental structuring requires few resources and relatively little planning compared with implementation of systematic instruction. Some examples of environmental structuring to teach language and communication include

- providing materials that encourage social play, cooperation, and interactive play themes;
- selecting and using materials and activities that are preferred by the children to encourage engagement;
- limiting and clearly defining activity and materials choices to encourage independent decision making;
- staying in close proximity to children to take advantage of opportunities to encourage engagement with peers; and
- providing activities and play areas that accommodate small groups so that there is the peer proximity conducive to social and play interactions.

Ostrosky and Kaiser (1991) outline seven environmental arrangement strategies to increase the number of opportunities to elicit communication. The seven strategies are: (1) making interesting objects, materials, and activities available; (2) placing desired objects out of reach or blocking access to objects and activities; (3) providing materials that require assistance to operate; (4) offering materials out of context; (5) providing inadequate portions; (6) failing to provide sufficient materials; and (7) doing something to elicit protest.

1. **Make interesting objects, materials, and activities available.** Because increasing the number of interesting objects, materials, and activities in the environment increases language use, it also increases the number of teaching opportunities. The teacher and the language interventionist determine children's object and activity preferences by noting the focus of their attention and by interviewing family members and other adults. An analysis of attention focus often reveals definite sensory preferences, for example, auditory feedback, visual stimulation,

tactile stimulations. Children with severe disabilities are most likely to attend to response-contingent materials (e.g., a battery-operated bear that marches and plays music when a switch is activated).

Some items should be made available because they give children access to interesting activities. For example, a communication board may not be particularly interesting, but it makes it possible for children to (1) request art materials and preferred centers, and (2) answer calendar and weather questions during morning circle (these interest them very much). A tape recorder with a loop tape that plays the repeatable refrain ("ee-i'-ee-'i-o") lets children join in singing of "Old MacDonald" at circle time.

2. **Place desired objects out of reach or block access to objects and activities.** Multiply opportunities for requesting by placing objects (toys, materials, games, foods) that the child finds desirable, attractive, and interesting in clear plastic bins or on a shelf out of reach (but within view). Also restrict access to high-interest activities. For example, if riding is a favorite outdoor activity, the rate of requests can be increased by placing a gate at the entry to the outside area where wheel toys are parked.

3. **Provide materials that are difficult to operate.** Providing toys that children cannot activate without assistance is another way to encourage requesting. A jack-in-the-box with a wind-up, a tightly capped bottle of bubbles, a mechanical toy with a hard-to-turn switch, and a swing are examples of toys and play equipment children may need to request assistance with. If a child does not request assistance, a verbal or nonverbal prompt (e.g., "What do you want?" or "Say 'help' ") is provided.

4. **Offer objects or materials out of context.** Offering objects or materials out of context is another strategy to elicit vocalizations, comments, or protests. Examples include attempting to put another child's (or an adult's) sweater on a child, or hanging a picture upside down. The idea is to create an absurd situation that violates children's expectations.

5. **Provide inadequate portions of needed or desired objects or materials.** Giving children only a small portion of what is needed or desired usually elicits a protest and/or a request. For example, at snack time, provide small servings of juice, fruit, and crackers with the understanding that more is available on request. Peer modeling often comes about as a bonus with this strategy. For example, a peer may say "Tell Miss Joy you need more" or a peer may even prompt with "Say 'more juice'."

6. **Fail to provide needed objects or materials.** Intentionally "forget" to provide the materials necessary or desired for a

favorite activity. This is similar to providing inadequate portions except that *no* portion of the needed materials—or none of the needed objects—is provided. For example, "forget" to put out crayons, paste, or scissors for an art activity or "mistakenly" provide a nonfunctional or inappropriate item (e.g., an empty paste container). An added benefit of this strategy is the need to problem-solve. Children must "figure out" what is wrong or missing.

7. **Do something that the child does not like.** Doing something that the child does not want or providing an item that she does not like creates an opportunity to prompt the child to say "No thank you" or "Don't do it that way." For example, when a child points to the top shelf and she is offered the container of Tinkertoys rather than the container with magnets that she wants, she can be prompted to say "No, I want magnets." Like the other strategies, this should be carried out in a warm, engaging manner so as not to frustrate the child. Adults must be extremely sensitive to prevent this strategy from becoming upsetting and intrusive to the point that the activity is no longer creative and spontaneous. The slightest indication that the child is becoming frustrated should be the signal to provide or do what the child wants.

Using the seven environmental arrangement strategies (together with milieu teaching techniques, described below) is a way to encourage the use of augmented communication systems (manual signing or a communication board) as well as oral language. Research suggests that, when teachers increase the frequency and variety of environmental arrangement strategies they use, there are associated increases in total child-communicative responses and in the spontaneous use of targeted signs (Kaiser, Ostrosky, & Alpert, 1993).

There are two caveats concerning these environmental arrangement strategies. One caveat has to do with the possibility of frustrating the child; the other has to do with fostering dependence. It is not possible to overemphasize the importance of adults being sensitive to children's tolerance for frustration. As noted above, if there is any indication that a child is feeling frustrated, he or she should be given the desired item or access and requests for communication should be *immediately* terminated. Do *not* upset and frustrate children with too many communication demands.

The second caveat has to do with fostering independence. Many adults are concerned that arranging the environment so that children must request desired objects and activities will foster dependency. This is a valid concern. Environmental arrangement strategies are used when language/communication objectives take precedence over independence objectives.

Activities and Routines

A routine is a sequence of interactive events that is repeated frequently and always in exactly the same way. Examples of routines include games (e.g., peekaboo); rhymes, jokes, and songs (e.g., "When you're happy and you know it . . . "); social amenities and courtesies (e.g., "please," "excuse me"); daily caregiving activities (e.g., toileting, dressing, bathing); storytelling; and activity formats (e.g., morning circle, show and tell, snack preparation, clean up). Over the past decade there has been a great deal of support for using routines to help teach language and communication skills. Routines teach sequences of appropriate behaviors because children learn to anticipate what will happen next, then they "fill in the slots."

Instruction within the context of routines relies on a prompting procedure that is also used in milieu teaching, **time delay.** The adult begins the routine and then interrupts the sequence at a point of maximum motivation. The adult simply waits, relying on the child's need and drive to move on to the next step. When a well-established routine is interrupted (particularly when the interruption is at a point where there is maximum anticipation of a positive next step), the child is very likely to either produce the behavior that is expected at the point of interruption or indicate a desire for the routine to continue.

In most environments there is no need to establish new routines to teach language and communication. There are already numerous routines in place throughout the day. Just take advantage of the opportunities for language teaching within existing routines. The following are steps in planning the use of routines to promote development and use of language and communication:

1. **Select a routine that the child enjoys.** Almost any routine can be used, but the best routines are those that involve a variety of objects and materials that children find attractive, interesting, and desirable and that require many repeated actions. Once instruction within the context of one routine is underway, other routines can be selected and used.
2. **List the specific steps in the routine and the language skills and/or concepts that can be elicited at each step.** You can teach new language forms and functions and provide opportunities to practice and thus generalize forms and functions learned in other contexts. For example, a simple toothbrushing routine provides an excellent opportunity for teaching new vocabulary (e.g., *toothbrush, toothpaste, water, spit, drink, up, down,* etc.) and requesting. When planning, it can be helpful to have a script of the routine. Figure 10.1 shows a sample script for snack preparation.

FIGURE 10.1   Sample script for snack preparation

	Time ___10:30___	
	Location __Snack Area__	
Routine __Snack Preparation__	Materials __Napkins, Cups, Food__	

Sequence of Events	**What You Might Say**	**What Child(ren) Might Say**
Announce snack time.	"It's time to eat! What do we need to do?"	"Wash hands."
Send children two or three at a time to wash hands.	"_____ and _____ go first to wash hands. Who is sitting next to _____ ?"	"_____ ."
	"Who is sitting next to _____ ?"	"_____ ."
	"Who will go when they return?"	"_____ and _____ ."
Remind children of designated leaders for snack time. Rehearse leader duties.	"Who are our hosts and hostesses today?"	"_____ , _____ and _____ ."
	"What do they do first?"	"Get out napkins and cups and food."
	"Then what?"	"Put napkins and cups on the table."
	"Then what?"	"Put apples on the plate."
By the end of leader duty rehearsal, all have returned from washing hands and all go to chairs at the snack table. Host/hostess prepares and distributes napkins and places crackers on a plate. When child asks, the apples are passed and/or the juice is poured when asked for.	"We're ready now. Why aren't you eating?"	"Want apple." "No food." "Pour juice." "No juice." "Thank you."

Developed by L. McCormick, 1990.

3. **Decide when and how the routine will be interrupted.** The possibilities for interrupting a routine are numerous (Halle, Alpert, & Anderson, 1984). You can simply halt the activity and wait or you may violate the child's expectations for the routine by
   • withholding or delaying provision of expected objects or actions;
   • providing an incomplete set of materials; or
   • making "silly" mistakes.

4. **Have a plan for eliciting the desired responses if time delay alone is not successful.** Possibilities include modeling the desired response (e.g., "Say 'I need a napkin' ") or providing a verbal direction (e.g., "Can you tell me what's wrong?").

The **interrupted chain strategy** is a variation of the interrupted routine strategy that is particularly effective with students with severe disabilities (e.g., Hunt & Goetz, 1988). The major difference is that with the interrupted chain strategy a *specific* instructional trial is inserted into the middle of the sequence. An example from a study by Hunt, Goetz, Alwell, and Sailor (1986) demonstrates this strategy. It was used with Nate, a 6-year-old nonverbal student with severe mental retardation. Prior to the intervention, Nate's primary mode of communication was gestural or physical. To request a hug, he walked up to the teacher or other familiar adult and reached out, putting his arms around the adult's neck or pushing his head against the adult's body. To request help with dressing or to go outside, Nate pulled at the nearest adult. To communicate opposition he cried, pushed objects away, blinked his eyes, or physically left the situation.

The goal of intervention was to teach Nate to use a picture communication book attached by a key clip to the waistband of his pants. The first objective was to teach him to point to the "want" card in his communication book. The initial step toward this objective was for Nate to pull the open communication book up to above waist level. The four response chains that were interrupted to teach this behavior were: (1) playing catch in the classroom or at recess; (2) preparing to go out to recess; (3) approaching and hugging an adult; and (4) playing with a See 'n Say during leisure time. The first three response chains were already performed independently and spontaneously; the fourth was taught through systematic instruction. In the first chain, an instructional trial was inserted after Nate threw the ball to his partner in the six-step ball-playing chain. In the second chain, a four-step chain for recess preparation, an instructional trial was inserted just after Nate's classmates were dismissed to go to recess. In the third chain (a three-step hugging behavior chain), an instructional trial was inserted while Nate's arms were around an adult. In the fourth chain (a five-step chain), an instructional trial was inserted while Nate was pulling on the cord of the See 'n Say.

The first instructional target for Nate—pulling his open communication book with the word "want" displayed to above waist level—was inserted into the "playing catch in the classroom or at recess behavior" chain at the predetermined point in the sequence. When Nate attained criterion on that target, a second target was taught within the second behavior chain, and so on until all of the target communication responses were acquired.

Activity-based intervention is a naturalistic teaching strategy developed and researched by Bricker and Cripe (1992). It is a somewhat more structured use of activities and routines as instructional contexts. Activity-based intervention is a systematic approach for teaching functional skills and generalizable skills in planned curriculum activities, routines, and child-initiated interactions. Functional skills are defined as skills that children need to be independent in self-care and social activities and routines in their environments. Generalizable skills are defined as skills, such as requesting, that can be practiced and used in many different settings throughout the day.

The teacher determines (1) how skill objectives for each child can be taught and/or practiced in the context of daily classroom activities, and (2) how the classroom environment will be made stimulating and interesting. For example, eating independently (a self-help objective), picking up a cracker (a fine-motor objective), and requesting more (a language objective) could be facilitated and practiced at snacktime. Children's individual goals and objectives would be incorporated into curriculum activities such as playing in the block center or participating in an art activity.

Transdisciplinary play-based intervention (TPBI), developed by Linder (1993), is an "inclusive curriculum" that integrates intervention strategies to strengthen developmental processes and increase functional skills across cognitive, social–emotional, communication and language, and sensorimotor domains. It is an outgrowth of Linder's (1990) transdisciplinary play-based assessment process. TPBI is a variation of activity-based instruction. It also incorporates aspects of milieu teaching and interactive modeling.

TPBI uses the objectives in the child's individualized program to generate specific intervention strategies that are then integrated into the child's daily routine. It integrates intervention in four domains: cognitive, social–emotional, communication and language, and sensorimotor. The recommendations, with respect to language and communication goals, are to incorporate instruction into play and routine activities such as mealtime and snacktime, bathing, hand washing, brushing teeth, dressing, and toileting. Designed to be used with children from infancy to age 6, the TPBI procedures can be implemented in almost any play environment using whatever play materials and opportunities are available in that environment. The most frequently used play environments are the home, infant and toddler programs, and preschool and kindergarten classes. Linder (1993) provides instructions for developing a play-based storybook curriculum but, generally speaking, the TPBI can be incorporated into almost any curriculum model.

Play

Play takes many forms with young children. There is *sensorimotor* play, during which children learn to use their senses to explore and manipulate objects. There is *functional play,* in which children explore and learn about relationships among objects and between objects and events, and *constructive play,* in which they learn to create. In *dramatic play,* they learn to make-believe, and in *game play* they learn about prescribed rules. Play can be child-initiated and child-directed or adult-initiated and adult-directed. Children may play alone, in proximity to others, or in interaction with others. However they play, the content and style of their play will reflect their development and their culture.

Play is possibly the most important and natural context for language learning and language instruction. It is not only a source of pleasure for young children, but also a way to learn and practice new behaviors. Children experiment with life experiences when they play, constructing their understanding of objects and events and learning how to talk about them. Cooperative play is the occasion for a variety of social and communicative interactions, a natural medium through which children learn acceptable modes of social interaction—sharing, taking turns, and accepting responsibility.

Cooperative play is not something that happens naturally for most children with disabilities. The skills needed for cooperative play are typically areas of difficulty for them. Because they are often delayed in their acquisition of play skills, they require support to develop the play behavior typical of their peers. The development of play skills may be especially important for young children with special needs because play encourages and sustains social engagement with family members as well as peers.

Many early childhood programs include play in the curriculum. Teachers view play as a rich opportunity for teaching cognitive, communicative, social, motor, and adaptive skills. Not until the past several decades, however, have interventionists begun to capitalize on the natural proclivity of children to play and use it as a setting for assessment (Linder, 1990), intervention and instruction (e.g., Linder, 1993; McGee, Krantz, & McClannahan, 1985), peer tutoring (Strain & Odom, 1986), and, specifically, language intervention (Warren & Gazdag, 1990).

Facilitate and Support

At the preschool level, the role of the adult (ECE teacher, ECSE teacher, language interventionist, or other support staff) is twofold: to provide an enriched environment, and to facilitate learning through natural interactions. Times when a child is interested in and manipulating objects are seized on as opportunities to name and label the objects and model conversational discourse and semantic and grammatical constructions. The initial focus is on increasing cognitive and pragmatic skills, with the idea that increased mean length of utterance and more advanced grammatical structures will follow.

The curriculum in most early childhood programs is based on the belief that the natural curiosity and exuberance of children should be nurtured in a meaningful and intellectually stimulating manner. Most curricula combine child-chosen play in a carefully arranged environment with planned developmentally appropriate activities (Feeney, Christensen, & Moravcik, 2000). Learning experiences are organized into thematic or topical units. The unit theme or topic is essentially the core around which appropriate activities are planned and organized so as to integrate learning in different developmental areas. It is selected or developed to reflect the interests, abilities, and specific concerns of the children in the program. The teacher engages the children in in-depth exploration of the theme by introducing a range and variety of theme-related materials, people, and experiences over a period of time, which can range from one or two weeks to several months. Learning experiences to help children relate information, knowledge, objects, and actions to the theme are provided in the contexts of child-initiated play activities, one-to-one instruction, small-group activities, and large-group activities. Activity descriptions are sent home on a regular basis, with suggestions for parents to provide experiences at home and talk about aspects of the theme. All themes include a variety of both familiar and new vocabulary.

Basic facilitation strategies are those procedures that early childhood educators use with all children to facilitate development and use of language forms and communication skills. They are typically used in the context of routine activities (e.g., snacks, washing hands before lunch, bathroom breaks, recess) and curriculum activities. The six most commonly used basic facilitation strategies are: (1) engaging the child; (2) commenting about the child's interests and activities; (3) responding to communicative attempts; (4) allowing time for the child to respond; (5) using rational modeling; and (6) expanding and extending child utterances. These strategies are listed and briefly described in Table 10.1.

Special facilitation strategies are procedures that are used with young children who are not acquiring language at the same rate as their peers. Special facilitation strategies include: (1) prompting a higher level of response; (2) promoting peer interactions; (3) encouraging use of particular materials; and (4) teaching communication to replace challenging behaviors. Table 10.2 describes and provides some examples of how these special facilitation strategies are used with preschoolers.

There are two language intervention procedures that apply the special facilitation strategies presented in Table 10.2: milieu teaching and responsive interaction interventions. They share the following basic characteristics (Kaiser, Ostrosky, & Alpert, 1993):

TABLE 10.1   Basic facilitation strategies

- **Engage the child.** Follow the child's attentional focus, show a sincere interest, and draw the child into interactions through actions or words related to the attentional focus. Initially accept any child behavior that is an indication of interest as a communicative effort.
- **Comment and ask questions about the child's interests and activities.** Use questions and comments to encourage children to talk about what they are doing and to express their feelings. Comment in order to provide a model of language describing what the child is doing or focused on. Use *wh*-questions and open-ended questions (e.g., "Tell me about _") to encourage children to formulate their thoughts and express them in a meaningful way.
- **Respond to all communicative efforts.** To teach the child how powerful communication can be, try to provide what is requested and/or continue the topic of the child's communication.
- **Allow time for the child to respond.** Wait at least five seconds after speaking, look expectantly at the child, and use verbal or gestural cues to encourage the child to take a turn and thus keep the conversation going. If the child does not respond, repeat or rephrase the previous utterance.
- **Use rational modeling.** Describe the relationships between objects, actions, people, and events over time and through space. For example, when the child says "Brendyn cry," say "Yes, Brendyn is crying because he hurt his knee when he fell."
- **Expand and extend child utterances.** Restate or rephrase the child's utterances, adding omitted words. Expansions are a means of modeling a structurally more complex utterance for the child while, at the same time, confirming for the child that his or her message and its intent was understood. Extensions add new information.

- teaching occurs in the child's natural environments (e.g., home, school);
- the environment is arranged to encourage and support child communication;
- teaching occurs in response to the child's interests;
- communicative efforts are acknowledged and rewarded by providing natural consequences.

Milieu teaching and responsive interaction interventions have been combined with environmental arrangement procedures to produce what Hemmeter and Kaiser (1994) label a *hybrid naturalistic procedure*. However, we will first consider the milieu teaching and responsive interaction separately.

TABLE 10.2   Special facilitation strategies

- **Prompt word retrieval and higher level of responses.** Prompt word retrieval with gestures, describing attributes, providing information about the function or category of the word, or by using a familiar phrase or sentence with the word omitted. Always try to elicit the most mature form of communication the child is capable of producing. Systematically fade prompts as the child demonstrates the target response.
- **Promote peer interactions.** Promote peer interactions through: (1) peer-mediated models whereby socially competent peers are taught to initiate interactions with less skilled classmates; (2) adult-mediated models whereby the adult encourages and prompts communicative responses toward less skilled peers; (3) direct instruction whereby children are taught to initiate communicative interactions; and (4) group models using cooperative learning or affection activities. (Affection activities are typical group games and songs such as "Simon Says" and "The Farmer in the Dell," which are modified to incorporate physical affection, e.g., a hug, pat on the back, high five, or handshake.)
- **Encourage use of particular materials.** Providing materials designed for two or more children sends a message about the importance of playing together. Similarly, providing duplicates of materials and toys sends a "play together and communicate" message. (Blocks foster cooperative building projects; housekeeping toys and clothing prompt children to act out familiar and meaningful routines.) How toys and other play materials are placed is a factor in communication. Placing materials so that children are face-to-face typically encourages communication. For example, there is considerably more communication across a dishpan full of sand or water when children are facing one another than with a large sand/water table (where children stand side by side). Easels are an exception. When placed so that children stand side by side there is more communication (than when they are arranged back-to-back).
- **Teach communication skills to replace challenging behaviors.** Sometimes young children who lack language skills use undesirable/disturbing behaviors (e.g., tantrums, hitting, screaming, crying, whining) to achieve their communication goals. What this tells us is that the child does not have appropriate ways to get his or her needs met. The teacher must identify the communicative intentions of the undesirable behavior (e.g., "I want attention," I want help," I don't want to do this") and teach more acceptable ways of expressing the intended messages.

Milieu Teaching

Milieu teaching is an umbrella term for a number of strategies that take advantage of a child's interest in material, activities, or other children to elicit particular behaviors. The basic difference between milieu teaching strategies and other language intervention procedures is not so much the nature of the strategies but *when* they are applied. The important defining characteristics are their incidental use in unplanned interactions and the fact that they are initiated by the child. Milieu teaching is based on observations of caregivers interacting with normally developing children. When parents interact with their children they (1) talk about objects, events, and/or relations that have attracted the child's attention; (2) model, imitate, and expand desired and actual child-communication efforts; (3) repeat and clarify words, statements, and requests that the child does not seem to understand; and (4) use such techniques as higher speech frequencies and stress to call the child's attention to important sentence elements.

Initial research with milieu teaching sought to facilitate acquisition of language and communication skills. It has since been expanded to include teaching of cognitive, social, motor, and adaptive skills (Brown, McEvoy, & Bishop, 1991; Nordquist, Twardosz, & McEvoy, 1991). Table 10.3 lists the basic assumptions of milieu language intervention (Alpert & Kaiser, 1992).

Milieu language teaching requires planning, preparation, and practice but there is no limit to the number of language targets that can be taught with milieu language teaching procedures. Typical intervention targets include increasing the frequency of communicative behaviors, production of longer and more complex utterances, and expression of familiar functions with more advanced forms. For example, the specific language targets for 5-year-old Lori are: (1) using labels to request desired foods at snacktime; (2) saying "more song," "more drum," and "more play" when appropriate during music time;

TABLE 10.3   Basic assumptions of milieu language intervention

- The child's natural environment(s) is the best setting for language intervention.
- The most effective language teachers are the significant others in the child's life.
- The child's focus of interest should set the occasion for language training episodes.
- The focus of training should be functional language.
- Language training should focus simultaneously on linguistic forms and their functions, and strategies for language learning.
- Training episodes should be brief and positive.

and (3) expression of familiar functions at snacks and at cleanup times (e.g., *wash, spill, wipe, dry, all done,* and *pick up*).

Some questions to assist selection of specific targets for milieu teaching are:

- What objects does the child come into contact with most frequently in routine activities in the classroom and other school environments?
- Who are the child's favorite people (possible communication partners)?
- What forms is the child expected to use (or respond to) most often in the greatest number of contexts? (Examples might include "yes" and "no," the child's name, food labels, names for family members, teachers, and favorite peers, a word for bathroom, labels of preferred activities, etc.)
- What functions would enable the child to be more effective in the greatest number of contexts? (Consider requesting, protesting, greeting, and questioning.)

The milieu teaching model differs from most other naturalistic intervention models in that it uses explicit prompts for specific communicative behaviors. The child is repeatedly prompted to use more advanced language forms and structures to request desired objects, activities, and assistance. The four milieu teaching procedures are: (1) modeling; (2) mand-modeling; (3) time delay; and (4) incidental teaching. All four procedures require the immediate presence of an adult to mediate between the child and the desired or needed object or activity.

In the **modeling procedure,** the adult first follows the child's attentional focus. When the child demonstrates an interest in an object or activity, a word or function is modeled for the child to imitate (e.g., "Say 'paint' " or "Say I want the puzzle' "). A correct imitation of the model is followed by praise, verbal expansion, and immediate access to the desired object and/or activity. If the imitation is not correct or the child does not respond, the model is repeated (and the child is given access to the desired object and/or activity).

The **mand-model procedure** adds one element to the modeling procedure, a mand or request. Skinner (1957) identified use of mands as one of two functions of verbal behavior; the other is describing or labeling. The child is presented with a request and, if necessary, a model of the desired communicative behavior. The mand-model procedure is used to teach children: (1) how to establish joint attention before addressing someone; (2) how to take turns in communicative exchanges; and (3) how to respond to verbal requests or instructions.

The **time delay procedure** uses a systematic wait procedure. When the child shows an interest in an object or activity, the adult delays responding until the child requests or comments.

The **incidental teaching procedure** is used to elicit more elaborate language and improve conversational skills. The child is prompted to provide a more linguistically complex request.

The language requirements placed on a child depend on the child's ability level and prespecified language/communication targets. Three activities in the typical preschool setting that afford particularly good opportunities for milieu language teaching are (1) eating times, (2) creative activities (e.g., free play, art, music, outside play, games, field trips, circle time), and (3) transition times. At eating times, food and drink are provided contingent on requesting behavior (depending on the child's capabilities). In addition to request forms, the names of foods and food-related items (napkins, dishes, silverware) and polite forms such as "please" and "thank you" can be taught at eating times. Objects and activities are *never* withheld; they are delayed as a tactic to teach language. If the child does not produce the desired language behavior after two or three prompts, the food or drink (or other object or activity) is always provided anyway. Creative activities provide numerous opportunities for adults to elicit requests and comments and encourage use of longer and more complex utterances. There are opportunities for children to communicate what they want to do, what they want to hear, what they want to play or work with, and where they want to go. Transitions between activities also provide numerous opportunities to prompt language use. Before transition to a new activity, children can be prompted to request assistance putting away materials, taking off outdoor clothing, or finishing a particular task. They can be asked and prompted to name the next activity and prompted to greet the adult and peers on entering the new activity.

Responsive Interaction

Similar to milieu teaching procedures, responsive interaction interventions are based on descriptions of interactions between parents and their language-learning children. The goal of responsive interaction intervention is to increase the contingent responsiveness of the child's conversational partner(s) and provide additional models of developmentally appropriate language. Research with responsive interaction intervention has taught mothers how to increase the amount of their speech that refers to their child's interest, to use more expansions of their children's utterances, to provide more opportunities for child turns, and to increase their overall responsiveness to their children (Mahoney & Powell, 1988: Tannock, & Girolametto, 1992; Weistuch & Lewis, 1985).

Responsive interaction procedures involve enhancement of conversational interactions and enrichment of the linguistic environment so they are appropriate for very young children at early stages of language as well as children who have already acquired some basic interaction skills (Kaiser, 1993). Adults must learn to (1) be more responsive to the child, (2) decrease their directiveness, (3) establish more balanced conversations, (4) follow the child's interests and conversational leads, (5) respond to the child's communicative attempts, and (6) increase the frequency of their contingent responses to the child.

Enhanced Milieu Teaching

Enhanced milieu teaching combines environmental arrangement, milieu teaching, and responsive interaction procedures (Kaiser, 1993; Hemmeter & Kaiser, 1994). This hybrid approach has demonstrated effectiveness when implemented by parents. Because it includes three well-documented sets of procedures, it should be equally effective in the preschool classroom.

Enhanced milieu teaching includes systematic arrangement of the environment as described earlier in this chapter, increased modeling of appropriate language by talking at the child's target level and expanding child utterances (responsive interaction), and the four milieu teaching procedures described above (modeling, mand-modeling, time delay, and incidental teaching).

The broad goal of environmental arrangement is to increase the child's engagement with the physical setting and the adults in the environment. Specifically, the objectives of environmental arrangement are to attract and sustain the child's interest in the environment; to increase opportunities for verbal and nonverbal communication; and to facilitate engagement between the child and adult(s). The focus is on providing as many opportunities as possible for communication with and by the child. There is continuous modeling of appropriate language forms and functions and immediate and contingent response to the child's verbal and nonverbal communication attempts. Actual environmental arrangement procedures are (as described earlier in the chapter):

- select toys and materials that interest the child;
- arrange the toys and materials to promote requests;
- mediate between the child and the toys and materials; and
- engage with the child in play and other activities with the toys and materials.

The broad goal of responsive interaction strategies is to develop a conversational style of interaction that promotes balanced communication between the child and adult(s). Specifically, responsive interaction seeks to facilitate engagement between the child and adults in the environment, turn-taking, sustained interactions, comprehension of spoken language, and spontaneous interactions. To accomplish these objectives, an adult should:

- follow the child's lead (his/her attention focus);
- balance turns;
- maintain the child's topic;
- talk about what the child is doing and joint activities being shared with the child;
- match the level of complexity of the child's language;
- expand and repeat the child's utterances; and
- respond communicatively to the child's verbal and nonverbal communication.

The broad goal of milieu teaching is to elicit elaborated and more sophisticated communicative responses from children. Specifically, milieu teaching facilitates responsiveness of adult requests for communication, generalized imitation skills, requesting, lexical and syntactic skills, communicative initiation, and improved conversational skills. It uses the four procedures discussed above: Modeling, mand-modeling, time delay, and incidental teaching.

As discussed above, in the modeling procedure the adult follows the child's attentional focus and models a request (either a verbal or nonverbal form) for the child to imitate. A correct imitation of the model is followed by praise, verbal expansion, and immediate access to the desired object and/or activity. If the imitation is not correct or the child does not respond, the model is repeated.

This is the sequence of steps to implement the mand-model procedure:

- When the child focuses attention on or approaches an object or activity, the adult says "Tell me what this is," or "Tell me what you want," or "Tell me what you want to do."
- If the child's response is less than he is capable of (or if he does not respond), present a model of the desired response (as in the modeling procedure) or, if the child provides a partial response, elaborate the mand (e.g., "Give me the whole sentence") and *then* provide a model.
- If the child responds appropriately, confirm the communicative attempt (e.g., "That's good"), provide a verbal expansion (e.g., "You want to work on the Beauty and the Beast puzzle today"), and give the child the desired object and/or activity.
- If the response is incorrect, provide a corrective model (e.g., "Say 'want puzzle' ") and then give the child the desired object and/or activity.

This is the sequence of steps to implement the time delay procedure:

- Face the child with an expectant look while displaying something that the child wants (e.g., a pitcher of orange juice, a favorite toy) or something that provides access to a desired activity (e.g., the gate to the sandbox area).

- Establish and maintain eye contact and wait a specified time (e.g., 4 to 15 seconds) for the child to attempt communication.
- If the child does not attempt to communicate, model the desired language (verbal or nonverbal) behavior.
- If the child responds, confirm the child's effort (e.g., "That's good"), provide a verbal expansion (e.g., "You want some orange juice"), and immediately provide the desired object and/or access to the desired activity.
- If the response is incorrect, provide a corrective model (e.g., "Say 'want juice' ") and then give the child the desired object and/or activity.

In summary, enhanced milieu teaching is a hybrid naturalistic intervention that includes environmental arrangement, responsive interaction, and milieu teaching. The procedures are not intrusive in an inclusive early childhood classroom because they include many of the developmentally appropriate practices for young children set forth by the National Association for the Education of Young Children (NAEYC) (Bredekamp & Copple, 1997). Most notable of these practices are: (1) following the child's lead, and (2) embedding instruction within activities and natural routines. Additionally, rather than providing contrived reinforcement such as praise or tokens, every effort is made to ensure that consequences for children's language use are natural and functionally related to the response.

PEER SUPPORT STRATEGIES

Language impairment has an enormous impact on peer interactions. Because children who are difficult or impossible to understand are not selected as social partners, they miss many opportunities for peer interactions. They are perceived as less popular, less smart, less attractive, and more insecure, more unpleasant, and "weird" by their peers (Windsor, 1995). The consequence of missed opportunities for interactions with peers is further language and communication problems, diminished social competence, and ultimately low self-concept. What occurs then is a self-fulfilling prophecy: Academic achievement suffers because students with low self-concept tend to be less motivated to achieve.

Missed opportunities for interactions with peers are also missed opportunities for learning because peers are not only natural partners: they are natural facilitators of language and communication. Children learn language from (and during) reciprocal social interactions with peers who are more experienced language users. Interactions with those who are experienced language users teach children how to

- express their needs and wants;
- exchange ideas, thoughts, and experiences;
- establish, maintain, and develop interpersonal relationships; and
- initiate and participate in conversations in a socially acceptable manner.

Children with disabilities interact with other children more frequently in inclusive settings than in segregated settings (e.g., Guralnick & Groom, 1988; Paul, 1985).

If more interactions between children with and without disabilities means more opportunities for language learning, then the challenge is increasing peer interactions. Interventions to increase peer interactions—sometimes called *peer support interventions*—may take the form of (1) teaching peers to initiate interactions with their classmates with disabilities, (2) teaching peers to respond to their classmates with disabilities, (3) peer modeling, and/or (4) cooperative learning practices. Most research has focused on the first: teaching peers to initiate interactions with their classmates with disabilities (Odom & Strain, 1984; Strain & Odom, 1986). Social initiations include play organizers (i.e., "Let's play with these blocks"), shares (i.e., "Here, you can play with this now"), physical assistance, and affection (e.g., hugging, patting, holding hands). Socially competent peers who have age-appropriate play skills, either no history with the child with disabilities or a positive history, and expressed willingness to participate are identified. Then they are taught how to initiate behaviors that elicit or support interactions with their classmates with disabilities.

Peers without disabilities also need to learn how to respond to their classmates with disabilities. Goldstein, Kaczmarek, Pennington, and Shafer (1992) describe a strategy for teaching peer responses. Past research suggested that (1) there is a high probability of language interactions when young children with and without disabilities are mutually attending to a particular object or activity, and (2) commenting (rather than requests or simple acknowledgment) seems to occur most frequently and to have the greatest probability of eliciting responses from communication partners. Preschoolers without disabilities were taught to attend to, comment on, and acknowledge the behavior of their classmates with disabilities in mutual activities. (The five preschoolers with disabilities who participated in this study exhibited significant linguistic, social, and cognitive deficits: four were diagnosed as autistic and the fifth was diagnosed as pervasive developmental delay.)

Peer training involved six direct instruction lessons focusing on three facilitation strategies: (1) mutual attention to a play activity, (2) commenting about ongoing activities, and (3) general acknowledgment of the partner's communicative behaviors. Each training session began with an overview of the step to be trained and a review of the previously learned steps. This was followed by descriptions of the requirements of the step, adult modeling of the step in isolation and within the complete sequence of steps, adult–child demonstrations with practice, and child–child practice. Posters were used to illustrate the strategies during the training and the demonstrations. The ten peers who participated in this study required between eleven and sixteen sessions to attain an 80 percent mastery criterion with the steps during triadic interactions (two peers without disabilities and a classmate with disabilities) in a free-play situation. Rates of interaction for four of the five classmates with disabilities significantly improved (Goldstein et al., 1992). Table 10.4 shows Goldstein and colleagues' format for teaching peer response strategies.

Peer modeling and observational learning are important advantages of group inclusive settings. In inclusive programs, children with disabilities learn a wide range of behaviors, including social, linguistic, and communication skills, by watching their peers. Teachers can increase the learning opportunities by prompting the "models." For example, the teacher might say, "Jordan, could you show Soo Jin what to say when she is the storekeeper?" or "Mark, when we go outside, will you remind Taylor how to ask when it is his turn to pull the big wagon?" According to the classic research of Bandura (1969), the effectiveness of modeling is increased when the sex, age, and other characteristics of the model closely resemble those of the imitator and when the modeled behavior is reinforced. For example, noting that Jordan received more juice when she said "More please," Sarah made an effort to produce the same request.

Group Interventions

Group interventions for promoting peer interactions fall into two categories: (1) cooperative learning arrangements, and (2) affection activities. The onus of responsibility for involving everyone in achieving the assigned task is on the group (rather than the teacher). Opportu-

TABLE 10.4   *Format for teaching peer-response strategies*

Teach peers to:
1. establish mutual attention by moving in front of the classmate with disabilities and looking at him, the toys he is playing with, or what he is doing;
2. say the name of the classmate;
3. say the classmate's name a second time and, if he does not respond, tap him on the shoulder and say his name again;
4. talk about what the classmate is doing and wait for him to respond (to take a turn in the exchange); and
5. talk about the activity again after the classmate responds.

---

nities for practice of social and communication skills occur naturally in the course of working together to reach their common goal so the group is the vehicle as well as the context for social interactions and friendships.

Cooperative learning arrangements are a powerful instructional method for promoting prosocial behavior and communication as well as academic achievement (Johnson & Johnson, 1991, 1994). Children learn (1) to encourage one another, (2) to celebrate each other's successes, and (3) to work toward common goals. The adult's role is to teach the necessary cooperative skills so that the group functions effectively. Gallagher (1991) describes a cooperative learning activity in which the group was asked to work together to draw a picture of a sunny day. Each child was given a different colored crayon. To ensure that he would have an important role in producing the final outcome, the peer with a language impairment was given the yellow crayon.

As a teaching strategy, cooperative learning has four basic elements: (1) positive interdependence, (2) face-to-face communication, (3) individual accountability, and (4) group process. Positive interdependence is working together and depending on one another to accomplish a common goal. Participants are expected to use some form of communication and appropriate interpersonal and small-group skills (e.g., turn-taking) and to feel individually responsible for the group's efforts.

Cooperative learning differs from other peer support strategies in that the emphasis is on fostering cooperative interactions. The dynamics of the groups and the cooperative interactions are viewed as the context for learning and practicing social, linguistic, and communicative skills. The focus on social skills, along with the structure that is inherent in cooperative learning lessons, provides an ideal context for language learning and practice of communication skills. The teacher and the language interventionist work together in developing and implementing cooperative learning lessons. Table 10.5 shows the steps in developing a cooperative learning lesson (Johnson & Johnson, 1991).

Affection activities modify well-known games and songs (e.g. "Simon Says," "The Farmer in the Dell," "If You're Happy and You Know It") in such a way as to increase opportunities for social exchanges. Several researchers have demonstrated positive effects on peer interactions from participation in these activities (Brown, Ragland, & Fox, 1988; Twardosz, Nordquist, Simon, & Botkins, 1983). Implementation is straightforward. Children are taught a new song or game or they participate in a familiar one. The first time through they sing and move in the usual manner. Then they are told "we are going to play/sing this a little differently next time." The song or game is modified so that children exchange some form of physical affection

TABLE 10.5 Steps in planning and implementing a cooperative learning lesson

Steps	Procedures
1. Select a lesson.	Select a lesson/activity that is simple, straightforward, motivating, and developmentally appropriate. Some examples for preschoolers include making jello, painting a mural, making a farm, fire station, or zoo.
2. Specify two objectives for the lesson.	Specify a cognitive objective and a social/language skill objective for the lesson. Ideally, one of these will be a new objective and the other will be a practice objective.
3. Assign children to groups.	Use small groups initially. *Gradually* move from pairs, to triads, and then to groups of four or five (in that order). Mix children of different ability levels, sexes, ethnic and cultural backgrounds, and language skills.
4. Introduce the objectives and what it means to be cooperative.	Discuss the objectives and how they will be used. Define cooperation and talk about cooperative behaviors that are appropriate and desirable (e.g., taking turns, asking for materials, sharing, looking at and listening to a speaker, saying nice things, helping others).
5. Model the steps and provide directions.	Explain the lesson with clear, step-by-step directions and demonstrations. If possible, show the steps in a sequence of pictures. Ask children to describe what they will be doing before beginning the lesson.
6. Observe and provide feedback.	Observe and provide positive feedback for cooperation. Provide assistance only if absolutely necessary. Clarify directions and/or answer questions related to the objectives.
7. Evaluate and debrief.	At the end of the lesson, take time to reflect on what they learned and what they said and did during the lesson. Especially talk about the cooperation and comment about how well they worked together.

(e.g., a pat on the back, "high five," or handshake). For example, instead of singing "the farmer takes a wife" or "the wife takes a child" in "The Farmer in the Dell," and then removing someone from the circle to stand in the middle, they would sing "the farmer *greets* a wife" and "the wife *greets* a child" and give high fives to one another.

Ostrosky, Kaiser, and Odom (1993) offer suggestions for facilitating peer interactions between children with and without disabilities, which serve as a summary of this discussion. These suggestions are presented in Table 10.6 as guidelines for facilitating social-communicative interactions.

TABLE 10.6   Guidelines for facilitating social–communicative interactions

---

- **Include peers without disabilities as facilitators,** not primary interventionists. They should not be expected to teach specific language/communication targets.
- **Teach social–communicative strategies to *all* children** (children with *and* without disabilities) during naturally occurring interactions.
- **Begin intervention activities with the children (with and without disabilities) who are most likely to be successful.** (Children with disabilities should be able to communicate consistently through either gestures, words, or signs.)
- **Focus preliminary individual instruction on developmentally appropriate initiation and response skills** for children *with* disabilities.
- **Teach the conversational strategies known to facilitate social–communicative interactions** (e.g., joint attention, establishing eye contact, commenting, responding, requesting information, turn-taking) to children without disabilities.
- **Use direct instruction and practice** (demonstrations, prompts, role-playing, and feedback) **to teach specific peer interaction skills** for individual children with disabilities *if needed*.
- **Program for maintenance and generalization** by:
  1. allowing adequate time for mastery of new skills;
  2. making skill training and opportunities for peer interaction a regular part of the classroom routine;
  3. systematically fading adult prompts and support; and
  4. concentrating on teaching those social-communicative skills that are likely to be most functional for the child.

Based on Ostrosky, Kaiser, & Odom (1993).

ECOLOGICAL ASSESSMENT

Early Childhood Education and Early Childhood Special Education both have a strong commitment to individualization. In the past, however, many have misunderstood individualization for children with disabilities to mean *one-to-one instruction*. Individualization is *not* one-to-one instruction: Individualization is:

- providing a learning environment that considers children's prior experiences and their present needs and interests (Bredecamp & Copple, 1997);
- ensuring availability of whatever supports, resources, and adaptations are needed for optimal learning; and
- continually adapting and expanding experiences in line with the individual needs of children.

Ecological assessment examines the environments in which children are expected to function to determine (1) what adaptations need to be made for children with disabilities, *and* (2) what children need to be taught to ensure participation with peers in ongoing activities. As described in Chapter 7, ecological assessment and planning is a strategy for individualization. The purpose is to determine children's strengths and exactly where and when extra help needs to be provided. The end result of this individualization process is:

- a clear picture of the expectations of the children's natural environments (e.g., preschool, home, playground);
- an understanding of the children's behavior in relation to the expectations; and
- ideas for ways to accommodate and enhance children's participation and communication.

Matrix Planning

Matrix planning is the last step in the planning (program-development) process. A matrix, as shown in Figure 10.2, shows how the objectives will be taught in the context of the routines and activities of the child's natural environment. The daily activity schedule is shown in the first column. Specific skill targets for each activity are written in the cells of the second column. The third, fourth, and fifth columns show planned environmental arrangements, instructional procedures, and peer support strategies, respectfully. Figure 10.2 shows planning for Josie, a 4-year-old with developmental delays who attends an inclusive preschool.

Another way to develop the matrix is to list the child's objectives in the first row. Then plans for how each objective will be taught—environmental arrangement, instructional procedures, peer supports—are written in the cells at the intersection of the activity and the target objective. (There is no expectation that all objectives can or should be addressed in each activity so, of course, some cells will be empty.)

PRESCHOOL INCLUSION MODELS

At the preschool level the possibilities for inclusion include a consultation model, an itinerant teacher model, or a co-teaching model. In a consultation model, the early childhood special education (ECSE) teacher and other professionals who provide specialized services consult with and advise the early education staff. They may also arrange or provide staff development activities. In the itinerant teacher model, the ECSE teacher and other specialized personnel visit the classroom on a regular basis. The ECSE teacher works with the team to develop

FIGURE 10.2   Example of matrix planning format

Weekly Planning Matrix

Child's name: _Josie_   Date:

Team Members Present: _Judy, Denise, Ferrell, and Christy_

Schedule	Behavior Target(s) in Routine/Activity	Environmental Arrangement	Instructional Strategies	Peer Support Strategies
Arrival/Free Play	Indicate (point + vocal) desired toy or center	Preferred toys placed out of reach	Time delay Modeling	Peers model toy and center requests
Morning Circle	Raise hand ("here"); gestures for songs	Place Josie between Ashley and Alice	Interrupt the routine Visual prompts Modeling	Peer modeling— Ashley and Jason
Art/Small Groups	Take turns and request (point + vocal) materials	Cut/paste activity Provide inadequate portions	Time delay Modeling Mand-Model	Cooperative learning structure
Transition	Participate in cleanup		Verbal prompt Physical assistance	Peer assistance Peer modeling
Bathroom	Follow the toileting and washing routines	Pull-up pants	Describe actions as performed + Partial physical assistance	
Outdoor Play	Request shoes Make play choices Take turns with buggy	Swing seat Wheel toys	Time delay Modeling Mand-mode	Peer (Ashley) to initiate play requests
Storytime	Respond to action requests in the story	Big books Other props	Verbal prompts Partial physical prompts	Peer (Alice) modeling
Bathroom	Follow the toileting and washing routines	Pull-up pants	Describe actions as performed + Partial physical assistance	
Lunch	Request choice of drink and food	Inadequate portions Food in plastic containers	Modeling Time delay	Peer (Ashley) modeling
Cleanup	Place containers in can		Verbal prompts Modeling	Peer modeling
Preparation for Home	Request help with sweater/coat Wave good-bye		Time delay Physical prompts	Peer modeling

IEPs for the children with disabilities. Itinerant teachers also work with the ECE teacher to establish activities and experiences that support acquisition of the IEP objectives and they may model specialized procedures and/or provide some direct services to the child or children with disabilities. However, the ECE teacher has the primary responsibility for following through with activities in the class.

Finally, a third model for inclusion is co-teaching (also called cooperative teaching). In the co-teaching model the ECSE teacher and the early childhood education (ECE) teacher plan together and share all teaching responsibilities. These classrooms often combine a public school-sponsored ECSE class and a Head Start class. The teaching team typically includes an ECE teacher, an ECSE teacher, and at least two aides or assistants, with consultation and some direct services provided by specialized professionals as required.

CHILDREN FROM CULTURALLY AND LINGUISTICALLY DIVERSE POPULATIONS

It is not difficult to imagine how confused and disturbed young children must feel when their earliest communication efforts are not recognized and valued. Sometimes, in their first experiences outside the family, people may even treat them as if they "do not have language."

Over the past several decades, there have been a number of descriptors used for second-language learners. The term *Limited English Proficient (LEP),* which was used in the nineties, is no longer in favor because it emphasizes what the child does *not* know rather than the positive aspects of bilingualism. The preferred term at the present time is *Potentially English Proficient (PEP)* (Quinones-Eatman, 2001). Preschoolers will learn English when they enter a classroom where English is spoken but it is equally important for them to continue the development of their native language and become bilingual individuals. This will happen *if* the home language is valued and incorporated into the curriculum.

Any disability that limits performance in the child's first language will also affect acquisition and performance in the second language. There is no support for the notion that linguistically diverse students who are academically at-risk should be exposed to as much English as possible (Quinones-Eatman, 2001). Some few may acquire the second language with maximum exposure but most will not succeed unless both languages are embedded in a meaningful communicative context with accommodations for the effects of their disabilities.

The needs of very young children with disabilities who come to the preschool or early intervention setting with limited English and limited knowledge of the content, roles, and rules common to such settings are especially challenging. The issue is not so much English-only instruction versus instruction that uses both English and non-English languages, as it is with older populations. In early childhood education, the issue is how to meet children's developmental needs. The challenges are: (1) how to make them feel emotionally secure, and (2) how to establish and maintain meaningful communication (Barrera, 1993). To feel emotionally secure, children must be able to express themselves as they have learned to at home. To learn, they must be able to understand the language being used around them.

Children cannot be expected to benefit from instruction that uses language to provide information and teach abstract concepts until their communication skills are well developed (Barrera, 1993). There should be a clear distinction between the development of language and the use of language as a medium for instruction. When children are learning language (either a first language or a second language), the emphasis should be on learning and practicing basic communication skills. Once the language system of these children is developed sufficiently, then they are ready to deal with the more complex demands of communication for learning.

How families interact with their children and the prelinguistic skills that develop from these interactions can be quite different across cultures (Richman, Miller, & LeVine, 1992). When working with young children from culturally and linguistically diverse populations, it is important to draw teaching materials directly from their homes and communities and capitalize on the communication skills that they bring to school, regardless of whether these skills are in English or in another language (Williams & De Gaetano, 1985). All children will see that community living is a balance between the needs of the individual and the needs of the group and that there are many ways to create and maintain that balance.

Quality inclusive preschool programs are structured to ensure that all of the children in the class are familiar with classroom routines and have ample opportunity to express themselves (whether they are fluent in English or not). Preschools may be more favorable settings for acquisition of a second language than elementary classrooms because most activities are child-initiated and children have almost continuous opportunities and encouragement to interact with one another and with the teachers.

Most important in classrooms that include children who are PEP is to be sure that verbal behavior is paired with gestures, actions, and/or directed gaze. The following strategies are useful and effective with these children:

- indicate acceptance and approval through warm smiles and greetings;
- respond to *all* verbal and nonverbal communication efforts;

- repeat directions without exaggerating tone or volume;
- talk about the "here and now";
- gently and sensitively expand and extend the child's utterances, taking into consideration the child's receptive and expressive capabilities in English;
- encourage the child in a sensitive manner to progress from non-verbal communication to verbal attempts at communication;
- revise and calmly restate your utterances until you are certain that they are understood;
- maintain set routines to make it easier for children to anticipate what is expected of them.

SUMMARY

This chapter began with an overview of the benefits of inclusion at the preschool level. Arguably, most important of these benefits is the opportunity to observe, learn, and practice age-appropriate social, communication, and cognitive skills. There is no way that these benefits can be simulated in environments that do not include nondisabled peers. I then discussed strategies for enhancing the benefits of inclusive settings. Specifically, I provided ways to increase opportunities to elicit language and communication by judicious environmental arrangement, and prudent selection and use of routines and activities. Procedures for enhanced milieu teaching and peer support strategies were described in some detail, followed by an overview of ecological assessment and matrix planning. The last section of the chapter discussed children from culturally and linguistically diverse populations. Intervention for this population is dealt with in depth in Chapter 14.

DISCUSSION QUESTIONS

1. The chapter states that learning experiences should be arranged along a continuum according to degree of intrusiveness when deciding which instructional approaches to try first. Why? What is the rationale for this recommendation?
2. Johnny is a 4-year-old boy with a speech and language delay. He loves playing with cars and trucks. What interventions would you use to promote his speech and language?
3. What is individualization? How do you go about individualizing the curriculum for a particular child?
4. Discuss the three types of collaborative teaching models for inclusive preschool classrooms. Give a rationale for selecting one over the other.

5. Discuss the challenges of teaching children who are PEP. What can you do in a classroom to facilitate their overall growth and development?

REFERENCES

Alpert, C. L., & Kaiser, A. P. (1992). Training parents as milieu language teachers. *Journal of Early Intervention, 16,* 31–52.

Bandura, A. (1969). *Principles of behavior modification.* New York: Holt, Rinehart & Winston.

Barrera, I. (1993). Effective and appropriate instruction for all children: The challenge of cultural/linguistic diversity and young children with special needs. *Topics in Early Childhood Special Education, 13,* 461–487.

Bredekamp, S., & Copple, C. (1997). *Developmentally appropriate practice in early childhood programs* (Rev. ed.). Washington, DC: National Association for the Education of Young Children.

Bredekamp, S., & Rosegrant, T. (1992). *Reaching potentials: Appropriate curriculum and assessment for young children* (Vol. 1). Washington, DC: National Association for the Education of Young Children.

Bricker, D., & Cripe, J. (1992). *An activity-based approach to early intervention.* Baltimore: Brookes.

Brown, W. H., McEvoy, M. A., & Bishop, N. (1991). Incidental teaching of social behavior. *Teaching Exceptional Children, 24,* 35–38.

Brown, W. H., Ragland, E. V., & Fox, J. J. (1988). Effects of group socialization procedures on the social interactions of preschool children. *Research in Developmental Disabilities, 9,* 359–376.

DEC recommended practices: Indicators of quality in programs for infants and young children with special needs and their families. (1993). Reston, VA: Division for Early Childhood of the Council for Exceptional Children.

Demchak, M. A., & Drinkwater, L. (1992). Preschoolers with severe disabilities: The case against segregation. *Topics in Early Childhood Special Education, 11,* 70–83.

Feeney, S., Christensen, D., & Moravcik, E. (2000). *Who am I in the lives of children?* (6th ed.). Columbus, Ohio: Merrill/Prentice-Hall.

Fewell, R. R., & Oelwein, P. L. (1990). The relationship between time in integrated environments and developmental gains in young children with special needs. *Topics in Early Childhood Special Education, 10,* 104–116.

Gallagher, T. M. (1991). Language and social skills: Implications for clinical assessment and intervention with school-age children. In T. M. Gallagher (Ed.), *Pragmatics of language: Clinical practice issues* (pp. 11–14). San Diego: Singular.

Goldstein, J., Kaczmarek, L., Pennington, R., & Shafer, K. (1992). Peer-mediated intervention: Attending to, commenting on, and acknowledging the behavior of preschoolers with autism. *Journal of Applied Behavior Analysis, 25,* 289–305.

Guralnick, M. J., & Groom, J. M. (1988). Peer interactions in mainstreamed and specialized classrooms: A comparative analysis. *Exceptional Children, 5,* 415–425.

Halle, J. W., Alpert, C., & Anderson, S. (1984). Natural environment language assessment and intervention with severely impaired preschoolers. *Topics in Early Childhood Special Education, 4,* 1–14.

Hemmeter, M. L., & Kaiser, A. P. (1994). Enhanced milieu teaching: Effects of parent-implemented language intervention. *Journal of Early Intervention, 18,* 269–89.

Hunt, P., & Goetz, L. (1988). Teaching spontaneous communication in natural settings through interrupted behavior chains. *Topics in Language Disorders, 9,* 58–71.

Hunt, P., Goetz, L., Alwell, M., & Sailor, W. (1986). Using an interrupted chain strategy to teach generalized communication responses. *Journal of the Association for Persons with Severe Handicaps, 11,* 196–207.

Johnson, D. W., & Johnson, R. T. (1991). *Learning together and alone: Cooperation, competition, and individualization* (3rd ed.). Englewood Cliffs, NJ: Prentice-Hall.

Johnson, R. T., & Johnson D. W. (1994). An overview of cooperative learning. In J. S. Thousand, R. A. Villa, & A. I. Nevin (Eds.), *Creativity and collaborative learning: A practical guide to empowering students and teachers* (pp. 31–44). Baltimore: Brookes.

Kaiser, A. P. (1993). Parent-implemented language intervention. In A. P. Kaiser & D. B. Gray (Eds.), *Enhancing children's communication:* Vol. 2. *Research foundations for intervention* (pp. 63–84). Baltimore: Brookes.

Kaiser, A. P., Ostrosky, M. M., & Alpert, C. L. (1993). Training teachers to use environmental arrangement and milieu teaching with nonvocal preschool children. *Journal of the Association for Persons with Severe Handicaps, 18,* 188–199.

Lamorey, S., & Bricker, D. D. (1993). Integrated programs: Effects on young children and their parents. In C. A. Peck, S. L. Odom, & D. D. Bricker (Eds.), *Integrating young children with disabilities into community programs* (pp. 249–270). Baltimore: Brookes.

Linder, T. W. (1990). *Transdisciplinary play-based assessment.* Baltimore: Brookes.

Linder, T. W. (1993). *Transdisciplinary play-based intervention.* Baltimore: Brookes.

Lipsky, D. K., & Gartner, A. (1997). *Inclusion and school reform: Transforming America's classrooms.* Baltimore: Brookes.

Mahoney, G., & Powell, A. (1986). Maternal communication style with mentally retarded children. *American Journal of Mental Deficiency, 92,* 352–359.

McGee, G. G., Krantz, P. J., & McClannahan, L. E. (1985). The facilitative effects of incidental teaching on preposition use by autistic children. *Journal of Applied Behavior Analysis, 18,* 17–31.

Miller, L., Strain, P., McKinley, J., Heckathorn, K., & Miller, S. (1993). *Preschool placement decisions: Are they predictors of future placements?* ERIC Reproduction Number 360-771. Pittsburgh, PA: Research Institute on Preschool Mainstreaming.

Montgomery, J. (1995). Inclusion, observation, outcome. *ASHA, 37,* 7.

Nordquist, V. M., Twardosz, S., & McEvoy, M. A. (1991). Effects of environmental reorganization in classrooms for children with autism. *Journal of Early Intervention, 15,* 135–152.

Odom, S. L., & McEvoy, M. (1988). Integration of young children with handicaps and normally developing children. In S. Odom & M. Karnes (Eds.), *Early intervention for infants and children with handicaps: An empirical base* (pp. 241–268). Baltimore: Brookes.

Odom, S. L., & Strain, P. S. (1984). Classroom-based social skills instruction for severely handicapped preschool children. *Topics in Early Childhood Special Education, 4,* 97–116.

Ostrosky, M. M., & Kaiser, A. P. (1991). Preschool classroom environments to promote communication. *Teaching Exceptional Children, 23,* 6–10.

Ostrosky, M. M., Kaiser, A. P., & Odom, A. L. (1993). Facilitating children's social-communicative interactions through the use of peer-mediated interventions. In A. P. Kaiser & D. B. Gray (Eds.), *Communication and language intervention services: Vol. 2: Enhancing children's communication: Research foundation for intervention* (pp. 159–185). Baltimore: Brookes.

Paul, L. (1985). Programming peer support for functional language. In S. Warren & A. K. Rogers-Warren (Eds.), *Teaching functional language* (pp. 289–307). Austin, TX: PRO-ED.

Peck, C., Odom, S., & Bricker, D. (Eds.). (1993). *Integrating young children with disabilities into community programs: Ecological perspectives on research and implementation.* Baltimore: Brookes.

Quinones-Eatman, J. (2001). *Preschool second language acquisition: What we know and how we can effectively communicate with young second language learners.* (CLAS Technical Report #5). Champaign, IL: University of Illinois at Urbana-Champaign, Early Childhood Research Institute on Culturally and Linguistically Appropriate Services.

Richman, A. L., Miller, P. M., & LeVine, R. A. (1992). Cultural and educational variables in maternal responsiveness. *Developmental Psychology, 28,* 614–621.

Schwartz, I. (1998, February). *Current findings of two early childhood research institutes.* Paper presented at the OSEP's Early Childhood Project Directors' Meeting, Arlington, WA.

Skinner, B. F. (1957). *Verbal Behavior.* New York: Appleton-Century-Crofts.

Strain, P. (1990). Least restrictive environment for preschool children with handicaps: What we know, what we should be doing. *Journal of Early Intervention, 14,* 291–296.

Strain, P., & Odom, S. L. (1986). Peer social initiations: Effective interventions for social skills development of exceptional children. *Exceptional Children, 52,* 543–551.

Tannock, R. M., & Girolametto, L. (1992). Reassessing parent-focused language intervention programs. In S. Warren & J. Reichle (Eds.), *Communication and language intervention: Vol. 1: Causes and effects in communication and language intervention* (pp. 49–79). Baltimore: Brookes.

Twardosz, S., Nordquist, V. M., Simon, R., & Botkins, D. (1983). The effect of group affection activities on the interaction of socially isolated children. *Analysis and Intervention in Developmental Disabilities, 13,* 311–338.

Warren, S. F., & Gazdag, G. (1990). Facilitating early language development with milieu procedure. *Journal of Early Intervention, 14,* 62–86.

Weistuch, L., & Lewis, M. (1985). The language interaction project. *Analysis and Intervention in Developmental Disabilities, 5,* 97–106.

Williams, L. R., & De Gaetano Y. (1985). ALERTA: A multicultural, bilingual approach to teaching young children. Reading, MA: Addison-Wesley.

Windsor, J. (1995). Language impairment and social competence. In M. E. Fey, J. Windsor, & S. F. Warren (Eds.), *Language intervention: Preschool through the elementary years* (pp. 213–240.) Baltimore: Brookes.

CHAPTER 11

Children with Culturally Diverse Backgrounds

Betty H. Bunce

Maria is informed that she will have a new child, José, in her first-grade classroom. José and his family have newly immigrated from Mexico and speak Spanish in the home. José has only limited proficiency in English. His vocabulary consists of a few words such as Coke, hamburger, car, hi, bye, and please. José will be the only child with a native language that differs from English in Maria's classroom. Marie is monolingual in English and has never taught a child who speaks a language other than English. Her immediate dilemmas are how best to incorporate José into the classroom and how to meet his language and academic needs while continuing to meet the needs of her 24 other students.

José is six years old and a competent speaker of Spanish. He has had one semester of schooling in Mexico. He is eager to learn about his new country, but, at the same time, apprehensive about his new school. José's dilemmas are how to gain acceptance in his new school, how to learn English, and how to do the academic work required of monolingual speakers of English.

With an estimated 2.5 million school-age immigrants in the mid 1990s increasing to a possible 9 million by 2010 (Fix & Passel, 1994; Jennings, 1988), this kind of scenario occurs and will continue to occur throughout the United States. In some cases, the class may have several language minority children from a variety of language and socioeconomic backgrounds. In other cases, there will be bilingual teachers and bilingual programming for several students of one language background. Another variation involves older children who may or may not have achieved facility in English and/or academic work. Still a different scenario is the child who is language-disordered in his first and/or second language. In any case, some of the concerns are the same. The teacher needs to be able to facilitate the language and academic achievement of the child, and the child needs to be accepted in the classroom and achieve both linguistic and academic competence.

This chapter addresses two specific concerns: how to facilitate the linguistic and academic achievement of the bilingual/bicultural child, and how to identify and provide the needed special programming for the bilingual child with a language impairment. There are several issues affecting both of these concerns. These issues are discussed at length in the following sections: (1) philosophies regarding second-language learning; (2) sociocultural factors; (3) language proficiency and academic achievement; (4) types of programs and instructional tactics; and (5) assessment and intervention.

Philosophies Regarding Second-Language Learning

Lindfors (1987) has delineated two viewpoints regarding the learning of a second language that have important educational implications. One approach, the audiolingual method, focuses on automatic mastery of utterance form. The second approach focuses on communication or on achieving communicative competence. Although people favoring the audiolingual method consider communication to be an eventual goal, an underlying assumption is that the second-language learner needs to develop some language structure and then learn to communicate. On the other hand, people favoring the communication viewpoint assume that such separation between form and use is not possible. They believe that the first language is learned in interactive contexts and that the second language is best acquired in the same manner. In both cases, beliefs about language learning affect teaching strategies and expectations.

For the audiolingual approach, oral pattern practice is an important instructional procedure. This is accomplished through structured drill with immediate correction of errors. The learner must memorize and recite sentences or passages as part of the drill. Procedures to facilitate the shift to a communicative situation are provided after practice on correct production of form. Correct phonological production is often emphasized. Therefore, much time is spent on discrimination activities between phonological systems of the first and second language. Sometimes the emphasis may be on sounds used in the second language, but not in the first. A major assumption involved in the audiolingual approach is that language learning is broken down into parts and practiced, and then the pieces are put together again. A second assumption of the audiolingual method is that the first language can interfere with the learning of the second language. Therefore, prohibitions against using the first language may be made. Finally, the audiolingual method emphasizes speech production.

Proponents of communicative competence place emphasis on communication from the beginning. This viewpoint assumes that language form and use cannot be separated; therefore, it is more global and context-oriented. Wholes are not broken down into parts (at least initially). Instructional procedures would emphasize interactive meaningful experiences rather than controlled pattern practice on correct form. Errors in form are tolerated, and corrections are made only if communication breaks down. Comprehension of language is emphasized and usually precedes production (see Krashen & Terrill, 1983, for further elaboration of the natural approach to second-language learning, particularly in classroom settings).

The communicative competence point of view is similar to prevailing views of how children acquire their first language (e.g., Bates, 1976; Berko-Gleason, 1993) and to the interactionist perspective as presented in this text. It is assumed that the children will acquire the rules of the second language much as they acquired rules in the first language. That is, through being immersed in the context, the child will construct novel sentences to communicate intent. A second assumption is that the child will adopt some of the same strategies used in acquiring the first language, so that overgeneralizations of rules and overextensions of vocabulary may occur. However, the first language is not expected to interfere with the learning of the second.

The two viewpoints represent the end points on a learning style scale. The audiolingual method utilizes a bottom-up approach, whereas communicative competence uses a top-down approach. The two viewpoints can also be divided on how language proficiency is perceived. The audiolingual (or interference) view appears to suggest that there are two distinct proficiencies that can interfere with each other (cf. Lado, 1957). The communicative competence position suggests one general language proficiency that can be represented by two different surface forms (Cummins, 1979, 1984).

In summary, these two positions or philosophies of second-language learning lead to different kinds of policies regarding instructional methods. The audiolingual favors pattern practice of correct oral productions, practice on parts before insertion into whole, sequential linear learning, and little facilitation of first-language usage. The communicative competence method favors using the second language within meaningful communicative situations, allows errors of form, starts with the global and then proceeds to parts, and supports further development of the first language. The focus in this chapter is on *facilitating communicative competence* of bilingual/bicultural children.

SOCIOCULTURAL FACTORS

A child learning English as a second language brings to the task knowledge of her first language and myriad other cultural and personal factors. These cultural and personal factors can affect the academic achievement of the child. Many of the factors contribute to academic achievement (e.g., broader understanding of concepts underlying word meanings, ability to analyze linguistic structure, broader understanding of different ways of interacting). However, other factors may be less positive due to what Iglesias (1985b) calls communication mismatch between teacher and child. This mismatch is due to linguistic differences and misunderstandings in ways of interacting. Teachers need to be aware of possible causes of communication failure in the school environment in order to circumvent misunderstandings and to facilitate academic achievement and acceptance of the bilingual/bicultural child in the school system. Teachers must be aware of their own cultural ways of interacting and how these may affect children who do not share their culture or language. Lynch and Hanson (1992) provide a summary of different cultures' beliefs, values, and practices as contrasted to the mainstream culture. For example, some cultures place importance on the group needs versus individual needs; some value observation as a way of learning versus overt explanations; still others may be less time-oriented than the mainstream culture. These overviews can help teachers and other professionals gain cross-cultural competence, at least in the broad sense of recognizing different ways of communicating, teaching, and learning. Teachers need to respect these differences as differences and not deficiencies.

Saville-Troike (1979) described the culture of the American school as one that "serves primarily to prepare middle-class children to participate in their own culture" (p. 141). This means that the classroom interactions extend to interactions already familiar to middle-class children. For example, these children are familiar with "test questions," where the adult asks a question, the child responds, and the adult then evaluates the appropriateness of the response ("What color is the box?" "Brown," "That's right"). To some children learning English as a second language, this is a peculiar interaction because adults in their culture do not ask questions about something they already know.

To the monolingual, monocultural teacher, this classroom conversation is a natural, obvious way to facilitate the learning of students. However, awareness that this interaction may not be a natural way of interacting for all students will help the teacher locate possible areas of confusion. The child's failure to respond may be due not to lack of knowledge, but to differences in styles of interaction. The child may be more familiar with learning by observation and indicating knowledge through demonstration. The child may also not be accustomed to responding individually or to the group at large.

How turn-taking is achieved in a classroom may also be an area of cultural difference. Raising a hand before responding may be strange to some children. It also may limit who responds to the teacher's questions or participates in the activities. Differential demands placed on students due to teacher expectations may also be a factor. For example, classroom interaction literature has indicated that teachers allow less time for responses to students they perceive as being low achievers (Rowe, 1969) and provide more explicit elicitations for high achievers (Cherry, 1978). Reasonable response time and explicit elicitations need to be provided to all children. By providing more explicit cues or by modeling a problem-solving procedure the teacher can teach more than just content. The students learn what are the important features of a problem and how to analyze a situation. They also learn what kind of response is expected.

Iglesias (1985a) also notes that children must learn to use language differently in different situations with different tasks and teachers. Heath (1986) suggests that success depends less on the specific language the children know and more on how they use the language they know. She lists some common teacher expectations of children's language use, which include the ability to: (1) use language to label and describe events; (2) participate in a test question format, in which the teacher asks a question, the child responds, and the teacher evaluates the response; (3) use language to recount past events or information in a predictable format and order; (4) use language to request and clarify information; and (5) follow oral and written directions with little sustained adult supervision. These expectations may not be realistic for all children, particularly children whose culture and language may be different from the teacher's. Therefore, the teacher needs to consider some of the assumptions behind classroom routine and recognize areas of possible conflict. The teacher may also need to provide more explicit examples or cues, to vary the way information is elicited, and to provide alternative ways to respond. Other aspects of school culture may also be unfamiliar. For example time, space, and materials are highly organized. A sequence of time blocks structures each day. Desks and other classroom furniture are usually organized in a linear fashion, either in rows or with several desks forming blocklike units. Areas of the room are designated for certain activities. Children are also organized into lines for moving outside of classrooms or into homogeneous (top, middle, bottom) groups for reading and other academic instruction.

The linearity of organization of time, space, and materials may not be difficult for a child from the mainstream culture who is accustomed to schedules and to using materials in prescribed ways. However, there are cultures within as well as outside the United States in which such order is not natural (cf. Garcia, 1992; Heath, 1983; Iglesias, 1985b). Thus, the organization and use of materials in a step-wise fashion may be inexplicable to a child who is accustomed to a more holistic, active, or associative learning style. The materials themselves may be unfamiliar and threatening. Children unfamiliar with boundaries around time, space, and materials may have difficulty adjusting to the school environment.

Individual differences in social interaction style may also be a factor in the acquisition of a second language. Children who are outgoing and who are allowed to interact with peers can increase the amount of meaningful input they receive. This in turn increases their second-language learning by providing additional practice in both comprehending and producing the new language. Some children make good use of a few routine phrases in order to initiate and maintain the interaction. Although many of the good second-language learners described by Wong-Fillmore (1983) were socially outgoing, another group also achieved good oral language skill: active observers. These children were participants, but their participation did not necessarily include being talkative. Other scholars have also noted that some children learning a second language have a silent period before they begin talking in the second language (Bunce, 1995; Tabors & Snow, 1994). Bunce estimated that the length of the silent period for some of the children in their program was three to five months. Teachers need to be aware of these individual differences in language-learning style and to provide opportunities for interaction and for observation of meaningful, comprehensible input within the classroom.

In summary, not all communication mismatches are due to linguistic differences and not every child knows the instruction conversational style. In addition, not all students learn best through individual instruction and responses or from a part-to-whole sequence. School linear organizational style may be unfamiliar and threatening to children. When there are sociocultural differences between teachers and children, there are many opportunities for miscommunication and for erroneous assessments of children's skills to occur (Garcia, 1992). Being aware of these possible areas of difficulty will help the teacher make adjustments and/or provide the necessary support to help the bilingual/bicultural child succeed. Teachers will need to find instructional methods that encourage children to learn both English and academic skills.

LANGUAGE PROFICIENCY AND ACADEMIC ACHIEVEMENT

Proficiency in language is difficult to determine. It is not an all-or-nothing situation, but rather a gradual process. One concern is the level of proficiency in the second language that is needed for the child to succeed academically. Studies of the French immersion programs indicate that students not only achieved proficiency in French and English but also reached high levels of academic achievement (Lambert & Tucker, 1972). Baetens-Beardsmore and Swain (1985) also document academic achievement by bilingual children attending various types of schools in Europe. Other scholars have documented the cognitive advantages to being bilingual (e.g., Ben Zeev, 1977; Ianco-Worral, 1972).

However, while positive effects of bilingualism are being documented, many bilingual children are not experiencing academic success (Cortes, 1986; Cummins, 1984; Iglesias, 1985a). Cummins suggests that a level of proficiency is needed before the cognitive advantages of being bilingual are realized. In addition, there are different kinds of language proficiencies. For example, some second-language learners have good oral language skills and yet do not succeed academically.

Cummins (1984) describes two language proficiencies that help explain the differences in achievement: *basic interpersonal communicative skills (BICS)* and *cognitive/academic language proficiency (CALP)*. To help explain the differences, Cummins conceptualizes language proficiency along two continuums. The first continuum concerns the amount of environmental or contextual support. At one end is context-embedded language where the language is supported by paralinguistic and situational cues. The other end is context-reduced language where the linguistic cues themselves must carry the message. Much of everyday conversation involves context-embedded language, whereas the language of the classroom is closer to the context-reduced end of the continuum.

The second continuum concerns levels of cognitive involvement in performing communicative tasks. At the top (this continuum is placed vertically) are relatively undemanding and largely automatic tasks requiring little cognitive involvement, while at the bottom are cognitively demanding communicative tasks. It is possible for a communicative task to be cognitively undemanding and context-embedded (e.g., routine greeting), or cognitively undemanding and context-reduced (e.g., writing a letter to a friend), or context-embedded and cognitively demanding (e.g., persuading another to your point of view), or both context-reduced and cognitively demanding (e.g., writing a research paper).

Chamot (1981, cited in Cummins, 1984) differentiates between BICS and CALP using Bloom's taxonomy (Bloom & Krathwohl, 1977). BICS involves *knowledge, comprehension* (basic understanding), and *application* (use in a particular concrete situation). CALP involves higher level cognitive skills of *analysis* (breaking down wholes into parts), *synthesis* (putting elements into a whole), and *evaluation* (judging adequacy of ideas).

Cummins's conceptualizations regarding BICS and CALP are important. Because children can converse in context-embedded situations does not mean they have the language skills needed to succeed in a decontextualized academic setting. It should be noted, however, that a person may have good academic language skills in the second language but not good oral interpersonal skills (as well as vice versa). This usually occurs when the CALP skills are already developed in the first language, as in the adult's learning a second language. It may be that BICS and CALP have somewhat independent development. This would mean that academic training does not depend on first developing oral language skills. Wong-Fillmore (1985) notes that immersion programs have shown that it is possible to develop academic and second-language skills simultaneously.

Cummins (1979, 1984) suggests that first- and second-language academic skills are interdependent. He conceptualizes a "dual iceberg" representation of bilingual proficiency. A common underlying proficiency can be represented by surface features of either language. Therefore, it should be relatively easy to transfer academic knowledge from one language to the other. He provides some evidence for this from studies of bilingual immersion programs.

In summary, because a child can use language in oral conversations does not mean the child can use language proficiently in an academic situation. If a general proficiency is represented by two surface forms, then developing academic skills in the child's first language should transfer to the child's second language. Pflaum (1986) describes just such an occurrence. In any case, educators must plan for acquisition of both kinds of language skills.

TYPES OF PROGRAMS AND INSTRUCTIONAL TACTICS

A variety of educational programs and settings have been devised to meet the needs of children who are learning English as a second language. In *immersion programs,* students are placed in classes where the instruction is in their second language. The classes consist of students at a similar level of proficiency in the language of instruction. The teacher is usually bilingual and knowledgeable about the culture of the students (cf. Lambert & Tucker, 1972, for description of French/English Immersion programs). Bilingualism is an educational goal in the immersion programs.

In the United States there are a variety of bilingual programs where the students use some combination of their first and second languages. Richard-Amato (1988) lists three types of bilingual programs: transitional, maintenance, and enrichment. In transitional programs, students learn most of the subject matter in their first language until they are ready to be placed into an all-English class. In the maintenance programs, students continue to have part of their education in their first language throughout their school years. In the enrichment programs, students are taught a second language to broaden cultural horizons or for some future visit to a foreign country (typical foreign language classes taught in junior or senior high school and usually not designed for language-minority groups).

Other types of programming for language-minority students involve submersion into the mainstream classroom with or without some support from English as a second language (ESL) classes. The educational goal is to enhance English and academic skills. There is no emphasis on the first language, though it may be used to teach some of the content. The ESL classes are similar to the transitional bilingual classes where the emphasis is on learning English for eventual placement in all English classes. Placement in special ESL classes may range from a few weeks to two or three years, depending on the school system involved and the student's proficiency in English.

Richard-Amato (1988) suggests that optimal programming for ESL students might be to combine ESL classes with various levels of mainstreaming. Students at beginning levels would be mainstreamed into courses in music, art, and physical education. High school courses might include home economics and industrial arts. During intermediate levels, more mainstream classes would be added but the remainder of the core courses would be taught in the first language. The advanced student would be mainstreamed into most subjects, though some classes might utilize what Richard-Amato calls *"sheltered" English* (p. 224). Sheltered English is an instructional approach that is used to make academic instruction in English understandable to students who speak a language other than English (Freeman, Freeman, & Gonzales, 1987). The students are "sheltered" in that they do not compete academically with native English speakers because the class includes only second-language learners. Teaching strategies would include using many extralingusitic cues such as props, visual aids, and body language. Additional strategies would employ linguistic cues such as the use of repetition and pauses, short sentences, and frequent comprehension checks. Some of the "sheltered" English strategies are similar to "motherese" strategies (e.g., repetition, short sentences, emphasis on joint attention, focus on comprehension, etc.) used to facilitate the acquisition of a first language.

A major problem for school districts is that only one or two students may speak any given language, and it is not feasible to hire bilingual teachers for only a few students. Also, qualified bilingual teachers may be difficult to find. Therefore, the teachers of ESL classes may be monolingual, but have special training in working with bilingual students. In this case the special programming would not include core content taught in the students' first language. Richard-Amato (1988) suggests that the mainstream classroom can be an appropriate environment for second-language acquisition if comprehensible, meaningful input is provided.

Programming for the individual student might take a variety of forms. For example, if José (returning to the case example in the introduction) was in a bilingual program, the instruction would be in Spanish for at least part of the day. Reading instruction might be in both languages. The more successful bilingual programs usually provide half-day or alternate day programs in which one language is used at a time. This is in contrast to programs that provide ongoing translations or an alternating back and forth between the two languages (Richard-Amato, 1988). Good communication between the bilingual teacher and the mainstream classroom teacher is needed. For example, Diaz, Moll and Mehan (1986) describe children who were at different reading levels in Spanish, but were put in the lowest reading groups in their English reading class. Much of what was demanded in English groups was letter-sound connections with little context support (CALP skills involving analysis, synthesis, and evaluation). With this type of instruction, all of the students appeared to be at the same low reading level. However, when tested on comprehension, many of the students demonstrated that they understood what they read in English in spite of their halting oral reading. The type of instruction did not reveal what some of the students were able to read and understand. Diaz and colleagues (1986) advocate using a bilingual reading approach that includes a focus on writing. For example, the child may dictate a story that is written down by the teacher and subsequently read her dictated story. Later on, the children can write their own stories using invented spellings, if necessary. The focus on writing allows active interaction within a specific context. All of these activities allow a pairing of BICS and CALP skills so that the child's knowledge is extended within a meaningful framework.

If José were in an ESL program with some mainstreaming into the regular classroom, then all instruction would be in English. ESL instruction would probably involve training vocabulary and syntactic structure in both comprehension and production. In addition, some tutoring of academic subjects may be included in the ESL instruction. In the first-grade classroom, the teacher, Maria, would focus on ways to integrate José into the classroom, to communicate with him, and to effectively teach him the academic content. Specific objectives might be: (1) to provide José with opportunities to interact with peers and teachers within a communication situation; (2) to increase his oral language skills; (3) to increase his literacy skills; and (4) to extend his knowledge of math, social studies, science, and other content area subjects.

A variety of activities and procedures could be used to achieve these objectives. An underlying concept would be that *meaningful input is most effective.* Some of the following procedures, summarized in Table 11.1 and then further described, involve classroom manage-

TABLE 11.1   Increasing communication opportunities for bilingual students

What To Do	What It Is	How It Helps
1. Set up a buddy system.	Designate a classroom peer.	Someone is available to help ESL students find materials and other resources.
2. Focus on communication.	Use gestures and short sentences.	Use of nonlinguistic as well as linguistic knowledge helps comprehension.
3. Use role-playing to provide contextual support.	Act out situation or dramatic play scenarios.	Stimulates language use and increases knowledge.
4. Use peer teaching and modeling of responses.	Have a peer demonstrate activities and provide explanations.	ESL student may comprehend better and be more likely to imitate a peer.
5. Use group work and cooperative learning.	Children working on assignments or projects in groups (usually 2–5 children in each group).	Group work may be the norm for a particular culture and more comfortable for a particular child; also it provides opportunities for ESL students to contribute to a project.
6. Record instructions on audiotapes.	Make recordings of important information.	Tape allows for repetition of instructions; repetition can aid in understanding word boundaries.
7. Allow observations.	Let the ESL student observe without pressure to respond.	ESL students often need an "input" phase or silent period before producing a new language.
8. Provide descriptions.	Describe what the student is observing.	Helps the student learn both language content and form within a specific context.
9. Provide opportunities for speaking.	Provide small-group or one-to-one activities where it is easy for the ESL students to talk but where they are not pressured to do so.	Students may feel more comfortable talking in a small group where they can choose when to speak.
10. Accept simplified syntactic forms.	Allow short sentences that may or may not be grammatically correct. Use expansions or recasts to provide information on form.	The focus is on communicating not on grammar; however, the use of expansions and recasts can aid in the learning of correct grammatical forms.

(continued)

TABLE 11.1   Increasing communication opportunities for bilingual students (*continued*)

What To Do	What It Is	How It Helps
11. Use global holistic activities.	Holistic activities begin with a top-down focus, starting with the whole and proceeding to the parts.	Nonlinguistic knowledge as well as linguistic knowledge can more easily be used in holistic activities. If a structure is learned within a context, it is more likely to be used appropriately than if learned in isolation.
12. Teach literacy skills through a whole-language focus.	Whole-language activities involve listening, speaking, reading, and writing in an interactive rather than sequential manner.	Literacy activities such as reading and writing may be taught simultaneously with oral language.
13. Use tutors who speak the child's first language.	Designate a volunteer adult or classroom peer who knows the child's first language.	Tutors may translate information between teacher and child or between children so that the ESL student can communicate with others and continue to develop academically while learning English.
14. Make content area books available in the child's first language.	Use literature, math, social science, and science books written in the child's first language.	Helps advance the academic skills of the child who is literate in her first language and is in the process of learning English.
15. Provide reading materials in the ESL student's linguistic or cultural group.	Use stories written in English, where the protagonist is from the ESL student's linguistic or cultural group, and available to all children.	Helps provide all of the children in the classroom some knowledge about and appreciation for different cultures.

ment techniques that foster communication in the classroom. Other suggested techniques focus on how the academic content could be taught. Also, most of the activities are appropriate for the non-ESL student and can be done within the classroom to facilitate the learning of all students. A few of the techniques may be more easily achieved within a preschool or kindergarten class; however, it is important to find ways to increase communicative opportunities for bilingual students in any classroom.

1. **Set up a buddy system.** The buddy is someone, usually a peer, who can be available to help the ESL student find materials and

places, and in general be a resource person who is available to explain instructions and answer questions. At first, this may be achieved through nonverbal means such as gesturing, pointing, or demonstrating. Having a buddy or buddies will increase the amount of language interaction the ESL child receives. Some teachers use a buddy system routinely so that all students have a resource peer/partner with whom to check work, to brainstorm ideas for projects, to help edit writing, and the like.

2. **Focus on communication.** The teacher may need to use more gestures and demonstrations and avoid using overly complex sentence structure when talking. However, use of single words without contextual support is not suggested. The child needs to be able to use her nonlinguistic knowledge to help in understanding the new language.

3. **Use role-playing as a way to provide contextual support.** Dramatic play activities are especially rich environments to stimulate language. Also, acting out stories (or historical events) can help make what has been read comprehensible to the ESL student.

4. **Use peer teaching and modeling of responses.** During or after explanations be sure to include a peer demonstration of what is to be done. Provide several practices so that understanding of the concept will more likely occur. In some cases, explanations given by peers will be more effective.

5. **Use some group work and cooperative learning.** Group work can be a way to employ peer demonstration and teaching. For some children, group work is more appropriate to their home culture. It also provides an opportunity for ESL students to contribute to a project.

6. **Record instructions on audiotapes.** Sometimes repetition will allow the student time to figure out what the instruction means. In oral language, it is not always clear where word boundaries are, and sometimes repeated listening will aid this process. Also, for some center activities, it is helpful to have audio instructions paired with written instructions and/or illustrations.

7. **Allow the ESL student time to observe without pressure to respond.** Remember that many children learning a second language have a silent period before they begin speaking.

8. **Describe what the student is observing.** This may help the student learn both language content and form within a specific context. Observation of real situations is more effective than rote memorizing of surface forms.

9. **Provide opportunities for the ESL student to speak, but do not pressure her to do so.** This can probably best be achieved through small-group activities where the student may be more comfortable in responding. However, one-on-one conversations with the teacher may also be effective.

10. **Accept simplified syntactic forms.** Focus on what is being communicated. Make corrections only indirectly by expanding or recasting. Expansions are restatements that expand the utterance by using correct grammar (e.g., child says, "Boy walk house," teacher says, "Yes, the boy walks *to the* house"). Recasts retain the basic information while syntactic structure is altered (e.g., child says, "Boy walk house," teacher says, "You're right, the boy *is walking* to the house. Where will he walk next?"). In both cases the conversational topic is maintained. The purpose of the expansions and recasts is incidentally to provide a model but to keep the focus on the communication.

11. **Use global, holistic activities that focus on meaning before using part-to-whole activities.** Holistic activities begin with a top-down focus. That is, they present the whole and then proceed to the part. A sociodrama, or choral reading, or a summary of a story all provide an overview or more holistic presentation so that the child can use nonlinguistic knowledge to understand (cf. Anim-Addo, 1992, for a description of the use of sociodrama in a classroom). The lack of contextual support in many oral drills or worksheets makes it difficult to use nonlinguistic knowledge. Also, transfer of rotely learned forms to conversation is difficult.

12. **Teach literacy skills through whole-language activities.** Whole-language activities involve listening, speaking, reading, and writing in an interactive rather than sequential manner (cf. Goodman & Goodman, 1986; or Norris & Hoffman, 1993, for description of whole-language activities; or Huddleson, 1985, on using a six-level ESL series that provides oral and written communication activities). That is, the child does not have to first engage in listening, then speaking, then reading, then writing. Therefore, the teacher does not have to wait for good oral control of the English language before teaching reading and writing. Some examples of whole-language activities include:

   a. *Language-experience stories*. These are stories dictated by the student(s) and written down by the teacher, often on a chart for later reference. The story is based on a shared experience. Often these stories are written following field trips. However, any shared experience can be used (e.g, film, film strip, guest speaker, favorite recess activity, class science project, etc.). After the stories have been written, the group (or individual) reads them. Often the children copy the story and read it again to themselves. Children are able to decode the story because it is written in their own words.

   b. *Choral reading and/or poetry activities*. The class can participate in choral reading activities by reading in unison or by having different groups read different lines. Often ESL children can join in even if they do not know all of the words. Reading and writing activities involving poetry also can improve literacy skills. Songs and fingerplays are appropriate activities within preschool and kindergarten classes. ESL children may first participate during songs and fingerplay activities. The repetitiveness of these activities helps provide support for the interaction.

c. *Predictable books or stories.* These books have recurring lines that can be predicted from earlier presentations. Allow the children to join in with the reading. (See the Appendix at the end of the chapter for a list of various titles.)

d. *A story that is read and retold by puppets.* First, the teacher could manipulate the puppets, later the children could do this. The story could be audiotaped and the tape, book, and puppets made available so that the children could listen, read, and retell the story later. Writing materials could be made available for the children to write their own stories involving the puppets. Invented spellings would be acceptable. (See Seawall as cited in Lindfors, 1987, for description of this type of activity used in a bilingual kindergarten.)

e. *Other writing activities.* The students can keep a journal, write a story from a story starter (e.g., "I like to play with . . . "), write a caption to a picture, or write a story on a topic of their choice. In all cases invented spellings would be acceptable.

13. **Use tutors who speak the child's first language.** This is not always possible, but if there are personnel available, make use of their knowledge to extend the teacher's knowledge of the child's language and culture as well as helping the child in content areas and other subjects.

14. **Make content area books available in the child's first language.** This is particularly helpful for the older ESL students who have literacy skills in their first language.

15. **Provide reading materials in which the protagonist is from the ESL student's linguistic or culture group.** (See Pisant, 1992 for resources.)

These are just a few of the instructional tactics that may help the teacher provide appropriate language and academic activities for the ESL child (or children) in the classroom. Many of these activities are also appropriate for use with special ESL classes. Of course there are many other activities that can facilitate acquisition of literacy and language skills. Many of the activities in the basal readers are appropriate or can be easily adapted. Again, the more context support, the more likely the ESL student will understand. Hands-on math and science activities are also important in facilitating learning for the ESL student.

ASSESSMENT AND INTERVENTION

There are many assessment issues involving children who are learning English as a second language. Some of these issues revolve around the testing instruments themselves. Other issues concern the use of tests for placement in special programs. For example, appropriate placement in ESL programs, bilingual classes, and mainstream classes may be facilitated by some assessment of skill levels. Also, assessment of communication skills is important in identifying handicapped bilingual, bicultural children who are in need of more specialized programming. Assessment is also important is determining appropriate intervention and in documenting progress. Finally, assessment can provide information regarding the student's progress in English and academic skills.

The development of nonbiased procedures for assessing bilingual, bicultural children is difficult. A book edited by Hamayan and Damico (1991) is devoted to ways bias can be limited in the assessment of bilingual students. As described by these and other scholars, some standardized test measures are available, particularly for the Spanish-English bilingual (see Cheng, 1987; Cole & Snope, 1981; Deal & Yan, 1985; Hamayan and Damico, 1991; Mattes & Omark, 1984, for listings of testing instruments). However, not all of these instruments are appropriate for all dialects of a particular language. Also, some tests are direct translations from English, which may alter the way certain concepts are expressed in the first language. Furthermore, there may not be appropriate norms provided. Finally, cultural factors may influence the assessment process.

In evaluating assessment instruments, Mattes and Omark (1984) suggest that the examiner note such features as:

1. *The purposes and construction of the tests.* Are the tests appropriate for the population to be tested? Is the test based on a theoretical model?
2. *Linguistic and cultural appropriateness.* Is the dialect of the tests appropriate? Are the types of required tasks and stimuli appropriate for the population?
3. *Adequacy of the norms.* How was the test standardized and on what population? Is the normed population an appropriate comparison group?
4. *Reliability and validity of the test instruments.*

Cheng (1987) underscores that care must be taken to ensure that test items are familiar to the children. She suggests that household objects such as items for baking; some kinds of furniture; sports such as football, hockey, skiing; buildings and signs such as hospitals, traffic signs; and historical events and people such as Thanksgiving, Halloween, George Washington, and Abraham Lincoln would not be appropriate test items for Asian-language minority children. These items may also be inappropriate test items for other ESL children.

A variety of scholars (e.g., Bernstein, 1989; Chamberlain & Medeiros-Landurand 1991; Lewis, Vang, & Cheng, 1989) caution that there can be cultural influences on assessment. For example, Chamberlain and Medeiros-Landurand list such factors as problems due to cultural misconceptions of the roles and expectations of a particular task. Although some children consider the assessment process as one linked to evaluation and promotion and work hard to demonstrate what they have learned, other children may not consider the assessment process a part of the learning process and may be less motivated to demonstrate their knowledge. Also, there may be stereotyping due to differences in cultural behavior. Some children may appear inattentive and be labeled as having comprehension difficulties; yet, they may be attending to the task but in a manner different than that expected by the evaluator. For example, children may be paying attention to the evaluator but have their eyes lowered as a sign of respect. The evaluator may expect the student to pay attention by maintaining eye contact and, therefore, may think the child is not attending and perhaps does not understand the task. Other cultural factors that could impinge on the assessment process include differences in viewpoints on competition and cooperation (individual versus group success); time (some children may not understand "speed" testing); proximity (some children may find the formal relationship of the testing situation to be stressful); gender of the participants (some children may respond differently to female versus male evaluators); and cognitive style (some children may use a global, intuitive style rather than the reflective, analytical style valued in many educational testing situations).

Another issue concerns the type of assessment instruments. Many of the language tests available are discrete point tests, which focus on knowledge of specific elements of phonology, grammar, and vocabulary, rather than integrative tests, which examine the ability of the student to utilize several skills at the same time (Oller, 1979; Damico, 1991). Also, some tests require integrative skills and yet evaluate only discrete items (e.g., having students write an essay in which only certain grammatical forms are judged). As yet, no comprehensive standardized instruments exist for testing children who speak English as a second language.

A variety of remedies for the assessment dilemmas have been suggested. Some of these include development of local norms for standardized tests, development of teacher-made checklists, and the use of criterion-referenced tests. It may be that qualitative assessment of the children's language skills within naturalistic settings provides the most relevant information. In particular, Richard-Amato (1988) suggests that test tasks should relate to the classroom communication situations.

The placement of students in bilingual or ESL classes depends on many factors. One is the availability of such classes. Another factor is English-language proficiency of the students. A third factor is how this proficiency is assessed and what criteria are used for placement. Cummins (1984), in discussing the differences between basic interpersonal communicative skills (BICS) and cognitive/academic language proficiency (CALP), estimated that it may take only two years for a child learning to speak English as a second language to reach peer-appropriate conversational skills, but may take five to seven years for the same child to reach grade norms on the language skills needed for academic work. If the children are judged to have reached English proficiency based on their conversational skills alone, then they may be dismissed prematurely from ESL classes.

The decision on placement may be made by reviewing students' scores on such tests as the Bilingual Syntax Measure (Burt, Dulay, & Hernandez-Chavez, 1976), by students' performance on criterion-referenced tests such as Assessment of Basic Skills, Spanish Edition (Brigance, 1984), or by teacher checklists. Teacher-made tests may be the most effective because they may include items particularly relevant to a specific situation.

Richard-Amato (1988) describes a checklist that may be helpful in grouping students within a classroom setting or in determining types of placement. She provides a description of typical language behaviors of students at beginning, intermediate, and advanced levels of second-language proficiency in a classroom setting. Within each grouping she has three levels ranging from low to high. For example, typical behaviors exhibited by the low beginner would include dependence upon gestures, facial expression, pictures, and even a translator. The middle beginner would demonstrate some comprehension, but only when the speaker provides gestural clues, speaks slowly, and uses concrete referents. He may show some recognition of written segments, and may speak haltingly and be able to write short sentences. The high beginner may comprehend more in social conversation and may be able to make wants known, though with frequent errors in grammar, vocabulary, and pronunciation. The high beginner may be able to read a simple test and write short sentences. Richard-Amato continues the checklist format describing behavior for the intermediate and advanced students. Behavioral descriptions included for the intermediate levels are: (1) has difficulty with idioms but has greatly increased vocabulary knowledge; (2) makes frequent errors in grammar and pronunciation; (3) comprehends substantial parts of conversations but may need frequent repetitions; (4) understands and uses more complex structures in reading and writing but still has difficulty with abstract language. For the advanced student, items included were: (1) comprehends conversational and academic discourse most of the time; (2) speaks fluently but makes occasional errors; (3) reads and writes with less difficulty; and (4) is able to comprehend and use both concrete and abstract language. In addition to language proficiency, Richard-Amato suggests that teachers should also test for competency in content areas. At first, the testing may be given in the student's first language by aides or tutors with appropriate language backgrounds. This information would be important in making placement decisions regarding sheltered or mainstreamed classes. Students are much more likely to succeed if they have appropriate background knowledge.

Assessment of Bilingual/Bicultural Children with Impairments

Kathy was a 3½-year-old girl who was the oldest of two children of a German-speaking mother and English-speaking father. Although both German and English were spoken by both parents in the home, German was the dominant language. Kathy was referred to a University speech and language clinic by her father, who was a doctoral student at the university. He was concerned about her German and English language acquisition. The family wanted her to be bilingual in German and English. At the time of the referral, Kathy spoke in two- to three-word sentences in German, but often omitted the sounds at the end of words. She spoke only a few English words. The dilemma for the speech and language clinic staff members was how to assess this child's speech and language development.

In developing an assessment plan, it is important to be careful not to misdiagnose the child's difficulty with language. For example, several scholars (Cummins, 1984; DeBlassie & Franco, 1983; Erickson & Walker, 1983; Mercer, 1983) have found inordinate numbers of language minority students placed in special education programs based on test scores normed on English-speaking students. As a result, many of the children were misdiagnosed as having mental retardation, learning disabilities, or language disorders. At the same time, some children with impairments may not have been identified because their difficulties were attributed to being speakers of English as a second language. In any case, Erickson and Walker suggest that if 8 percent to 12 percent of the school-age population have impairments then there must be a sizable number of bilingual children who also have impairments. Therefore, procedures for identifying and treating these children need to be developed. All of the issues raised earlier regarding the use of different types of assessment measures need to be addressed.

DeBlassie & Franco (1983) suggest that it is not necessary to throw out the standardized tests, but teachers should remember that many of these tests have been standardized on middle-class monolingual speakers of English. Tests should be used in conjunction with other measures (e.g., observations, teacher checklists, adaptive behavior data, personality assessment, medical and developmental data). De-Blassie and Franco's model for nondiscriminatory assessment involves the collection of history, current characteristics, and specific treatments or interventions. It is important to compare behavior in both languages. For Kathy, the child referred to earlier in this section, there was information from her parents that she deleted important grammatical endings from words in both languages.

Roussel (1991) has provided an annotated bibliography of communicative ability tests that have been used with children learning English as their second language. Some of the tests screen for language dominance (particularly between Spanish and English); whereas other tests assess English language proficiency. Roussel cautions that many of the tests do not provide reliability or validity measures. Also, for some tests, normative information is not available.

This lack of reliable and valid testing instruments makes it especially difficult to identify a bilingual child with speech and language impairments. The surface deviations may be due to a disorder or to a stage in development of the second language. Damico, Oller, and Storey (1983) believe that the assessment of the student's ability to use language for communication is more helpful in identifying the bilingual child with language impairments than are assessments of morphological and syntactical structures. Specifically, they examined language samples for non-normative patterns using surface-oriented syntactic criteria and the following pragmatic criteria: (1) linguistic nonfluencies; (2) revisions; (3) delayed responses; (4) nonspecific vocabulary; (5) inappropriate vocabulary; and (6) poor topic maintenance. The different criteria identified different subgroups as language-disordered. The results indicated that the pragmatic criteria were better predictors of achievement and teacher ratings seven months later than were the syntactic assessments. Earlier, Damico and Oller (1980) demonstrated that teachers trained to look for pragmatic difficulties made significantly more appropriate referrals than did teachers trained to use traditional morphological and syntactic deviancies as the basis for referrals.

Mattes and Omark (1984) developed an inventory for rating bilingual childrens' communication skills in both the first and second languages. The inventory, Bilingual Oral Language Development (BOLD), uses a + or – to rate 20 different behaviors (e.g., comments on own actions and other's actions, describes experiences, attends to speakers, follows directions, initiates interactions). It is recommended that these behaviors be evaluated on direct observations and on information from teachers and parents. This type of inventory can help determine the language in which the child functions best. The inventory can be modified if some behaviors are not typical of the child's culture. Cheng (1987), in her book on assessing Asian children's language, also provides a variety of checklists that rate functional communication, nonverbal behavior, and overall behavioral patterns. Adler (1991) provides an Assessment Instrument for Multicultural Clients for use by a speech-language pathologist. This instrument involves different rating scales of the client's language proficiency including structure, intelligibility, and comprehension.

Another instrument that can be effective for evaluating young children's skill in both languages is the Speech/Language Assessment Instrument (SLASS, Hadley & Rice, 1993). This observational tool evaluates the child's use and understanding of language and is completed by an adult familiar with the child (e.g., a parent or teacher). The adult rates the child on a variety of skills using a one- to seven-point rating scale with one being very low ability, four being the normal ability for age, and seven being very high ability. Although this instrument was developed primarily as a way to rate the skills of children with speech and language impairments in English, it can be used to rate these abilities in two languages by having the parent or an adult familiar with the child and both languages rate the child in both languages. For Kathy, this would be accomplished by having her parents rate her language skills in English and in German. Such a rating scale may reveal that the child is communicating appropriately in the home language but is not in English, or, as was the case for this child, not communicating effectively in either language.

As part of a comprehensive evaluation, Mattes and Omark (1984) suggest that standardized tests may be used; however, in many cases there are no tests available. Therefore, an inventory of communication skills may be an appropriate first step. In addition, adaptive behavior inventories may be used. One such measure that has normative data on nonwhite children is the Adaptive Behavior Inventory for Children (Mercer, 1979). Other informal measurements include language samples and criterion-referenced tests (e.g., Brigance Comprehensive Inventory of Basic Skills, 1983; Spanish Language Assessment Procedure, Mattes, 1984). Story retelling tasks may also be helpful in judging children's comprehension of content and effectiveness in describing events. The most appropriate measures are often assessment instruments developed at a local level (cf. Mattes & Omark, 1984, for suggestions for developing local assessment instruments). These instruments are developed for a target population with a specific content and focus and are normed using the local population. Bilingual children are thus compared to local peers rather than to a national sample.

Shipley and McAfee (1992), in their handbook on assessment, provide information on phonemic, grammatical, and pragmatic contrasts between Hispanic English and standard English and between Asian English and standard English. These contrasts can help the clinician become aware of possible confusions that children learning English as a second language may have between the structures of the two languages. The knowledge is helpful is determining what pattern or structure might be typical of some speakers and what pattern might signal an impairment.

Finally, another procedure that can help determine if a child's difficulty is due to a difference or a disability is using dynamic assessment procedures (Gutierrez-Clellen & Peña, 2001). In their article, Gutierrez-Clellen and Peña provide a tutorial on how to use the test-teach-retest procedures with culturally and linguistic diverse children. After the initial assessment, the specific learning experiences that teach the principles of a task are provided. The examiner can then retest to see if the child made gains. It is suggested that, if the child made gains, then the difficulty may be due to differences, not a disability. The gains may be measured by qualitative changes, a variety of quantitative changes, or by ratings of modifiability.

Other sources (e.g., Battle, 1998; Cheng, 1989, 1995; Lynch & Hanson, 1992; Screen & Anderson, 1994; Wyatt, 1998) provide information on speech and language services in multicultural settings. Battle suggests that speech-language pathologists must become culturally sensitive to the changing natures of families and the ways different families view child-rearing practices and the expectations they have for the development of communicative skills. Wyatt (1998) suggests that interventionists must be careful in gathering information for a case history. There may be culturally based differences in what are considered appropriate topics, in concern over confidentiality, in familiarity with proposed clinical procedures or recommendations, and in views regarding health and disabilities. Cultural mistrust may cause the clients to refuse to participate in assessments or intervention activities. Professionals may need to rely on interpreters or informants who know the culture to help them in learning to work appropriately with children who have communication disorders and with their family members.

It is also important to understand family roles and relationships (Lynch & Hanson, 1992). For example, in many Native American cultures the concept of family includes many extended family members; it may not be the parents but older members of the family who have authority over a child. If interventionists talk only to the parents, they may make less of an impact and gain less information than if they had talked to the family elder. Also, developmental milestones are not necessarily important in some cultures, so exact information about the child's language development may not be available. Parents of a child who does not talk by age 2 may not seek help for the child if it is not customary to be concerned until the child is 4 years old. Also, the child may be viewed as a well-behaved child rather than a child with a communication difficulty because silence in the presence of adults is seen as being respectful.

In the case of Kathy, her father was the family spokesman. However, both of her parents were very concerned about her difficulty in

German as well as in English and questioned whether they should stop speaking German to her. They thought that maybe trying to teach her two languages was causing her problem. They decided that, if she could learn only one language, then it should be English because she would be attending school in the United States. However, they really wanted her to know both languages because they made frequent trips back to Germany to visit relatives. Her mother was very interested in knowing how to work with Kathy. She currently would demand that Kathy imitate what was said to her and then would try to correct the imitation. Kathy was beginning to refuse to imitate and would withdraw from the interaction. Her mother was concerned that Kathy would never learn to speak well if she didn't try.

Assessment of Kathy at the clinic involved observation of the child playing with her parents. During that time, a language sample was taped, and an informal communication inventory was completed noting how Kathy communicated her needs and thoughts. This inventory was similar to the SLASS (Hadley & Rice, 1993). Because of the parents' concern about their daughter's deletion of final sounds from words, a phonological inventory was completed. In addition, the parents completed the MacArthur Communicative Development Inventory: Words and Gestures (Fenson, Dale, Reznick, Thal, Bates, Reilly, & Hartung, 1993) to document words and phrases Kathy understood and produced in English and in German. Although, Kathy had a history of ear infections, hearing testing completed at the time of the evaluation indicated hearing was within normal limits.

Results of the evaluation of Kathy's language skills indicated that she primarily used one- and two-word utterances to communicate. Words usually consisted of consonant–vowel syllables. Longer utterances were in German (2 to 3 words). Sometimes the sentences appeared to be a mixture of English and German. Much of her communication depended on gestures. The phonological inventory indicated she used the following English consonant sounds: *m, p, b, n, t, w, h, sh,* and *f.*

Recommendations for general intervention goals for Kathy were

1. to increase her understanding and production of English vocabulary (her parents were to continue speaking German in the home to allow for improvement in German language skills);
2. to increase the length of her utterances;
3. to increase intelligibility by decreasing the number of open syllables produced (consonant–vowel syllables) and increasing the number of closed syllables (consonant–vowel–consonant syllables); and
4. to increase correct production of /k/.

Other recommendations included that she be enrolled in a language preschool classroom with intervention provided in the classroom, if possible. Alternatives included receiving therapy at the clinic setting three times per week and attending a preschool or play group where she would be interacting with other children her age.

In summary, the bilingual exceptional child needs to be identified and to have an appropriate intervention program provided. To attain needed services, information concerning language abilities in the first language is necessary. Also necessary is information on adaptive functioning, educational achievement, and language abilities in the second language based on integrative and communicative functions. Discrete point assessments of surface morphological and syntactic functions are not enough.

Language Intervention with Bilingual Children Who Have Language Impairments

Intervention programs for bilingual children who have language impairments will depend on several variables including age and severity of the disability, attitude and goals of the family, resources and available social interactions, and vocational expectations (Erickson & Walker, 1983). The availability of programs is also a factor. Evans (1983) describes several programs for bilingual children under the age of six with language impairments. Some programs involve parents extensively, whereas others encourage parental involvement but do not require it. Some programs also serve nonhandicapped children. The content of the intervention and the extent to which the first language is incorporated into the programming also vary. Most infant and preschool programs focus on basic self-help and language skills rather than academic instruction.

For some of the programs, the language of instruction was the child's first language. However, according to Erickson and Walker (1983), most programs do not provide intervention in the child's first language because further schooling in the United States will require knowledge of English and it may be better to have the child focus on one language rather than two. Also, a continuing problem is the lack of personnel proficient in languages other than English. Bilingual paraprofessionals may be a solution. Paraprofessionals can be used as interpreters, referral sources and, to some extent, providers of intervention.

LAP: A Model Program

Rice and Wilcox (1995) describe a model preschool at the University of Kansas that provides programming for children who have language impairments, who are developing language in a typical manner, and who are learning English as their second language. The language skills of all children are facilitated within an inclusive classroom setting. The children are 3 to 5 years old. All children attending the Language Acquisition Preschool (LAP) receive an initial screening to document their language development. Assessment instruments include the Peabody Picture Vocabulary Test, Revised (Dunn & Dunn, 1981), the Reynell Test of Language Development (Reynell, 1985), an articulation test, and a language sample. For the ESL children, interpreters are available to provide translations for the children. Periodic retesting of the children is done to document progress.

The LAP, as described by Rice and Wilcox (1995), is designed to develop language skills in a naturalistic preschool group setting. The curriculum is language-focused, whereby language skills are facilitated throughout all curriculum activities. This language-focused curriculum model views children as active learners who learn best when they plan and carry out activities. The overall purpose of the classroom is to provide a language-rich environment conducive to language learning. The schedule of activities includes those that are routine (e.g., calendar time), and those that change daily (e.g, dramatic play). There is also a balance between activities that are child-centered (e.g., center activities where the children can choose between activities and the level of their participation in the chosen activity) and activities that are more teacher-directed (e.g., large-group activities). The schedule is organized in the following manner:

Entry and Free Play	with children arriving and playing until all have arrived
Circle Time	with greetings, calendar, roll call and special announcements
Center Time	where the child chooses to participate in one of four available centers (art table, dramatic play, blocks area, and quiet area)
Story Time	
Sharing Time	where children respond to questions from other children about "show and tell" items
Outdoor Play	
Snack Time	
Large-/Small-Group Time	a teacher-directed time where problem solving, classification, and pre-academic activities are presented
Music and Fingerplay Time	

The longest scheduled period is the play center time where the children are free to choose and plan their activities. Adults are present to respond to and interact with the children. In the quiet area, the adult is available to read stories or play with puzzles with the child. There is plenty of adult input, and less talking is expected from the child. At the art table the adult may use modeling and narration to provide ongoing descriptions of what the child is doing. For example, at the art table the adult might say, "This play dough feels soft and squishy, . . . or . . . I need some glue to paste the hat on the man . . . or . . . You need some glue, too." The block area is where a moderate amount of verbal activity from the children takes place. Again, the adult may model or provide narration of what the child or the adult is doing. Verbal output from the children is usually highest in the dramatic play center. It is the area where the child can act out a situation such as making dinner, being a doctor, going to the store, and playing dress-up (for further elaboration see Bunce & Watkins, 1995; Bunce, 1995a; Rice, 1995).

For the new ESL children, interpreters are initially available to help each child adjust and to provide explanations to the child concerning LAP classroom activities and routines. They also provide the teachers with needed information regarding cultural differences. For the language-delayed children, speech-language graduate students plan therapy programs under the supervision of the classroom teacher, who is a certified speech-language pathologist. Therapy is conducted within the classroom setting while the child is interacting with the materials and other children. Intervention is achieved through a concentrated normative model (CNM). As described by Rice (1995), the normative aspects emphasize the commonalities of development across children and conform to normative models of language development. They also recognize that language is a specific domain of development. The concentrated aspect of the model: (1) recognizes the need to emphasize or highlight specific language skills; (2) focuses on language in the classroom; and (3) allows for special techniques to direct children's attention to specific language forms. It also allows for much redundancy (e.g., the child is surrounded by language focusing on the child's interests and activities). Operational guidelines as described by Rice (1995) for the CNM model include:

1. Language intervention is best provided in a meaningful social context.
2. Language facilitation occurs throughout the entire curriculum.
3. Language curriculum is rooted in content themes.
4. Language intervention begins with the child.
5. Verbal interaction is encouraged.
6. Passive language learning and overt responses are encouraged.
7. Children's utterances are accorded functional value.
8. Valuable teaching occasions can arise in child-to-child interactions.

9. Parents are valuable partners in language intervention programming.

10. Routine parent evaluations are an integral part of the program (pp. 32–37).

Specific intervention techniques used within the concentrated normative model, described by Bunce and Watkins (1995), include (1) providing many opportunities for language use; (2) using focused contrasts; (3) modeling appropriate sounds, structures, and functions; (4) providing event casts; (5) using open questions, expanding and recasting children's utterances; (6) providing redirects and prompted initiations; and (7) using scripted play.

For example, to facilitate the acquisition of vocabulary, Kathy would be surrounded by language describing what she is doing. Comments, not questions, would be used by the adult. If she were at the block area and playing with a dollhouse, an adult could describe her actions, pausing for comments from Kathy. Kathy would not be required to make a response. If /k/ was to be facilitated, words such as wal*k*, li*k*e, tal*k*, could be inserted into the conversation (e.g., the doll is wal*k*ing, she li*k*es to tal*k* to her mother). To facilitate production of longer sentences and to highlight the importance of grammatical forms, sentences involving focus contrasts could be used. For example, the adult could say, "The mommy *is* walk*ing* to the house. Look, she walk*ed* in," as the child plays with the dolls. The close proximity of the two grammatical forms allows the child, over time, to begin to understand the differences in meaning. If the child comments, the adult can expand on the child's utterances. For example, if the child said, "Baby cry," the adult can respond, "Yes, the baby is crying." Different techniques can be used within one interaction. The resulting conversation may look like the adult is just "playing" with the child. However, the conversation is tailored to meet the child's communication needs.

These intervention techniques can be used anytime there is opportunity for interaction between a child and adult or between children. There may be more opportunity for such interaction during the dramatic play activity. Here, the play theme supports the child's knowledge, but also elaborates on it. For example, a grocery store scenario is often familiar to the child but it also allows for expansion of the child's knowledge, particularly of the words associated with it (e.g., food items, phrases such as "How much does this cost?" or "That is five dollars," etc.). Again, an emphasis can be placed on highlighting appropriate grammatical forms. A further advantage of providing intervention in the classroom is that interactions between children can be facilitated. For example, an adult can prompt a child to initiate to another child by saying, "Ask Jay how much the banana is," or "Ask Lisa if you can have a turn," or "Say, 'Lisa, my turn now.' " Therefore, a major advantage of providing language intervention within the classroom is that appropriate form, function, and use can be taught at the same time. There is no need to teach a form in isolation and then provide for generalization to an appropriate context. The context is learned with the form (see Bunce, 1995b; or Bunce & Watkins (1995) for further elaboration of how the intervention techniques are embedded into the different preschool activities).

Most of the ESL children attending the LAP preschool have not been delayed in their first language development. Typically these children have approached monolingual norms after 14 months in LAP (Bunce & Shirk, 1993). However, several children, such as Kathy described above, have been both language impaired and learning English as a second language. These children receive intervention following the techniques described above. Research on the development of language skills of these children is just beginning. So far, the children have all made progress in their English language skills, and parents report much improvement in their first language skills as well.

School-Based Intervention

Intervention in the public school setting has been provided by a variety of specialists including speech-language pathologists and special education teachers. However, a bilingual child with language impairments may receive only ESL services because the language problem is assumed to be due to a language difference. Not much has been written regarding specific instructional or intervention techniques for bilingual children with language impairments. However, techniques already discussed as being helpful for second-language learners are appropriate, especially those that include: (1) focusing on meaning; (2) teaching vocabulary and syntax within a context; (3) allowing time for comprehension to develop before insisting on production; (4) using a peer buddy; (5) using predictable books; and (6) incorporating parents and significant others in the teaching.

A variety of techniques used with monolingual children with language impairments may also be helpful. These interventions involve various aspects of language including pragmatics (use in context), semantics (meaning), morphology and syntax (grammatical forms and word order), and phonology (sound system). The specific focus of the intervention depends on the child's needs. However, the most effective programming involves all aspects. When possible, the intervention should not focus only on basic interpersonal communicative skills (BICS), but should also include skills that foster cognitive/academic language proficiency (CALP) as discussed by Cummins (1979, 1984).

PRAGMATICS.   The appropriate use of language within a context is the goal of any language intervention program. It does not matter that a child can understand and produce language forms in a clinical setting if the child does not use language to get needs met, to make routine greetings, to follow turn-taking rules, and to make repairs when communication breaks down. Routine activities are a starting point. Allowing the child to observe and take part in appropriate interactions is important. A peer buddy may provide a model. (Remember that active, though silent, observation may play an important role in language development for many children.)

Within a kindergarten or preschool setting, activities such as show and tell can teach question-and-answer routines (e.g., "What do you have?" "A truck," "Where did you get it?" etc.). Snack time can also be used to teach and practice appropriate language to get needs met ("Please pass the juice," "I need more crackers," "More cookie," etc.).

Within an elementary classroom, routines such as lunch count, roll call, and procedures for passing out and handing in materials can be used to teach specific responses to a specific situation. For example, during roll call, the child who is learning English as a second language may first respond nonverbally by raising his hand; later the appropriate classroom verbal response may be required. If this child is the helper and responsible for passing out papers, the teacher can demonstrate what is needed and at the same time provide a verbal description. The child can, at first, perform the task without speaking but later may use language while doing the task. Other classroom activities can provide opportunities for children to observe and take part in classroom discourse. It is very important for children learning English as a second language to know the classroom procedure for asking questions on assignments, for requesting help, and for requesting additional information. How to ask clarifying questions may be a particularly important skill for all the children to learn. Teachers also need to be aware of each child's culture and ways of interacting within the culture. The test question format in which the teacher asks a question, the child answers, and then the teacher evaluates the response may be new to the child. Cultural mismatches need to be avoided when possible.

SEMANTICS.   As children learn to use language to get their needs met, they learn meanings of words and concepts. Some activities may be specifically focused to enhance vocabulary. Various activities can be used to teach vocabulary, ranging from object and picture labeling to reading stories. When possible, new vocabulary should be used in context so the child can understand the use as well as the meaning of the word or concept. This may be particularly important if the concept is not marked in the child's first language. Various kinds of classification activities are also helpful in improving conceptual knowledge. Activities such as matching, categorizing, and choosing the different item in a set can help extend the child's academic language proficiency.

SYNTAX AND MORPHOLOGY.   Many procedures facilitate syntactic and morphological development. Sentence rearrangement games help focus the student on the various ways in which content could be said. Question games provide practice in asking and answering questions. Role playing and story retelling provide practice with syntactic structures within a certain context. Various sequencing activities, including sequence patterns and sequential story games or puzzles, can be used. Having the child generate a story that is written down for later rereading improves oral language and literacy skills. For the primary (and older) students, writing activities may be helpful, particularly if the emphasis is on the process, not a perfect product. Invented spellings would be allowed so the child can focus on the content (cf. Edelsky, 1982; Lloyd, 1992, for description of writing in a bilingual program).

The child who, after an initial period of adjustment, does little or no combining of words to form sentences may need help learning word-order rules in English. One way to provide a focus on the demarcation of word boundaries and word order rules is to use a miniature linguistic system (MLS) procedure (e.g., Bunce, Ruder, & Ruder, 1985; Goldstein, 1983). The MLS focuses on syntax, but also on teaching a system so that generalization to nontrained items is facilitated. The MLS can be used to train any structure that can be broken into two components. Examples include:

verb | object

preposition | object

adjective | object

adjective | subject

subject | verb-object

adjective-subject | verb-object

A matrix of 16 or 25 squares (depending on whether it is a 4 by 4 or 5 by 5 matrix) outlines the training steps. For example, if the verb + object construction is to be taught, then all of the nouns are placed across the top of the matrix (see Figure 11.1) and all of the verbs are listed on the side of the matrix. In the case of a 4 by 4 matrix there are four different nouns and four different verbs. The first verb is paired with each noun to form four different combinations. Each combination is taught separately. For example, if the verbs chosen were *touch, push, drop,* and *wash* and the nouns were *car, ball, chair,* and *truck* then the first training item would be "touch car." After the child can indicate the correct item, the next structure consisting of the first verb and the second noun is trained (i.e., "touch ball"). In a similar manner "touch chair" and finally "touch truck" are trained. After the first verb

Figure 11.1   MLS training matrix for verb-object combinations

	Noun 1 (car)	Noun 2 (ball)	Noun 3 (chair)	Noun 4 (truck)
Verb 1 (touch)	Training 1	Training 2	Training 3	Training 4
Verb 2 (push)	Training 5			
Verb 3 (drop)	Training 6			
Verb 4 (wash)	Training 7			

has been paired with the four nouns, the first noun is paired with the rest of the verbs. In this case, the fifth, sixth, and seventh training steps would be "push car," "drop car," and "wash car." A check of the comprehension of other possible structures within the matrix (e.g., *push, drop, wash,* paired with each of the nouns) usually indicates generalization to untrained structures. This means that after training seven combinations, the child learns 16 combinations. In addition, children often understand verb-noun combinations utilizing different lexical items so they usually have learned many more than 16. The miniature linguistic system provides a systematic way for children to distinguish between word boundaries.

Once the child has learned some verb-object combinations, subjects may be added and a new matrix formed. For example, four nouns can be listed along the side of the matrix (e.g., boy, girl, man, woman) and four verb-object combinations across the top (e.g., touch car, push ball, drop chair, wash truck). Again, the margins of the matrix are trained. That is, the first subject is paired with all the verb-object combinations, and then the first verb-object combination is paired with all of the subjects. The training items are "boy touch car," followed by "boy push ball," "boy drop chair," "boy wash truck," "girl touch car," "man touch car," and "woman touch car." Again, each training item is trained to criterion before the next item is taught. Generalization to untrained combinations is expected. Theoretically, the child should be able to understand any combination of subject-verb-object, which is now a total of 64 different combinations. This is not including any other vocabulary words the child may know and could insert into the subject-verb-object construction. The use of articles can be added relatively easily once the basic subject-verb-object pattern is established. Adjective-noun constructions, prepositional phrases, and other constructions can be trained and the basic subject-verb-object pattern expanded (e.g., becoming adjective-subject-verb-preposition-object).

In using the MLS, Bunce and colleagues (1985) suggest three important training procedures: (1) initial training should focus on comprehension because generalization to production without further training sometimes occurs; (2) a variety of exemplars should be used to represent the components (e.g., several different cars are used so the child understands that the term refers to a class of objects not just one particular referent); and (3) training should involve the use of contrasts (e.g., if the target item is "touch car," then foils include a different verb paired with car and a different object paired with touch). The use of contrasts ensures that the child focuses on both aspects of the construction, learning the concept of "touch" as well as of "car." Just pointing to a picture of someone "touching" is not enough because there are two pictures of someone "touching" something. Likewise, just pointing to a picture with a car is not correct because there are two pictures with cars. The training can be done using pictures representing the constructions or by using objects with the teacher or clinician performing the actions.

Using a miniature linguistic system is an example of working with a particular component of language. It provides a means for the child to analyze syntactic rules and note word boundaries, and it also teaches some vocabulary. The effectiveness of the miniature linguistic system is that generalization to untrained structures is planned and expected. However, the child then needs to use the structures within a naturalistic setting, such as a classroom. Training the structures is only the beginning. Generalization to settings outside the training situation is the main goal. The teacher who is aware of the child's abilities can do much to foster this transfer through conversations, stories, songs, role playing, and other activities.

PHONOLOGY.   In the case of the bilingual child who is language impaired, the primary focus should be on developing communication. As the child's ability to use language improves, often pronunciation also improves. However, some children may need specifically tailored intervention in order to learn the sound system of a language. Providing children with good speech models may help. Articulation therapy provided by a speech-language pathologist may be necessary to help some children discriminate between the sound systems of the two languages. This discrimination may be aided by teaching the alphabet or phonic skills (or the articulation therapy may aid the learning of the alphabet and phonic skills).

If José were a 5-year-old kindergarten child with a language impairment, what kind of programming might he receive? Several options may be available. For example, José might be placed in a language classroom where he would receive intensive language therapy as well as academic work, he might be placed in a preschool setting to enhance his language skills before focusing on academic skills, or he might be placed full or part time in an ESL class. It is also possible that José's language problems would be assumed to be due to his lack of exposure to English and he would be placed in a kindergarten class with or without ESL programming.

In any case, the classroom teacher would need to seek ways to help José achieve in the classroom. Again, utilization of a buddy system and use of peer models would be helpful. Teacher observation of José's communication skills (as well as language skills) would be important. The use of the Bilingual Oral Language Development (Mattes & Omark, 1984) could be a starting point in assessing José's language skills, as well as procedures described earlier by Damico and colleagues (1983) that focus on pragmatic criteria (poor topic maintenance, delayed responses, nonspecific vocabulary, etc.). Language samples also can provide information on José's use of both English and Spanish. Information from the parents concerning José's development would be important to consider, as well. More formal assessment involving standardized and criterion-referenced testing might then be done. Formal testing in Spanish may depend on availability of Spanish-speaking professionals.

While observations and testing are being completed, the classroom teacher will be providing programming through routine activities in the classroom. Singing, show and tell, story time, snack time, and center time with a variety of pre-academic activities are rich environments for language learning. In addition, the speech-language pathologist, special education teacher, and/or ESL teacher may be involved in setting up programming. The kind of programming will vary depending on the setting and the needs of the child.

Many of the language intervention activities described earlier may be appropriate for José. However, these are just a few of the many activities possible in a classroom or clinical setting. In any case, the emphasis needs to be on improving both basic interpersonal communication skills and cognitive and academic language skills. In addition, when developing appropriate intervention activities, the following intervention principles, summarized in Table 11.2, should be considered:

1. Begin intervention where the child can be successful. Train through strengths, not weaknesses; that is, make sure the child can respond correctly at least 30 percent to 50 percent of the time with support. If the child can respond correctly 60 percent of the time with no support, then monitoring of the skill may be important but the target is not necessarily an intervention target. The child is already well on the way to mastery. If the target is not produced correctly with support at the 30 percent level, then be

TABLE 11.2   Intervention principles

Principles	Guidelines
1. Begin intervention where the child can be successful.	a. Train through strengths. b. Begin training where the child can respond correctly 30–50% of the time with support. c. Don't practice error responses. d. Some simplification of the response may first need to be taught.
2. Base intervention on testing (formal and informal) and observations.	a. Assess child's skills using formal and informal testing. b. Develop intervention plan based on child's needs and strengths. c. Continue to assess needs and progress through observations and additional testing.
3. Choose to remediate those items that will have the greatest effect on the child's life.	a. Focus on communication first. b. Teach vocabulary and structure that is important for academic achievement.
4. Plan for generalization.	a. Use a variety of contrasts in order to highlight the discrimination between components. b. Train in a variety of contexts. c. Vary the interactants (when the child can do the task for you, set up the task to be done with others). d. Train strategies that work in more than one situation.
5. If training on isolated features is done, end training at a more global level.	a. First train the isolated form, (e.g., question reversals), then use in "real" conversations. b. Use role play as an intermediary step to "real" conversations, if necessary.
6. Simplify target structures only as far as needed to get the appropriate response.	a. If you can get correct production of a sound at the syllable level, don't train at the sound level. b. If child can produce the target form (with cuing) in a sentence, don't practice at the word level.
7. Assess as you remediate.	a. Attend to gains and losses within each session. b. Use probes periodically to assess progress. c. Use formal testing as needed.
8. Train first in comprehension, then in production.	a. Model appropriate responses within a context. b. When possible, have children make nonverbal responses (e.g., pointing, responding to directions, etc.) to target items. c. Probe for production; may not need to train.
9. Follow the child's lead.	a. Attend to child's focus. b. Let child's interests provide the content to be trained.
10. Let the child be the teacher.	a. Child can demonstrate new knowledge when playing teacher. b. Teacher can assess child's competencies. c. Child is motivated to do the task.

careful in choosing that target because what will be practiced is error responses. Some simplification of the response may first need to be taught.

2. Base intervention on testing (both formal and informal) and observations.

3. Choose to remediate those items that will have the greatest effect on the child's life (e.g., help most in making the child a competent communicator, help in academic achievement, etc.)

4. Plan for generalization from the very beginning:

   a. Have a variety of contrasts available in order to highlight the discrimination to components you want the child to make. For example, if you want the child to focus on the preposition "in," have the one object pictured *in* another object, then *on* the same object (and maybe *beside* it, too). This presentation forces the child to attend to the location of the object rather than focusing on either of the two objects as the component being trained.

   b. Train in a variety of contexts (including the classroom— you may have to set up situations to provide the extension activities).

   c. When the child can perform for you, set up the task so it can be done for others.

   d. Train strategies that make sense and work in more than one situation.

   e. Train concepts, rather than rote memory.

5. If training on isolated features is done (sometimes this is both needed and effective), be sure to end training at a more global level. For example, if work is on syntax involving question reversals (e.g., "Did you go?" versus "You did go?"), be sure to eventually have the question used in a real conversation. Sometimes this can be achieved through role playing. Just being able to respond appropriately when asked to do so is only one step. The next step is to produce the response when needed in "real life."

6. Break things down into smaller components only as far as needed to get the response, particularly if the tasks need to become automatic. For example, if you can get a child to produce the correct sound at the syllable level, don't work at the sound level. Later, as part of training analysis skills, it may be appropriate to focus on part-to-whole activities.

7. Continue to assess as you remediate. This does not mean a multitude of formal testing, it means you attend to gains (and losses) within each session. Procedures need to be changed if progress is not being made. What is appropriate for one child is not always appropriate for another.

8. If possible, train first in comprehension, you may get transfer to production without training.

9. Take advantage of "teachable" moments. This means following the child's lead. Let the child's interest provide the content to train. For example, if the child is involved in building with the blocks, describe what she is doing. Also, join in and build with the child or provide additional props and describe the action. For an older child, reading or discussing the book the child has selected, or getting the child to tell about the story she has written or what has happened in ballgames at recess, are all opportunities to teach language.

10. Let the child be the "teacher." Sometimes you can better assess what a child understands about a task if you switch roles.

SUMMARY

Bilingual/bicultural children have special educational needs. These needs can best be met by teachers and special educators who are aware of both linguistic and cultural factors influencing educational achievement. Appropriate programming depends on flexibility in designing ways to facilitate their learning of both linguistic and academic skills. Achieving this flexibility is not easy, but must become a goal if the educational needs of bilingual children are to be met.

QUESTIONS/ACTIVITIES:

1. Divide into groups of four to five people. Discuss the different ways you celebrate a holiday such as a birthday or other special event. Note the similarities and differences in the ways each person views the event and the kinds of "rituals" that are done.

2. Discuss or write an essay about the following scenario: Picture yourself in a country where you don't know the language or the customs. What are some of the first words or phrases you want to learn and why?

3. If you were in a foreign country trying to learn the language and customs, describe how you would like people to teach you (e.g., by making you memorize phrases, by demonstrating as well as providing the words, by writing down the words, by giving you choices as they say the words, etc.). Discuss with others or write your answers.

4. If you are a English-speaking speech language pathologist who is to evaluate a seven-year-old child whose first language is Vietnamese to determine if she has a speech and language impairment, what are some of the ways you will do this? Discuss or write as an essay.

5. How can you find out what cultural issues may need to be considered when doing an evaluation of a child with cultural and linguistic differences? Discuss or write as an essay.

REFERENCES

Adler, S. (1991). Assessment of language proficiency of limited English proficient speakers: Implications for the speech-language specialist. *Language Speech & Hearing Services in Schools, 22,* 12–18.

Anim-Addo, J. (1992). Drama with young learners in school. In P. Pisant (Ed.), *Language, culture and young children: Developing English in the multi-ethnic nursery and infant school* (pp. 110–122). London: David Fulton.

Baetens-Beardsmore, H., & Swain, M. (1985). Designing bilingual education: Aspects of immersion and "European School" models. *Journal of Multilingual and Multicultural Development, 6,* 1–15.

Bates, E. (1976). *Language and context: The acquisition of pragmatics.* New York: Academic Press.

Battle, D. E. (1998). *Communication disorders in multicultural populations.* Boston: Butterworth-Heinemann.

Ben Zeev, S. (1977). The influence of bilingualism on cognitive strategy and cognitive development. *Child Development, 48,* 1009–1018.

Berko-Gleason, J. (1993). *The development of language* (3rd ed.) New York: Macmillan.

Bernstein, D. K. (1989). Assessing children with limited English proficiency: Current perspectives. *Topics in Language Disorders, 9*(3), 15–20.

Bloom, B. S., & Krathwohl, D. R. (1977). *Taxonomy of educational objectives: Handbook I: Cognitive domain.* New York: Longman.

Brigance, A. H. (1983). *Comprehensive inventory of basic skills.* North Billerica, MA: Curriculum Associates.

Brigance, A. H. (1984). *Assessment of basic skills: Spanish edition.* North Billerica, MA: Curriculum Associates.

Bunce, B. H. (1995a). *Building a language-focused curriculum for the preschool classroom (Vol. II): A planning guide.* Baltimore: Brookes.

Bunce, B. H. (1995b). A language-focused curriculum for children learning English as a second language. In M. L. Rice & K. A. Wilcox (Eds.), *Building a language-focused curriculum for the preschool classroom (Vol. I): A foundation for lifelong communication* (pp. 91–103). Baltimore: Brookes.

Bunce, B. H., Ruder, K., & Ruder, C. (1985). Using a miniature linguistic system in teaching syntax: Two case studies. *Journal of Speech and Hearing Disorders, 50,* 247–253.

Bunce, B. H., & Shirk, A. (1993, November). *Children learning English as a second language: Classroom language facilitation.* Poster session presented at the American Speech-Language-Hearing Association Convention, Anaheim, CA.

Bunce, B. H., & Watkins, R. V. (1995). Language intervention in a preschool classroom. In M. L. Rice & K. A. Wilcox (Eds.), *Building a language-*

focused curriculum for the preschool classroom (Vol. I): A foundation for lifelong communication (pp. 39–71). Baltimore: Brookes.

Burt, M., Dulay, H., & Hernandez-Chavez, E. (1976). *Bilingual syntax measure*. New York: Harcourt Brace Jovanovich.

Chamberlain, P., & Medeiros-Landurand, P. (1991). Practical considerations for the assessment of LEP students with special needs. In E. B. Hamayan & J. S. Damico (Eds.), *Limiting Bias in the assessment of bilingual students* (pp. 111–156). Austin: PRO-ED.

Cheng, L. (1987). *Assessing Asian language performance*. Rockville, MD: Aspen.

Cheng, L. (1989). Service delivery to Asian/Pacific LEP children: A cross-cultural framework. *Topics in Language Disorders, 9*(3), 1–14.

Cheng, L. (1995). *Integrating language and culture for inclusion*. San Diego: Singular.

Cherry, L. (1978). A sociolinguistic approach to the study of teacher expectations. *Discourse Processes, 1,* 373–394.

Cole, L., & Snope, T. (1981). Resource guide to multicultural tests and materials. *ASHA, 23,* 639–649.

Cortes, C. E. (1986). The education of language minority students: A contextual interaction model. In *Beyond language: Social and cultural factors in schooling language minority students* (pp. 3–34). Los Angeles: Evaluation, Dissemination and Assessment Center, California State University.

Cummins, J. (1979). Linguistic interdependence and the educational development of bilingual children. *Review of Educational Research, 49,* 222–251.

Cummins, J. (1984). *Bilingualism and special education: Issues in assessment and pedagogy*. Clevedon Avon, England: Multilingual Matters.

Damico, J. S. (1991). Descriptive assessment of communicative ability in limited English proficient students. In E. B. Hamayan & J. S. Damico (Eds.), *Limiting bias in the assessment of bilingual students* (pp. 157–217). Austin: PRO-ED.

Damico, J. S., & Oller, J. W. (1980). Pragmatic versus morphological/syntactic criteria for language referrals. *Language, Speech and Hearing Services in Schools, 11,* 85–94.

Damico, J. S., Oller, J. W., & Storey, M. E. (1983). The diagnosis of language disorders in bilingual children: Surface-oriented and pragmatic criteria. *Journal of Speech and Hearing Disorders, 48,* 385–394.

Deal, V., & Yan, M. (1985). Resource guide to multicultural test and materials, Supplement II. *ASHA, 26,* 6, 43–49.

DeBlassie, R. R., & Franco, J. N. (1983). Psychological and educational assessment of bilingual children. In D. R. Omark & J. G. Erickson (Eds.), *The bilingual exceptional child* (pp. 55–68). San Diego: College Hill Press.

Diaz, S., Moll, L. C., & Mehan, H. (1986). Sociocultural resources in instruction: A context-specific approach. In *Beyond language: Social and cultural factors in schooling language minority students* (pp. 187–230). Los Angeles: Evaluation, Dissemination and Assessment Center, California State University.

Dunn, L. M., & Dunn, L. M. (1981). *Peabody picture vocabulary test—revised*. Circle Pines, MN: American Guidance Service.

Edelsky, C. (1982). Writing in a bilingual program: The relation of L1 and L2 texts. *TESOL Quarterly, 16,* 211–228.

Erickson, J. C., & Walker, C. L. (1983). Bilingual exceptional children: What are the issues? In D. R. Omark & J. G. Erickson (Eds.), *The bilingual exceptional child* (pp. 3–22). San Diego: College-Hill Press.

Evans, J. (1983). Model preschool program for handicapped bilingual children. In D. R. Omark & J. G. Erickson (Eds.), *The bilingual exceptional child*. San Diego: College-Hill Press.

Fenson, L., Dale, P. S., Reznick, J. S., Thal, D., Bates, E., Reilly, J. S., & Hartung, J. P. (1993). *MacArthur Communicative Development Inventory: Words and Gestures*. San Diego: Singular.

Fix, M., & Passel, J. (1994). *Immigration and immigrants: Setting the record straight*. Washington, DC: Urban Institute.

Freeman, D., Freeman, Y., & Gonzales, G. (1987). Success for LEP students: The Sunnyside sheltered English program. *TESOL Quarterly, 21,* 361–367.

Garcia, G. E. (1992). Ethnography and classroom communication: Taking an "emic" perspective. *Topics in Language Disorders, 12,* 54–66.

Goldstein, H. (1983). Training generative repertoires with agent-action-object miniature linguistic systems with children. *Journal of Speech and Hearing Research, 26,* 76–89.

Goodman, K., & Goodman, Y. (1986). *What is whole about whole language?* Portsmouth, NH: Heinemann.

Gutierrez-Clellen, V. F., & Peña, E. (2001). Dynamic assessment of diverse children: A tutorial. *Language, Speech and Hearing Services in Schools, 32,* 212–224.

Hadley, P. A., & Rice, M. L. (1993). Parental judgments of preschoolers' speech and language development: A resource for assessment and IEP planning. *Seminars in Speech and Language, 14,* 278–288.

Hamayan, E. V., & Damico, J. S. (1991). *Limiting bias in the assessment of bilingual students*. Austin: PRO-ED.

Heath, S. B. (1983). *Ways with words*. Cambridge: Cambridge University Press.

Heath, S. B. (1986). Sociocultural contexts of language development. In *Beyond language: Social and cultural factors in schooling language minority students* (pp. 143–186). Los Angeles: Evaluation, Dissemination and Assessment Center, California State University.

Hudelson, S. (1985). *Hopscotch*. New York: Regents Publishing Co.

Ianco-Worrall, A. (1972). Bilingualism and cognitive development. *Child Development, 43,* 1390–1400.

Iglesias, A. (1985a). Communication in the home and classroom: Match or mismatch. *Topics in Language Disorders, 5,* 29–41.

Iglesias, A. (1985b). Cultural conflict in the classroom. In D. N. Ripich & F. M Spinelli (Eds.), *School discourse problems* (pp. 79–96). San Diego: College-Hill Press.

Jennings, L. (April, 27, 1988). Panel: School must aid immigrants in "struggle to succeed". *Education Week, 7*(31), 1–2.

Krashen, S., & Terrill, T. (1983). *The natural approach: Language acquisition in the classroom.* Oxford: Pergamon.

Lado, R. (1957). *Linguistics across cultures.* Ann Arbor: University of Michigan Press.

Lambert, W. E., & Tucker, G. R. (1972). *Bilingual education of children: The St. Lambert experiment.* Rowley, MA: Newberry House.

Lewis, J., Vang, L., & Cheng, L. (1989). Indentifying the language learning difficulties of the Hmong: Implications of context and culture. *Topics of Language Disorders, 9,* 21–37.

Lindfors, J. W. (1987). *Children's language and learning* (2nd ed.). Englewood Cliffs, NJ: Prentice-Hall.

Lloyd, P. (1992). Children's developmental writing. In P. Pisant (Ed.), *Language, culture and young children: Developing English in the multi-ethnic nursery and infant school* (pp. 98–109). London: David Fulton.

Lynch, E. W., & Hanson, M. J. (1992). *Developing cross-cultural competence: A guide for working with young children and their families.* Baltimore: Brookes.

Mattes, L. J. (1984). *Spanish Language Assessment Procedures: A Communication Skills Inventory.* Oceanside, CA: Academic Communication Associates.

Mattes, L. J., & Omark, D. R. (1984). *Speech and language assessment for the bilingual handicapped.* San Diego: College-Hill Press.

Mercer, J. R. (1979). *SOMPA: System of Multicultural Pluralistic Assessments.* New York: Psychological Corporation.

Mercer, J. R. (1983). Issues in the diagnosis of language disorders in students whose primary language is not English. *Topics in Language Disorders, 3,* 46–56.

Norris, J. A., & Hoffman, P. R. (1993). *Whole language intervention for school-aged children.* San Diego: Singular.

Oller, J. W. (1979). *Language tests at school.* London: Longman.

Pflaum, S. W. (1986). *The development of language and literacy in young children.* Columbus, OH: Merrill.

Pisant, P. (1992). *Language, culture and young children: Developing English in the multi-ethnic nursery and infant school* (pp. 110–122). London: David Fulton.

Reynell, J. K. (1985). *Reynell Development Language Scales.* Los Angeles: Western Psychological Services.

Rice, M. L. (1995). The rationale and operating principles for a language-focused curriculum for preschool children. In M. L. Rice & K. A. Wilcox (Eds.), *Building a language-focused curriculum for the preschool classroom (Vol. I): A foundation for lifelong communication* (pp. 27–38). Baltimore: Brookes.

Rice, M. L., & Wilcox, K. (1995). *Building a language-focused curriculum for the preschool classroom (Vol. I): A foundation for lifelong communication.* Baltimore: Brookes.

Richard-Amato, P. A. (1988). *Making it happen: Interaction in the second language classroom.* New York: Longman.

Roussel, N. (1991). Annotated bibliography of communicative ability tests. In E. B. Hamayan & J. S. Damico (Eds.), *Limiting bias in the assessment of bilingual students* (pp. 320–343). Austin: PRO-ED.

Rowe, M. (1969). Science, silence, and sanctions. *Science, 6,* 11–13.

Saville-Troike, M. (1979). Culture, language, and education. In H. T. Trueba & C. Barnett-Mizrahi (Eds.), *Bilingual multicultural education and the professional: From theory to practice* (pp. 139–148). Rowley, MA: Newberry House.

Screen, R. M., & Anderson, N. B. (1994). Multicultural perspectives in communication disorders. San Diego: Singular.

Shipley, K. G., & McAfee, J. G. (1992). *Assessment in speech-language pathology: A resource manual.* San Diego: Singular.

Stanford Working Group. (1993). *A blueprint for the second generation.* Stanford, CA: Stanford University.

Tabors, P. O., & Snow, C. E. (1994). English as a second language in preschool programs. In F. Genesse (Ed.), *Reading, writing, and schooling* (pp. 103–125). New York: Cambridge University Press.

Wong-Fillmore, L. (1983). The language learner as an individual. In M. Clake and J. Handscombe (Eds.), *On TESOL '82: Pacific perspectives on language learning & teaching.* Washington, DC: Teachers of English to Speakers of Other Languages.

Wong-Fillmore, L. (1985). Teacher talk as input. In S. Gass and C. Madden (Eds.), *Input in second language acquisition* (pp. 17–50). Rowley, MA: Newberry House.

Wyatt, T. (1998). Assessment issues with multicultural populations. In D. E. Battle (Ed.), *Communication disorders in multicultural populations* (pp. 379–425). Boston: Butterworth-Heinemann.

Appendix
Selection of Predictable Books

(Predictable books have limited text per page, repeated patterns, strong rhythms, and supportive illustrations.)

Bayer, A. (1984). *My name is Alice.* New York: Dutton.

Brett, J. (1985). *Annie and the wild animals.* Boston: Houghton Mifflin.

Brown, R. (1984). *If at first you do not see.* London: Anderson Press.

Carle, Eric. (1982). *What's for lunch?* New York: Putnam.

Gibbons, G. (1981). *Trucks.* New York: Crowell.

Ginsburg, M. (1980). *Kittens from one to ten.* New York: Crown.

Goss, J. L., & Hardste, J. (1985). *It didn't frighten me.* Worthington, OH: Willowisp.

Lobel, A. (1981). *On Market Street.* Toronto: Scholastic.

Lobel, A. (1984). *A rose in my garden.* New York: Greenwillow.

Mayer, Mercer. (1983). *Just Grandma and me.* Racine, WI: Golden Books.

Parish, P. (1980). *I can, can you?* New York: Greenwillow.

Wildsmitih, B. (1982). *Cat on the mat.* Toronto: Oxford Press.

Zolotow, C. (1983). *Some things go together.* New York: Crowell.

CHAPTER 12

Special Needs of Students with Severe Disabilities or Autism

Mary Jo Noonan and Ellin B. Siegel

As discussed throughout this text, the trend in service delivery for students with disabilities is intervention in natural environments, or "full inclusion." Until very recently, full inclusion was available primarily for some students with mild disabilities who received most of their education in the mainstream of general education classes. Special education professionals believed that students with more significant disabilities would be better served in smaller, more controlled school settings that allowed intensive, one-to-one instruction. We have now learned that it is possible to fully include students with severe disabilities as well as those with autism. With proper supports, all students can participate in the general education setting, and all students benefit.

For students with disabilities, **full inclusion** means that they are served in natural environments, such as their home or day-care center, and preschool and elementary age students are enrolled in general education classrooms in their neighborhood schools. For elementary age students with severe disabilities or autism, special education may include **community-based instruction,** that is, instruction in home and other community locations to teach daily living and life skills. Together, full inclusion and community-based instruction are considered "recommended practice." This chapter will discuss strategies for assessing communication needs and designing appropriate interventions for students with severe disabilities or autism in natural school and community settings.

STUDENTS WITH SEVERE DISABILITIES OR AUTISM

The primary purpose of communication intervention for students with severe disabilities or autism is to provide them with an effective means to participate in family and community life. Communication allows social participation when it enables students to influence the people and events around them. Students influence people and events when they communicate their choice of playmates, ask their parents for a kiss, or tell their teacher that they have had enough to eat. Effective communication provides freedom and independence to students who are otherwise very dependent because of the severity of their disabilities.

Students with severe disabilities have diverse characteristics, but they share the need for extensive and ongoing supports (e.g., personal assistance, special equipment) in order to participate in school, home, and community activities. They also exhibit a wide array of disabilities. For some, mental retardation is their primary disability. Others have physical and neurological disabilities that interfere with their ability to demonstrate their intellectual capacity so that they appear to have mental retardation; this is referred to as "functional retardation" (Guess & Mulligan, 1982). Still others have mental retardation in addition to physical, neurological, visual, and/or hearing impairments that compound the debilitating effects of mental retardation. Behaviorally, students with severe disabilities have obvious delays in basic skills associated with everyday living (dressing, eating, toileting, etc.).

Students with autism are also a diverse group with a wide range of abilities and needs (cf. Simpson & Myles, 1998). Autism is characterized by significant delays and/or differences in social interaction and communication. Many students with autism are socially withdrawn and make little or no eye contact with others. Developmental delays in addition to social/communication disabilities may or may not be present. Students with autism frequently engage in nonfunctional repetitive behaviors (stereotypy) and are often preoccupied with sameness.

Communication characteristics of students with severe disabilities are as diverse as their general characteristics. Some learn to talk in simple phrases and understand most of what is said to them, but their development of speech is delayed. Some understand speech and communicate through pointing, gesturing, or using an augmentative communication system, but do not speak. Others communicate primarily through emotional responses, such as crying or smiling, and do not seem to understand speech, nor do they attempt to use language verbally or nonverbally. Students with severe disabilities or autism may have a range of speech, language, and communication difficulties. For example, their speech may be unintelligible due to oral-motor coordination difficulties associated with cerebral palsy or behavioral problems (e.g., speaking too rapidly) or they may demonstrate echolalia, repetition, perseveration, irrelevant speech, or distortions in pitch or intonation.

Many students with autism seem unaware of their surroundings and others' attempts to communicate with them. Some do not use speech and may not even attempt to communicate with gestures. Others learn to speak, but their speech may be echolalic (imitative) or they may not know how to use their speech to communicate their wants and needs. Although students with severe disabilities or autism have diverse characteristics and difficulties, a number of common educational needs have been identified:

Communication interventions and/or supports are needed by the vast majority of students with severe disabilities or autism. Given the presence of mental retardation (actual or functional) and a likelihood of multiple disabilities among students with severe disabilities, it is difficult to imagine a student with severe disabilities who does not have significant communication needs. By definition, students with autism have extensive communication needs.

Systematic and consistent intervention is needed to provide sufficient opportunities to learn the relationship between natural cues, the communication skill being taught, and natural consequences (Snell & Brown, 2000). Students with severe disabilities or autism sometimes focus on irrelevant stimuli ("stimulus overselectivity") and fail to recognize natural cues (Lovaas, Schreibman, Koegel, & Rehm, 1971). Effective teaching techniques focus the student's attention on stimuli that indicate when a skill is needed/appropriate (natural cues) and the reinforcement that results from a correct response. Errorless or near-errorless instructional procedures should be used to minimize confusion when learning new skills.

Teaching techniques must emphasize independence. Although prompting is a necessary component of teaching, all prompts must eventually be eliminated. Eliminating prompts ensures that students do not become "prompt dependent" and unable to use their communication skills independently (Reichle & Sigafoos, 1991). Furthermore, students who are unable to use speech effectively should be provided with an augmentative communication system as a means to independent communication.

Intervention should occur in actual settings where the communication skills are required to reduce the need for generalization (Kaiser, 2000). Typically, students with severe disabilities or autism do not generalize learned skills to new situations. Teaching techniques that facilitate generalization should be included in all intervention programs.

ASSUMPTIONS

An important assumption of this chapter is that *all students communicate in some way,* even if they are not intentionally trying to do so. For example, an infant winces when she is uncomfortable, or a student says "ah" when an activity stops. Recognizing that all students communicate means that there will always be a starting point for intervention.

A second assumption of this chapter is that *communication intervention should enhance participation in natural environments.* This second assumption influences the nature of communication goals, the selection of priorities, and intervention methods. For example, new vocabulary words may include the names of foods to enhance a student's social participation during family mealtimes, or printed words may be included on a communication board of photographs so that a wide range of people can understand the augmented communication system.

Communication assessment and intervention techniques described in this chapter are relevant to students who use speech, augmentative communication systems, and/or other nonverbal/gestural means of communication. Specific considerations for selecting and teaching augmentative communication systems are described in detail in Chapter 13.

FORMULATING COMMUNICATION GOALS

Communication goals for students with severe disabilities or autism are established following the ecological assessment and planning process described in Chapter 7. The purpose of this process is twofold: first, to determine present and future communication needs associated with home, school, and community activities prioritized by the student's family and other members of the intervention team; second, to determine present abilities associated with communication needs. The procedures described in Chapter 7 for determining present and future communication needs (i.e., creating a vision and conducting discrepancy analyses) are recommended for identifying broad communication goals for students with severe disabilities or autism. Additional assessment procedures, however, may be required to identify present communication abilities and obtain information needed to formulate specific short-term communication objectives and corresponding intervention plans to address each objective. For example, if a student is using one-word utterances, and most of the utterances seem to be requests, a more detailed assessment of pragmatic functions may be desired. This additional assessment will provide information on the variety of pragmatic functions in the student's repertoire and how frequently the functions are used. A complete assessment of these functions would not have been obtained through the discrepancy analysis. Four assessment approaches may be used to provide information about a student's present level of communication associated with the goals identified through the ecological assessment and planning process. These approaches are particularly relevant to students with severe/multiple disabilities.

Identifying Present Communication Abilities

As noted above, information concerning a student's present communication abilities is often necessary to formulate specific, short-term instructional objectives. The approaches for assessing present communication abilities are: communication/language sample, behavioral assessment/functional analysis, ABC analysis, and motor assessment. A thorough assessment will probably require two or more approaches.

Communication/Language Sample

The language sample (Miller, 1978) was described in detail in Chapter 6. For students with severe disabilities or autism, it is particularly useful for assessing the adequacy of their communication repertoires. For example, a communication/language sample analysis of the functions associated with language *use* may reveal that a student communicates to make simple requests (e.g., asking for a toy) or to protest and express dissatisfaction (e.g., saying, "no more"), but rarely answers questions and does not contribute to conversation.

The language sample can be used with students who are nonverbal to evaluate the functions and effectiveness of gestural communication. One such communication/language sample indicated that a nonverbal student communicated a wide range of requests, but had frequent difficulties in communicating the exact nature of his request. When the interventionist tried to guess what he wanted, the student often changed his request if something equally appealing was mentioned. For example, he wanted help retrieving something he had dropped, but indicated he wanted a drink of water when the interventionist attempted to discern his request and asked if he was thirsty.

Behavioral Assessment/Functional Analysis

Behavioral assessment is a direct observation technique. Its main purposes are to measure a behavior of interest and to identify what seems to be controlling or maintaining it (Nelson & Hayes, 1979). The first step is to operationalize the behavior by writing a behavioral definition (e.g., "A *nonverbal request* occurs when Tommy points to something, with or without vocalizing"). Next, the behavior is quantified by observing and recording a relevant and measurable characteristic of it, such as frequency of nonverbal requests. Other types of measurement used in behavioral assessment include percentage, duration, latency, rate, interval recording, and time sampling. (For a more extensive discussion of measurement techniques see Brown & Snell, 2000.)

In addition to measuring behavior, events that occur before (antecedent) or after (consequent) may be altered to determine what may be controlling the behavior (Baer, Wolf, & Risley, 1968). For example, a student's favorite game can be placed out of reach to determine whether the arrangement will result in the student making requests. Altering antecedent and consequent events illustrates what *may* be maintaining (reinforcing) a behavior and allows the interventionist to evaluate potential intervention strategies.

Functional assessment is a behavior assessment approach to determine what use or purpose a behavior serves for the student (Iwata, Dorsey, Slifer, Bauman, & Richman, 1982). This is an important part of communication assessment because some students use socially unacceptable behaviors, such as tantrums or self-injury, to communicate when they lack appropriate communication skills.

Functional assessment yields hypotheses about what purposes an inappropriate behavior is serving. For example, several days of data collection might indicate that a preschooler bites her hand at about 11:00 each morning. The observations also indicate that, when she begins to bite, classroom staff give her some of her lunch. One plausible hypothesis is that the student bites her hand to get food. Teaching an appropriate communication skill that serves the same purpose as the behavior of concern will test this hypothesis. The student may be taught to ask for food. If the hypothesis is correct (both behaviors serve the same purpose), reinforcing only the appropriate communication behavior will result in a decrease in the inappropriate behavior.

ABC Analysis

This assessment strategy is a behavioral assessment technique utilizing continuous recording (Bijou, Peterson, & Ault, 1968; Brown & Snell, 2000). The evaluator lists each student behavior ("B"), the events that precede the behavior ("A," antecedents), and those that follow the behavior ("C," consequences). Typically, the evaluator records the observations in a three-column A-B-C format (see Table 12.1). The ABC analysis may include several short segments (e.g., six ten-minute intervals) or one or more lengthier segments (e.g., two one-hour intervals).

Following the observation(s), the data are reviewed to identify patterns of behavior; antecedent-behavior relationships, behavior-consequent relationships, and/or antecedent-behavior-consequent relationships. This information allows the evaluator to assess communication/language behavior *in context*. Contextual informa-

TABLE 12.1   Sample Portion of an ABC Analysis

Antecedent	Behavior	Consequences
T. lifts Frank and carries him to tilt table	Licks upper lip	
Places Frank supine on tilt table	Head right, right arm extended, left arm flexed, increased tone	
	Head hyperextended to right, moans, appears to be biting lip (?)	T. says, "Relax, relax. What's the matter?" & fastens knee strap (T. leaves)
	Tone decreases	
Another child calls out	Mouth opens, head extends back and to the right	
The other child whines and whines	Head moves slowly back and forth	
T. returns, unstraps Frank, puts her arms behind Frank's shoulders	Lifts head and chest up (anticipates being picked up?)	T. pauses to talk to aide, lifts Frank and places Frank prone in the block area
	Moves head slowly side to side	

tion (noted in the antecedent and consequent columns) is helpful in identifying the content and use functions of the student's communicative responses (e.g., when the student said "me," and pointed to a juice box in response to a peer getting a soda; "me" was probably serving the function of a request).

The communication/language sample, behavioral assessment, and ABC analysis are observational assessments. They should focus on the individual's typical and spontaneous behavior, be conducted by familiar persons, and employ real-life materials and situations. This will result in relevant information regarding activities at home, at school, and in the community.

Motor Assessment

Information on motor development must also be considered in a thorough communication assessment of students with severe disabilities, particularly those who have multiple disabilities. Physical therapists may conduct the assessments or, preferably, collaborate in transdisciplinary assessment (see Chapter 5). Three areas of motor development are important to communication assessment (Morris & Klein, 1987):

> *Head control,* including neck and shoulder stability, is evaluated to identify whether there is effective operation of the muscles that support articulation and respiration.
>
> *Respiration and phonation* are assessed to determine the extent to which the student is able to coordinate them. Coordination of respiration and phonation enables the student to produce a steady vocalization that may eventually be modified to articulate speech sounds.
>
> *Development of oral motor patterns for eating* coincides with acquisition of oral-motor skills necessary for articulation. For example, the articulation of *m, p,* and *b* is based on the oral-motor patterns of lip smacking and lip rounding for sucking. While *babbling,* infants practice vowel and consonant sounds of speech. Eventually, intonation patterns are added, and adults assign meaning to the speech sounds (e.g., *mama* and *hi*).

In addition to assessing the acquisition of motor skills, atypical motor responses, particularly those associated with neuromotor disabilities such as cerebral palsy, must be evaluated because they often interfere with speech development. Three motor patterns that may be atypical in students with neuromotor disabilities are (1) postural tone, (2) movement patterns, and (3) secondary or compensatory movement patterns.

POSTURAL TONE.   Postural tone refers to muscle tenseness throughout the body. If a student's muscle tone is too low (hypotonic), chest stability required for deep, regular breathing may be lacking; head control is likely to be poor, and there will be limited phonation. If the student's muscle tone is too high (hypertonic), breathing will be inhibited by stiffness in the chest. Tone that is too high, too low, or fluctuating is also likely to affect the lips, tongue, and palate, making oral-motor movements for articulation difficult.

PATTERNS OF MOVEMENT.   Atypical motor patterns, such as extraneous movements caused by fluctuating muscle tone or primitive reflex patterns, interfere with oral-motor movement necessary for speech. One atypical pattern is the asymmetrical tonic neck reflex (ATNR). When the head is turned to one side, there is a significant increase in muscle tone and the arm and leg extend on the face side. The student's jaw may deviate to the face side, and there may be tongue thrust and jaw thrust.

LACK OF SELECTIVE MOVEMENT.   Selective movements refer to movements that are isolated or differentiated from larger patterns of movement (e.g., pointing with the index finger rather than reaching out with the arm and hand). Selective movements are more mature and sophisticated as compared to gross, undifferentiated movements. Differentiation in oral-motor patterns allows for independent tongue, lip, and jaw movement. Students with neuromotor disabilities often lack selective oral-motor movement, and thus have difficulties with the refined oral-motor patterns required for articulation.

SECONDARY OR COMPENSATORY MOVEMENT PATTERNS.   Students with atypical reflexes and motor patterns frequently develop secondary or compensatory patterns that affect speech. For example, a student with a strong flexion pattern may sit with a rounded back that eventually results in a sunken chest deformity. In turn, the sunken chest results in shallow breathing patterns.

As noted earlier, the assessment of normal and atypical oral-motor patterns is best conducted by a transdisciplinary team, including a physical therapist, occupational therapist, and/or speech-language therapist. Specific guidelines for assessing oral-motor functioning are beyond the scope of this chapter. An excellent oral-motor assessment, *Pre-speech Assessment Scale* (Morris, 1984), provides thorough directions for assessing each area of oral-motor behavior described above (see also Morris & Klein, 1987).

Communication Profile Assessment

Assessment information for students who are communicating non-symbolically may be organized across cognitive, social, communicative, and motor domains. The Communication Profile Assessment (Siegel & Wetherby, 2000) is a strategy for organizing this information in six areas.

Communicative Forms
Assessment data on communicative forms include a comparison of vocal and gestural forms. Consideration should be given to both conventional forms recognized by most people and those that are idiosyncratic. Initial communicative forms might include generalized movements, vocalizations (undifferentiated vowels, laughs, cries), facial expressions (smiles, grimaces), head and eye orientation to object/actions of interest, reaching toward desired objects, movement of the body to request action, and withdrawal to avoid activity.

Communicative Functions
Communicative functions are the reasons a student communicates. There are three broad categories of communicative functions: using

TABLE 12.2   Communication Functions and Samples

Communicative Function	Examples of Forms
Behavior Regulation: To get others to do something or to stop doing it	
Request Object/Action	Child looks at or reaches toward objects
	Child gives object when assistance is needed to open or activate it
	Child holds up empty cup for refill
Protest Object/Action	Child pushes other's hand away to stop getting tickled
	Child cries when toy is pushed away
	Child throws unwanted toy
Social Interaction: To draw attention to self	
Request Social Routine	Child taps other's hand to request continuation of game
	Child looks at others and laughs to keep interaction going
Request Comfort	Child reaches toward mother when upset
	Child raises arms to get picked up
	Child wiggles in chair to get another to adjust his position
Greet	Child waves "hi" or "bye"
	Child extends arm in anticipation of other shaking hand to say goodbye
Call	Child tugs on other's pants leg to get notice from other
	Child vocalizes to get other to come
Show Off	Child vocalizes, looks at other, laughs to get reaction
	Child hides under jacket and laughs until other notices
Request Permission	Child holds up cookie to ask permission to eat it
Joint Attention: To draw attention to object or event	
Comment on	Child shows book to get other to look at it
Object/Action	Child points to photograph to get other to look at it
Request Information	Child holds up box and shakes it with questioning expression to ask what's inside
	Child points to picture and vocalizes to ask what it is

Adapted from Siegel-Causey & Wetherby (1993).

communication (1) to regulate the behavior of others, (2) to engage in social interaction, and (3) to reference joint attention. Table 12.2 lists communicative functions and provides examples. It should be determined whether the student uses any of these communicative functions and how messages are conveyed.

Degree of Intentionality

The degree of intentionality in a student's communication responses must be inferred from observable behavior displayed during interactions. One approach to inferring intentionality at the preverbal level is to define intentional communication using behavioral criteria, such as (1) alternating eye gaze between goal and listener, (2) persistent signaling until the goal is accomplished or failure indicated;

or (3) changing the signal quality until the goal has been met (Bruner, 1978). The more such behaviors are displayed, the more confident the interventionist can be that the behavior was intentional communication.

Readability of Signals or Forms

Readability refers to the clarity of a communicative signal and ease with which a signal can be interpreted. For students who communicate nonsymbolically, readability is influenced by the degree of familiarity of people interacting with the students as well as the conventionality of the communicative signals.

Repair Strategies

Students who do not use symbolic communication may be faced with frequent communication breakdowns because of the more limited readability of their signals. Repair strategies describe the student's ability to modify communication when desired effects are not obtained. An absence of repair strategies would be reflected in abandoning a communicative goal if it is not immediately achieved. Repairing communicative breakdowns promotes successful social exchanges.

Capacity for Symbols

Although some students do not use symbols expressively, they may understand words or nonverbal symbols (e.g., pictures, sign language). Therefore, receptive language and comprehension response strategies should be evaluated. It is also important to evaluate cognitive skills that are correlates of language (i.e., tool use, causality, imitation, and functional object use). In other words, the student's communicative strategies should be considered in reference to other problem-solving and learning strategies.

As one completes the student's profile, it is important to consider the influence of the activities, and the patterns of interaction currently used by staff within these activities. From the student's perspective, what is there to communicate about in each familiar activity? These considerations may help the interventionist to discover the potential content that the student could communicate about.

Assessment techniques—communication/language sample, behavioral assessment, oral-motor assessment, and the Communication Profile Assessment—are used to provide detailed information on students' present levels of performance. The next step is to gather these assessment data, along with information on parent priorities and the discrepancy analysis results (refer to the planning and assessment process described in Chapter 7). All of this information will be reviewed and discussed when formulating communication goals.

Formulating Communication Goals

The list of priorities identified through person-centered planning and the parent interview should be reviewed by the parents and professionals. The most important of these should be identified as intervention goals (Snell & Brown, 2000). Determining which are most important can be facilitated by considering a set of functional criteria:

- is preference of parent;
- is preference of student;
- is age appropriate;
- is immediately useful and functional;
- increases ability to control environment/make decisions;
- is needed throughout the day and across multiple settings;
- allows greater access to age-appropriate activities and natural environments;
- enhances social interaction with peers; and
- facilitates the performance of many other skills ("tool skill").

Once communication goals have been established, assessment information pertinent to the selected goals is reviewed. This information includes performance levels on goals, adaptations that may be needed (alternative or augmentative approaches), and/or possible intervention techniques that may aid in designing interventions. For example, if a goal is for the student to request assistance, ABC analysis results indicate when and where the student might need assistance, as well as the percentage of time when the student currently requests assistance. Such detailed information will help the intervention team develop three to five short-term objectives for each communication goal.

Given that students with severe disabilities or autism learn slowly and frequently fail to generalize, *an ideal communication objective is one that targets a generalized skill*. According to Horner and McDonald (1982), a generalized skill is one that is performed in natural situations when appropriate and is not performed when inappropriate. Generalization occurs when a student uses a skill correctly in situations where intervention did not occur. It is not necessary to wait for a student to acquire a skill in one teaching situation before addressing the concern of generalization: Generalization can be promoted when a student is *first learning* a skill rather than afterwards.

Objectives are developed to address one of three types of generalization: (1) stimulus generalization, (2) response generalization, and (3) stimulus and response generalization. A communication objective that addresses stimulus generalization teaches a student the various antecedent conditions (people, settings, or situations) when/where the skill would be appropriate, for example, "Tommy will say, 'stop please,' when he is bored or finished with an activity in the classroom, cafeteria, or on the playground." In objectives that address response generalization, the communication behavior itself is broadened: a group of skills that serve the same purpose (a "response class"), rather than a discrete skill, is taught (e.g., Deana will point to *fine* on her communication board, smile and nod her head, or say "OK" when someone asks how she is). In objectives that address both stimulus and response generalization, a response class is demonstrated across stimuli (e.g. Lily will point to *want,* a photo on her communication board, or to the item itself to initiate a request to the teacher, physical therapist, or a peer at recess).

TEACHING FUNCTIONAL COMMUNICATION SKILLS

Communication intervention in natural settings *ensures* that communication skills are functional and demonstrated when and where they are needed. When the natural setting is a home or regular classroom, instruction does not occur during a "communication training" period. Instead, it occurs throughout the day, when the communication skills are required and meaningful. For example, rather than teaching a new communication board picture (a cup to indicate *drink*) in isolation, the student is taught to point to the picture to request a drink during breakfast or when arriving at school. Teaching in the natural situation eliminates the need to generalize from the teaching setting to a natural one. Teaching across several natural situations throughout the school day promotes generalization to other untrained natural settings.

A matrix format (adapted from Mulligan & Guess, 1984) is helpful for identifying multiple teaching opportunities for communication skills (see Figure 12.1). In the first column, the student's daily schedule of activities is listed. Communication objectives are noted across the top of the matrix and are infused into the schedule with checkmarks indicating activities that provide meaningful contexts for instruction. Because these communication objectives were identified through discrepancy analysis (see Chapter 7), at least one activity is appropriate for each communication goal. Embedding communication skills into other instructional activities teaches functional relationships among skills and promotes generalization.

Establishing a Symbolic Communication Repertoire

For students without symbolic skills (i.e., words, sign, communication board symbols) or with very limited symbol usage, the general goal is to teach one or more signals or symbols for controlling the environment. (Potential communicative signals include behaviors such as vocalizations, changes in muscle tone, eye gazing, or body

FIGURE 12.2 Sample matrix for integrating communication and other basic skill objectives into a child's preschool schedule

Student __Carrie Y.__

Semester __Fall__

Year __2002__

Daily Schedule and Activity Objectives	**Communication**							**Fine motor**						**Gross motor**		
	greet familiar persons	request needed items	request assistance	indicate task completed	answer single questions	comment to continue conversation	identify sight words	maintains grasp	points with index finger	grasps small items	moves wheelchair forward	pulls self to stand	full elbow extension	transfers to chair		etc.
7:45–8:00 Arrival/Put away personal items	√	√	√		√		√			√	√					
8:00–8:30 Grooming																
Toothbrushing		√					√		√	√		√				
Face washing		√														
Hair brushing			√													
8:30–8:50 Circle time																
Socialization	√			√	√		√									
Songs				√	√	√		√	√							
Daily Schedule		√		√	√	√	√	√	√							
8:50–9:30 Centers																
Select items	√			√			√	√		√			√			
etc.																

422

movements). Because communication is a reciprocal process, intervention may address the behavior of the interventionist or the student. A dual focus on student and interventionist recognizes that interactions are influenced by what both the initiator and responder do rather than assuming that one partner has deficits to remediate (Siegel & Wetherby, 2000).

Communication and language intervention should match the student's skills regardless of the nature or the mode of expression. There are five intervention strategies that are tailored to the student's skill levels and allow the student to experience control of interactions as she initiates, maintains, and/or terminates communication exchanges: enhancing sensitivity to the student's nonsymbolic communication, increasing opportunities for communication, structuring routines in a predictable order, augmenting input provided to the student, and modifying the environment (Siegel & Bashinski, in press; Siegel & Cress, in press; Siegel & Wetherby, 2000).

Enhancing Sensitivity

Studies of early communication interactions between the caregiver and infant show that caregiver sensitivity is vital to the infant's acquisition of communication skills (Snow, 1984). Caregivers of nondisabled infants typically are sensitive to signals of readiness to communicate (e.g., the infant's direct gaze or leaning forward). Furthermore, they allow the infant to take turns during interactions, and they wait until the infant has finished responding before taking their turn (Clark & Seifer, 1983). The caregiver's ability to discern the infant's signals and to assign meaning to the infant's expressions promotes communication exchanges.

Interventionists can enhance their sensitivity to students' signals and capitalize on opportunities for communication in two ways. First, the interventionist should recognize the student's nonsymbolic behavior. Some students with severe disabilities or autism communicate at a nonsymbolic level in a manner similar to students without disabilities. These students may move unintentionally in ways that can be communicative, such as opening their mouth, turning their head, or touching an object. The interventionist can observe and use an ABC analysis to help identify the student's nonsymbolic behaviors that may be communicative in nature.

Second, the interventionist should assign meaning or intentionality to the student's nonsymbolic behaviors. Although it is not always clear if a student's nonsymbolic behaviors are intentional, it is important that the interventionist respond to nonsymbolic behaviors as though they are intentional. For example, the student may smack her lips when she has finished a bite of food. If the interventionist gives the student a bit of food each time she smacks her lips, the student learns to smack her lips to request more food.

Increasing Opportunities

In order to learn to communicate, students must have opportunities to interact with others. For many students with severe disabilities or autism, however, their need to communicate seems to have been eliminated. In home and at school, these students are usually dressed, fed, and cared for with minimal participation expected or required from them (MacDonald, 1985). Furthermore, interventionists may view the students as responders, not initiators. Changing the views and expectations of adults toward individuals with severe disabilities or autism may greatly improve interactions (Affleck, McGrade, McQueeney, & Allen, 1982). Four intervention techniques are recommended for increasing opportunities for communication:

1. *Utilize motivating situations.* In designing instructional programs, interventionists should take note of situations that are highly motivating and/or likely to promote communication. Highly motivating situations, such as activities with favorite peers or games, can provide natural reinforcers for targeted communication behaviors. Group activities in which adult attention is given contingent on each student's communicative responses promotes communication through modeling and reinforcement.

2. *Create communication opportunities and need to make requests.* Interventionists can create opportunities for communication by delaying their anticipation of the student's needs and desires. Halle (1984) focused on arranging the environment to increase the need and motivation to communicate. For example, a student may expect a teacher to provide a snack, a gesture with a fingerplay game, or a certain object at a certain moment. If the teacher hesitates (time delay), the student may become impatient and demand that the teacher follow through. The student is thus motivated to communicate a need/desire.

3. *Interrupt behavior chains.* Stopping a student in the midst of a task and requiring a communicative response (e.g., requesting to continue the activity) is very effective in teaching students an initial communication response (Goetz, Gee, & Sailor, 1985). For example, after a student looks at a book and starts to put it away, the interventionist physically blocks the student from placing it on the book rack. The student must point to a communication card that says *want* to be permitted to complete the task.

4. *Provide choices.* The right to choose and express self-determination are highly valued. Many sources for teaching choice are available (e.g., Bambara & Koger, 1996; Brown, Belz, Corsi, & Wenig, 1993). It is important to consider the student's level of receptive understanding and it may be helpful to implement choice-making instruction on a continuum from simple to complex.

In addition to providing instruction on how to make choices, it may be helpful to extend the manner in which choices are offered by examining the student's natural routines (Brown et al., 1993). According to Brown et al., there are seven categories of choice available during daily routines: within activities, between activities, refusal, where, when, who, and terminate. Each routine could by analyzed by team members and the aspects of choice making to provide (e.g., within, who, terminate) would be selected for an individual activity or time of day.

Structuring Routines

Organizing daily activities into a regular, sequential format allows students to become familiar with recurrent patterns and to assume a definite role in the activity (Yoder & Reichle, 1977). This is sometimes referred to as "scripting." For example, a mother's utterances repeated several times in a game with her infant establishes a predictable, familiar pattern. Games, familiar routines, and community activities such as ordering food in restaurants or grocery shopping with a friend often can have a component of "your turn—my turn" that helps students learn to express themselves.

Two suggestions for structuring routines are:

1. *Provide natural, recurring events.* There are numerous daily activities when successive routines are possible, such as self-help activities (bathing, dressing, mealtime), leisure activities, and transition times (between activities, between environments). The redundancy of routines and recurring events encourages the student to anticipate what may occur next (Writer, 1987).

2. *Provide turn-taking.* Routines can be established to help ensure consistency and opportunities for communication across the day. Examining the routines can help provide structure for the many partners the student communicates with. The goal is to allow turn-taking so that communication from the student is expected and the adult interventionists respond in a similar manner. For example, an interventionist can establish a give-and-take play with an electronic game, stop the game, and then begin the game again contingent on any type of "impatient" behavior (e.g., whining). Later, restarting the game can be made contingent on a more specific communication behavior, such as the student's making eye contact with the interventionist.

Augmenting Input

This strategy focuses on the use of verbal input to the student paired or "augmented" with another mode of communication. This may help the student understand the messages received. Enhancing the meaning of a message, commonly used by interventionists, may help the student receive information more clearly because verbal (symbolic) input is elaborated on with another mode. This alternative mode should be matched to the student's level of understanding and may include concrete gestures, touch cues, real objects, or photographs. The use of an object schedule for a student with severe disabilities or a picture schedule for a student with autism are examples of augmenting input when the interventionists pair these with verbal or sign language descriptions.

Modifying the Environment

This strategy takes into consideration how the environment may influence the communication interactions. Students with severe disabilities or autism may require additional physical and social supports to promote learning. The use of ecological assessment, discussed in Chapter 7, would be the first consideration to identify the factors that contribute to the difference between the student's participation and that of an age-matched peer. Interventionists can adjust the environment to assist the student to interact with others and display more alert, responsive behavior. Two suggestions for modifying the environment are:

1. *Altering the physical orientation of the student.* It is important to consider the student's body position and body movements. Interventionists may find it helpful to consider tempo or movement of body parts and the student's body tilt and position during specific activities. Minor changes or manipulation of environmental characteristics could be easily implemented and are likely to increase alertness (Ault, Guy, Guess, Bashinski, & Roberts, 1995). For example, while in the stander is Jessie at eye level with her peers during the music activity? If the educational assistant helped move Jessie's arm using more quick, short strokes to the tambourine would she be more involved when it was her turn?

2. *Adjusting the sensory qualities of materials.* Sensory qualities that can be modified encompass visual, auditory, tactile, gustatory, and olfactory stimuli. The interventionist determines whether certain features of sensory stimuli in the activity (or that could be added to the activity) would have an activating or soothing effect on the student. For example, materials highlighted with bright or reflective backgrounds or a change from light to deep pressure may produce more responsive behavior in the student.

Expanding the Communication Repertoire

When students demonstrate one or more symbolic communication responses reliably (i.e., repeatedly and across several situations) they have met the goal of *establishing a symbolic communication reper-toire*. The next major goal is to *expand the student's communication repertoire* across the dimensions of form, content, and use. As noted in Chapter 7, generalized communication objectives are determined through person-centered planning and are modified with considera-tion of the assessment information. This approach to developing in-structional objectives results in form, content, and use goals referenced to home, school, and community activities.

Communication *forms* are expanded by building grammatical structures, such as two-word combinations (e.g., noun-verb, verb-noun, adjective-noun) and three-word combinations (e.g., noun-verb-noun, adjective-noun-verb). Expansion of communication *content* focuses on developing the student's vocabulary, semantic functions (e.g., agent, action, object, possession), and combinations of seman-tic functions. Expanding communication use involves increasing prag-matic functions in frequency (i.e., a function is used more often), type (i.e., new functions are added), and across situations (e.g., school, home, one-to-one, in groups). Goals for expanding communication repertoires will frequently focus on form, content, and use *concur-rently*. A student's grammar is built in the context of an expanding vo-cabulary and an increasing number of semantic functions, and interventions to build grammar, vocabulary, and semantic functions occur as the student uses communication more frequently, for more purposes, and in an increasing number of situations. Several instruc-tional approaches are recommended for expanding the communica-tion repertoires of students with severe disabilities or autism: direct teaching, general case instruction, incidental teaching, script-fading, and conversation skill training. These approaches are appropriate for students who use speech or an augmentative communication system.

Direct Teaching

As noted in Chapter 8, direct teaching refers to instructional tech-niques that present the student with a consistent stimulus-response-consequence (S-R-C) arrangement (Snell & Brown, 2000). In other words, the same prompt(s), correction if necessary, and reinforce-ment are provided each time the skill is taught. Students with severe disabilities or autism must learn to recognize the S-R-C relationships that naturally occur. The intent of direct teaching is to *highlight* these relationships by assisting the student with prompts, corrections, and motivational techniques. As learning occurs, instructional assistance is gradually eliminated and the student uses the skill in the presence of natural stimuli and consequences. For example, if a student is being taught to ask a peer to play with her, when she approaches a peer the teacher may prompt her by modeling, "Want to play?" If the student repeats the model (correct response), the teacher assists the peer to share a toy or offer the student a turn (reinforcing consequence).

Once the student is responding correctly on a consistent basis, the prompt must be faded. An initial step in fading the model, "Want to play?" may be to change to a gestural prompt in which the teacher taps his or her own lips. When the student responds to this prompt consistently, the teacher may shift to simply raising his or her index finger. Finally, the teacher may fade the prompt by waiting five to ten seconds before raising his or her finger. This will allow the student time to respond correctly before the prompt is given, thereby producing an unprompted correct response.

General Case Instruction

Teaching generalized skills means that generalization is taught during skill acquisition rather than later. It incorporates the generalization strategy of "train sufficient exemplars" (discussed in Chapter 8) in the instructional program by teaching more than one stimulus or response variation concurrently (Horner, Sprague, & Wilcox, 1982). It is particularly helpful for students who display the characteristic of stimulus overselectivity and respond to a limited number of cues (Koegel, Koegel, Harrower, & Carter, 1999).

Implementing general case instruction begins by identifying the range of stimuli (stimulus class) to which the student is expected to generalize. For example, in teaching a student to take conversational turns, the stimulus class could be a list of people the student would be expected to converse with and the home, school, and community activities where conversation would be expected. Once a stimulus class is identified, three stimuli ("exemplars") from the class that represent the various types of stimuli in the class are selected for instruction. In the conversational turn-taking example, if a stimulus class of people was identified for instruction, a classmate of the opposite gender, the recess monitor, and an older sibling of the same gender might be selected to represent the characteristics of familiar/less familiar people, gender, and ages. Direct instruction is then provided on conversational turn-taking each day with each of the three selected people. Once conversational turn-taking has been demonstrated across exemplars (the three people), one or two exemplars who were not included in the training are presented to assess generalization.

Incidental Teaching

Although direct teaching requires consistency, it is most effective when implemented in the course of naturally occurring activities. *Incidental teaching* (or "milieu teaching"), described in detail in Chapter 8, is one approach for doing this. The hallmark of incidental teaching is that communication skills are taught at times throughout the day when the skills are needed (Kaiser, 2000). These natural times for instruction are determined by a student action (e.g., "when the student stops working because assistance is needed" or "when the student looks at mom or dad") rather than at times predetermined by the teacher. When incidental teaching occasions occur, instruction is implemented consistent with the direct teaching plan. The consistent instruction promotes learning and facilitates generalization through instruction across multiple situations and natural stimuli. Incidental teaching also helps students learn to initiate communication because occasions for instruction are natural events rather than verbal prompts from an adult.

Conversation Skill Training

One approach to teaching students with severe disabilities or autism to participate in conversations is to use a communication book of photos. The photos are selected to suggest topics to talk about (Hunt, Alwell, Goetz, & Sailor, 1990). They should be of people, objects, places, and activities that the student enjoys and labeled with short phrases identifying/explaining them. The photos may be grouped by setting and/or special event (e.g., birthday party). A small photo album (5" × 7") works well as a communication book. Using a prompt fading technique (described above under Direct Teaching), the student is taught to point to a picture and say something about it. Conversation partners (e.g., peers without disabilities) are taught to respond to the student's comment or answer the student's question, and then to provide another question as a prompt to continue the conversation. Conversation partners must be sure to wait and allow the student an opportunity to respond or comment on another photo. As students and conversation partners become independent in following the conversation procedures, the teacher should back away from the situation. Multiple conversation partners are involved in this training to promote generalization.

Script-Fading

Similar to conversation training, script-fading is an instructional approach that teaches students to initiate a social/communication interaction (Krantz & McClannahan, 1993). Students must be able to read at a first-grade level. Scripts are developed by printing up to ten simple statements and questions about recently completed, current, and future activities on a piece of paper. For example, "Tommy, did you like the swing today?" or "Sally, would you like a cookie?" At least three peers' names should be included in the script. The teacher stands behind the student and guides the student to point to an appropriate line of the script with a pencil. The student is prompted to read the line of the script as the pencil moves along. If the student doesn't look at the peer to whom the statement or question was addressed, the teacher may physically guide the student's head to face the peer. The script and other prompts are faded as quickly as possible. Script-fading is accomplished by presenting less and less of the written statements and questions as training sessions proceed.

SUMMARY

Students with severe disabilities or autism have diverse characteristics but share a need for interventions directed at establishing or expanding their communication repertoires. Working from the assumption that all students communicate in some way, goals aimed at establishing a communication repertoire focus on teaching symbolic communication skills. For students who already communicate symbolically, goals are to build the communication repertoire by increasing communication forms and functions. For all students with severe disabilities or autism, the goal of communication intervention is to enable them to communicate more effectively and across a wider range of situations.

DISCUSSION QUESTIONS

1. Why are the communication needs of students with severe disabilities and students with autism addressed together in this chapter?
2. What role does the environment play in identifying communication goals and objectives for students with severe disabilities or autism?
3. What is the purpose of functional analysis? How are the data from functional analysis used?
4. Discuss a number of ways in which physical disabilities can interfere with speech development.
5. Studies of caregivers and infants show that caregiver sensitivity is vital to the infant's acquisition of communication skills. How can caregivers and interventionists enhance their sensitivity to students' signals and capitalize on opportunities for communication?
6. Leilani is a fourth-grade student who is learning to use a communication board. She has a communication board with thirty symbols and can point to each of them when named. She can also answer simple questions by pointing to a symbol. Although her communication board has the necessary symbols to construct simple sentences (subject-verb-object), Leilani only uses her board to answer questions. Discuss how each strategy for *Expanding the Communication Repertoire* (direct teaching, general case instruction, incidental teaching, conversation skill training, or script-fading) could be applied to teach Leilani to use her communications board for simple conversations with her peers.

REFERENCES

Affleck, G., McGrade, B. J., McQueeney, M., & Allen, D. (1982). Promise of relationship focused early intervention in developmental disabilities. *Journal of Special Education, 16,* 413–430.

Ault, M., Guy, B., Guess, D., Bashinski, S., & Roberts, S. (1995). Analyzing behavior state and learning environments: Application in instructional settings. *Mental Retardation, 33,* 304–316.

Baer, D. M., Wolf, M. M., & Risley, T. R. (1968). Some current dimensions of applied behavior analysis. *Journal of Applied Behavior Analysis, 1,* 91–97.

Bambara, L. M., & Koger, F. (1996). *Opportunities for daily choice making.* Washington DC: American Association on Mental Retardation.

Bijou, S. W., Peterson, R. F., & Ault, M. H. (1968). A method to integrate descriptive and experimental field studies at the level of data and empirical concepts. *Journal of Applied Behavior Analysis, 1,* 175–191.

Brown, F., Belz, P., Corsi, L., & Wenig, B. (1993). Choice diversity for people with severe disabilities. *Education and Training in Mental Retardation, 28,* 318–326.

Brown, F., & Snell, M. E. (2000). Measurement, analysis, and evaluation. In M. E. Snell & F. Brown (Eds.), *Instruction of students with severe disabilities* (5th ed., pp. 453–492). Upper Saddle River, NJ: Prentice-Hall.

Bruner, J. (1978). From communication to language: A psychological perspective. In I. Markova (Ed.), *The social context of language* (pp. 17–48). New York: Wiley.

Clark, G. N., & Seifer, R. (1983). Facilitation of mother-infant communication: A treatment model for high-risk and developmentally delayed infants. *Infant Mental Health Journal, 4,* 67–81.

Goetz, L., Gee, L., & Sailor, W. (1985). Using a behavior chain interruption strategy to teach communication skills to students with severe disabilities. *The Journal of the Association of Persons with Severe Handicaps, 10,* 21–30.

Guess, D., & Mulligan, M. (1982). The severely and profoundly handicapped. In E. L. Meyen (Ed.), *Exceptional children and youth: An introduction* (2nd ed., pp. 263–303). Denver: Love.

Halle, J. (1984). Arranging the natural environment to occasion language: Giving severely language-delayed children reason to communicate. *Seminars in Speech and Language, 5,*(3), 185–197.

Horner, R. H., & McDonald, R. S. (1982). Comparison of single instance and general case instruction in teaching a generalized vocational skill. *Journal of the Association for the Severely Handicapped, 7,* 7–20.

Horner, R. H., Sprague, J., & Wilcox, B. (1982). General case programming for community activities. In B. Wilcox & G. T. Bellamy (Eds.), *Design of high school programs for severely handicapped students* (pp. 61–98). Baltimore: Brookes.

Hunt, P., Alwell, M., Goetz, I., & Sailor, W. (1990). Generalized effects of conversation skill training. *Journal of the Association for Persons with Severe Handicaps, 15,* 250–260.

Iwata, B., Dorsey, M., Slifer, K., Bauman, K., & Richman, G. (1982). Toward a functional analysis of self-injury. *Analysis and Intervention in Developmental Disabilities, 2,* 3–20.

Kaiser, A. P. (2000). Teaching functional communication skills. In M. E. Snell & F. Brown (Eds.), *Instruction of students with severe disabilities* (5th ed., pp. 453–492). Upper Saddle River, NJ: Prentice-Hall.

Koegel, L. K., Koegel, R. L., Harrower, J. K., & Carter, C. M. (1999). Pivotal response intervention I: Overview of approach. *Journal of the Association for Persons with Severe Handicaps, 24,* 174–185.

Krantz, P. J., & McClannahan, L. E. (1993). Teaching children with autism to initiate to peers: Effects of a script-fading procedure. *Journal of Applied Behavior Analysis, 26,* 121–132.

Lovaas, O. L., Schreibman, L., Koegel, R., & Rehm, R. (1971). Selective responding by autistic children to multiple sensory input. *Journal of Abnormal Psychology, 77,* 211–222.

Miller, J. F. (1978). Assessing children's language behavior: A developmental process approach. In R. L. Schiefelbusch (Ed.), *Bases of language intervention* (pp. 269–318). Baltimore: University Park Press.

Morris, S. C., & Klein, M. D. (1987). *Pre-feeding skills.* Tucson, AZ: Therapy Skill Builders.

Morris, S. E. (1984). *Pre-speech assessment scale.* Clifton, NJ: Preston.

Mulligan, M., & Guess, D. (1984). Using an individualized curriculum sequencing model. In L. McCormick & R. L. Schiefelbusch (Eds.), *Early language intervention* (1st ed., pp. 299–323). Columbus, OH: Merrill.

Nelson, R. O., & Hayes, S. C. (1979). Some current dimensions of behavioral assessment. *Behavioral Assessment, 1,* 1–16.

Reichle, J., & Sigafoos, J. (1991). Establishing spontaneity and generalization. In J. Reichle, J. York, & J. Sigafoos (Eds.), *Implementing augmentative and alternative communication* (pp. 157–171). Baltimore: Brookes.

Siegel, E., & Bashinski, S. (in press). *Enhancing interactions with learners who communicate without symbols.* Baltimore: Brookes.

Siegel, E. B., & Cress, C. (in press). Overview of the emergence of early communication and symbolic behaviors. In J. Reichle, D. Beukelman, & J. Light (Eds.), *Volume X: Implementing an augmentative communication system: Exemplary strategies for beginning communicators.* Baltimore: Brookes.

Siegel, E., & Wetherby, A. (2000). Enhancing nonsymbolic communication. In M. Snell & F. Brown (Eds.), *Systematic instruction of persons with severe disabilities* (5th ed., pp. 411–442). Columbus, OH: Merrill.

Simpson, R. L., & Myles, B. S. (1998). Understanding and responding to the needs of students with autism. In R. L. Simpson & B. S. Myles (Eds.), *Educating children and youth with autism* (pp. 1–23). Austin, TX: PRO-ED.

Snell, M. E., & Brown, F. (Eds.). (2000). *Instruction of students with severe disabilities* (5th ed.). Upper Saddle River, NJ: Prentice-Hall.

Snow, C. E. (1984). Parent-child interaction and the development of communicative ability. In R. L. Schiefelbusch & J. Pickar (Eds.), *The acquisition of communicative competence* (pp. 69–107). Baltimore: University Park Press.

Writer, J. (1987). A movement-based approach to the education of students who are sensory impaired/multihandicapped. In L. Goetz, D. Guess, & K. Stremel-Campbell (Eds.), *Innovative program design for individuals with dual sensory impairments* (pp. 191–223). Baltimore: Brookes.

Yoder, D., & Reichle, J. (1977). Some current perspectives on teaching communication functions to mentally retarded children. In P. Mittler (Ed.), *Research to practice in mental retardation, education, and training* (Vol. 2, pp. 199–205). Baltimore: University Park Press.

CHAPTER 13

Supporting Augmentative Communication

Linda McCormick and Jane Wegner

Communication is at the core of the school experience. For the student with significant disabilities, the educational experience is compromised if communication differences are not addressed. Augmentative and alternative communication (AAC) is the area of support that focuses on this need. AAC refers to any means that helps a person communicate when conventional speaking, writing, and/or understanding others are not possible. AAC systems are personalized to include gestures, signs, communication boards, and books with line drawings or photographs, and/or voice output communication aids or devices (VOCAs) as well as any speech or vocalizations an individual might have.

While the history of AAC as a field spans only a little more than four decades, the sum of its accomplishments is impressive (Zangari, Lloyd, & Vicker, 1994). In the early 1970s, there were fewer than a dozen published reports of hearing individuals with severe expressive communication disability using manual signs, communication boards, or modified typewriters to augment or replace speech. Today there are hundreds of books, chapters, periodicals, and newsletters devoted exclusively to AAC information and research reports. Most university personnel preparation programs now have at least one AAC course, and there is a professional organization for people interested in the AAC field that publishes a quarterly journal.

Two trends in the 1980s contributed to the dramatic growth in AAC research and applications. One of these trends was a direct consequence of passage of PL 94-142, The Education for All Handicapped Children Act (EHA): the public schools began serving increasing numbers of students with severe disabilities, many of whom had little or no functional speech. The EHA was renamed Individuals with Disabilities Act (IDEA) in 1990. In the 1990 amendments to IDEA, the terms *assistive technology devices* and *assistive technology services* were introduced. IDEA describes an assistive technology device as

> *any item, piece of equipment, or product system, whether acquired commercially off the shelf, modified, or customized, that is used to increase, maintain, or improve the functional capabilities of children with disabilities* (Federal Register, 1992).

The IDEA regulations describe assistive technology services as

> *any service that directly assists a child with a disability in the selection, acquisition, or use of an assistive technology device* (Federal Register, 1992).

These services include evaluation of assistive technology needs, selecting and adapting devices, procuring devices, maintaining them, coordinating and using therapies, and training or technical assistance to the child, family, and other individuals who provide services.

The importance of assistive technology devices and services as a means of curriculum access continued to be supported and strengthened by PL 105-17, the 1997 reauthorization of IDEA. The 1997 Amendments retained the earlier definitions but require that assistive technology and services be considered for each student when developing or revising his or her IEP. The regulations also include a provision that stipulates, on a case-by-case basis, the use of school-purchased devices in a child's home or other settings if the IEP team determines that access to the devices in those settings is necessary for the child to receive a free and appropriate education.

The second trend that contributed to the growth in AAC research and applications was theoretical: a shift in the field of speech-language disorders from narrow conceptualizations of language to a focus on the broader phenomena of communication. Moving away from preoccupation with trying to determine the cause of speech difficulties and teaching sound and word production to considering the effect of communication difficulties and working to develop the ability to communicate at a level adequate to meet the individual's communication needs in home, educational, vocational, and community environments was a major paradigm shift. This shift is exemplified by the *Guidelines for Meeting the Communication Needs of Persons with Severe Disabilities* (National Joint Committee for the Communicative Needs of Persons with Severe Disabilities, 1992). These guidelines focus on communication as a social behavior, multimodal communication, communicative functions, modification of the environment to promote successful communication, intervention in natural contexts, and collaborative service delivery.

Initially, there was some concern that the introduction of an AAC system would interfere with acquisition of speech. The many reports describing increased speech following implementation of an AAC system have finally put these concerns to rest (e.g., Daniloff, Noll, Fristoe, & Lloyd, 1992; Millar, Light, & Schlosser, 2000; Romski, Sevcik, & Ellis-Joyner, 1984; Silverman, 1980). There is now a substantial literature (reviewed by Abrahamsen, Romski, & Sevcik, 1989) indicating that, in addition to acquiring communicative use of an AAC system, AAC users demonstrate positive gains in (1) speech production and comprehension (if they are exposed to speech in conjunction with corresponding nonspeech symbols), (2) attention span, (3) task orientation, and (4) social skills.

Underlying AAC systems and their use are the two important concepts of multimodal communication and the collaboration needed to support the use of AAC. Multimodal communication refers to the idea that most communication involves a combination of techniques including residual speech, vocalizations, facial expressions, and/or gestures. Collaborative teaming is needed among the AAC users, their families, and professionals from a variety of disciplines if the AAC system is to be successfully integrated to support social and academic participation in school. These concepts are integrated throughout this chapter. The remainder of this chapter will focus on AAC systems, assessment and instructional strategies, and the supports needed for AAC users to be successful.

AAC Systems

An AAC system is "an integrated group of components, including the symbols, aids, strategies, and techniques used by individuals to enhance communication" (ASHA, 1991, p. 10). An AAC system can be aided or unaided. Unaided AAC components are those that do not require anything external to the communicator, such as gestures, sign language, vocalizations, or speech. Aided AAC components are external such as a communication board or a dedicated electronic communication device. Though discussed separately, it is likely that most AAC users will have an unaided technique as part of their AAC system even if they use an aided component as their predominant mode of communication. This is due to the multimodal nature of communication, the need students who use AAC have for an unaided system when their aided components are not available, and the distinct advantages and disadvantages of both systems. See Table 13.1 for a summary of AAC system components.

Unaided AAC

Two common unaided AAC techniques are gestures and manual signs. Similar to their speaking partners who use natural speech, most AAC users employ gestural communication. Gestures that are more conventional and communicative in nature include pointing, reaching,

TABLE 13.1   AAC Systems

	Unaided	**Aided**
Representing the Meaning	Speech Vocalizations Demonstrative gestures Symbolic gestures	Objects Tangible symbols Photographs Representational symbols Abstract representational symbols
Selecting the Message	Memory	Direct Selection Scanning
Sending the Message	Visual Verbal	Voice output Visual display Voice output + visual display Print

showing, offering, and giving objects, touching others, and head movements. Other gestures such as body movements are not as conventional and as easily understood. Mirenda (1999) suggests the use of a gesture dictionary to assist communication partners unfamiliar with an AAC user's communicative gestures.

Amer-Ind is a gestural system based on American Indian Hand Talk (Skelly, 1979). It falls somewhere in the middle between conventional, generally understood gestures and manual language systems. The Amer-Ind system has 250 concept labels, each with multiple meanings. The basic features of Amer-Ind that make it appropriate for some AAC users are: (1) concreteness, (2) flexibility, and (3) lack of grammatical structure.

Manual sign systems are symbolic in nature. The three types of manual sign systems are (1) systems that are alternatives to (rather than paralleling) spoken language; (2) systems that parallel spoken English, and (3) systems that supplement other means of transmitting language (Beukelman & Mirenda, 1992).

American Sign Language (ASL) is the language system used by people who are deaf or hard-of-hearing in North America. ASL is an example of an alternative system. ASL is not a manual version of English. It does not use English word order, there is no form of the verb *to be,* no passive voice, no articles, and there are no signs for pronouns. With ASL, it is possible to convey an entire statement with a single sign.

Other manual sign systems used in AAC systems include *Signed English* (Bornstein, Saulnier, & Hamilton, 1983), *Signing Exact English* (Gustasaon, Pfetzing, & Zawolkow, 1980), and *Sign English*

(Woodward, 1990), also known as Pidgin Sign English. These systems directly code English word order, syntax, and grammar and incorporate ASL signs. Signs are typically accompanied by gestures and vocalizations.

Aided AAC

Aided AAC components can take several forms but all include a way to represent meaning, a way to select or access the meaning represented, and a way to share or transmit that information with others. Aided AAC components can be "low-tech," involving no electronics, or more "high-tech," incorporating electronic equipment.

REPRESENTING THE MEANING.   Both low- and high-tech aids utilize a variety of symbols to representing meaning. Symbols range from exact representations that are easy to understand to abstract representations that may be difficult for communication partners to interpret. Some collections of symbols are properly termed *symbol sets* while others, because they are rule-governed, can be called *symbol systems*.

   Iconicity refers to the ease with which the meaning of a symbol can be recognized. The greater the iconicity, the easier it is to recognize the symbol's meaning. At one end of the continuum are symbols that, because they allow for total iconicity (they resemble their referents), are said to be transparent symbols. The meaning of a transparent symbol is easily recognized or can be easily guessed. At the other end of the iconicity continuum are opaque or arbitrary symbols. When there is only an arbitrary relationship between the symbol and its referent, the symbol's meaning is not immediately apparent or easily guessed and must be learned. The written word *tree* is an opaque symbol. At some point near the middle of the iconicity continuum there are symbols that can be recognized *if* additional information is available or with minimal training; these symbols are translucent (Reichle, York, & Sigafoos, 1991). An example of a translucent symbol is a heart, referring to love.

   Real objects, parts of objects, miniature objects, photographs, and line drawings fall under the heading of "exact representational symbols." For the most part, these symbols are transparent. Objects or parts of objects that feel or sound like what they represent are called *tangible symbols* (Rowland & Schweigert, 1989). Tangible symbols are particularly useful for students with dual sensory impairments. Examples of tangible symbols might be a spoon to represent hunger or a piece of terrycloth to represent washing or bathing.

   Photographs are often used on communication boards. Digital cameras and editing software have made it easier to utilize photographs in AAC systems because they can be printed immediately and are easily edited for size and content. Photographs can be imported into some electronic communication devices. Several investigators have considered the characteristics of photographs that have implications for their use as communication board symbols. One study found an advantage for color photographs over black-and-white photographs (Mirenda & Locke, 1989). Another (Dixon, 1981) found some advantage for using objects cut out from color photographs rather than the entire photograph. On the other hand, Reichle and colleagues (1991) note that the context in which an item appears in a photograph may affect its recognizability. For example, a photograph of a light switch may be recognized more readily if it is photographed with a lamp next to it.

Line drawings may be very detailed and realistic representations of concepts or sketchy outlines. They can represent actual things (milk) or ideas or concepts (feelings). Rebuses are pictures that represent words or syllables. They were originally designed to teach reading to children (Woodcock & Davies, 1969) but have been adapted and expanded for use as communication symbols. There are many types of rebuses, but the most readily available collection is available from American Guidance Service.

There are several commercial symbol sets available (see Figure 13.1). Picture Communication Symbols (PCS; Johnson, 1985) includes more than 3000 symbols and is available in a number of formats including notebooks with prepared boards, stickers, and computer software from the Mayer-Johnson Company. Picsyms is a symbol set developed by Carlson (1985). This symbol set has been adapted to create the DynaSyms symbol set originally for use with the DynaVox augmentative communication device. The symbol set is available in paper form as well (Carlson, 1994). Minspeak is a set of icons used with Prentke Romich communication devices such as the VanGuard, DeltaTalker, and Pathfinder. The symbols are organized and sequenced based on semantic associations. For example, the sequence of the symbols rainbow and lemon would refer to the color yellow.

Blissymbols is a semantically grounded symbol system based on 100 basic elements that are combined together to create many different meanings. Some Blissymbols are pictographic in that they depict

FIGURE 13.1   Commercially Available Symbol Systems

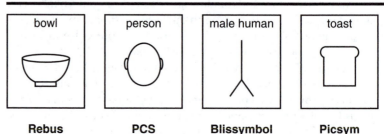

the outline of the concept represented, others are ideographic, and still others are arbitrary. Blissymbols are available in many forms from the Blissymbolics Communication International in Toronto and can be used with some electronic devices.

Students who cannot use speech but are functionally literate typically use traditional orthographic symbols. When provided with a display (electronic or nonelectronic) of printed letters, words, syllables, phrases, or sentences, the AAC user can create an unlimited number of messages. Traditional orthography may be used alone or in combination with other symbols.

Other alphabet-based symbol systems are Morse code and Braille. When used in AAC applications, the Morse code dots and dashes are transmitted via microswitches to an emulator that translates them into letters and numbers (Beukelman & Mirenda, 1998). Morse code can be used with a number of communication devices.

SELECTING THE MESSAGE. In addition to having a symbol set or system that matches the user's abilities and preferences, the AAC user needs a way to select the message he or she wishes to deliver. With unaided components, the user relies on memory to select the message. For AAC users with aided systems, selection of the message is done through direct selection or indirectly through scanning.

With direct selection the AAC user chooses the item he or she wants. Direct selection can be through touch, pointing, use of a pointer, a switch, eye gaze, or a mouse. An example of direct selection with a communication board is when the AAC user touches the picture of a glass to get a drink. Direct selection is the fastest and most efficient way to select a message, but for some individuals with poor motor control this may not be possible.

Scanning involves the sequential presentation of the symbols or messages to the AAC user who chooses from those presented. The symbols or messages can be presented by a communication partner or an electronic device. The selection can be made through the use of a switch or a head nod when scanning is facilitated by a partner. Most electronic communication devices have a scanning option. Scanning is slower than direct selection and more cognitively difficulty (Ratcliff, 1994).

SENDING THE MESSAGE. Once a symbol has been selected, it is transmitted or sent to the communication partner. With unaided AAC components, the message is presented for the partner to receive visually or verbally. With aided AAC components, the message may be transmitted visually through a display, with voice output from an electronic device, through print, or a combination of all three. Voice output can be synthesized or digitized. Synthesized speech is computer-generated and -produced. Digitized speech is produced when a voice is recorded and digitized. Synthesized speech is not as natural sounding as digitized speech, but is intelligible. Some electronic AAC devices offer a combination of synthesized options.

Nonelectronic Communication Aids

The most common low-tech aids are communication boards or charts, communication books, communication cards, communication vests, communication aprons, and E-trans.

A communication board or chart typically has a flat surface with an array of two-dimensional symbols in a matrix format. The size of the communication boards depends on the AAC user's needs and abilities. The boards range from lapboard-size single-sheet displays to smaller miniboards. Single-sheet display may be fitted beneath plexiglass or some other protective covering on a lap tray, or folded in half and equipped with carrying handles (similar to a brief case). Some communication boards have symbols that are attached with Velcro. These boards are often used as calendar or schedule communication aids.

Photo albums and three-ring notebooks are often modified to be used as *communication books,* with the number of pages and the number and arrangement of the symbols determined by the AAC user's needs and preferences. There are a variety of commercially produced notebooks available in different sizes, construction materials and colors. *Communication cards* with symbols can be carried in wallets with windows such as those designed for credit cards or business cards or attached to a wristband or keychain. A *communication vest* or *apron* with objects or symbols attached may be worn by the student's communication partner or the student him- or herself (see Figure 13.2).

An *E-tran,* or eye-transfer aid, is a clear Plexiglas rectangle with a square or circle cut out in the center. Objects, pictures, symbols, alphabet, numbers, or words and phrases are attached to the frame with Velcro, clear contact paper, or plastic pockets. The student uses eye gaze to indicate a desired selection, or possibly a series of eye gazes to encode and expand message selections. An E-tran can be purchased commercially or cut at a local hardware store.

Electronic Communication Aids

There are many electronic or voice output communication aids (VOCAs) available today and the field is constantly advancing. Electronic devices come in a variety of sizes, complexities, and costs. VOCAs range from one-message portable switches such as the BIGmack (AbleNet) to sophisticated devices with large memory capacity and wide vocabulary options such as the Vanguard (Prentke Romich) or the DynaMyte (DynaVox Systems).

Single-level devices are easy to program and operate but are limited in the number of messages available at any one time. An example

FIGURE 13.2   Non-Electronic Communication

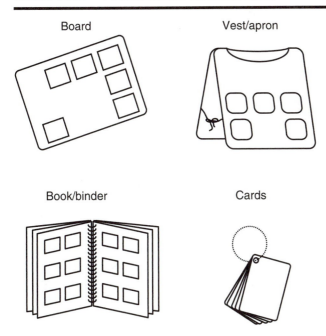

of this is the Tech/Four (Advanced Multimedia Devices). Four symbols are displayed in 2½-inch grids. Messages are recorded and, when the symbols on the grid are activated, the message is spoken. Up to twenty seconds of recording can be done. New messages can be recorded over old messages. Other examples of single-level VOCAs include Partner/Four (Advanced Multimedia Devices) and Parrot (Zygo Industries).

Other VOCAs have multiple levels on which to store vocabulary. Some of these aids, such as the AlphaTalker (Prentke Romich), allow for expanded vocabulary without changing symbol displays while others, such as the Macaw (Zygo Industries) and Tech/Speak (Advanced Multimedia Devices), require manual changing of the symbol display to access the various levels. There are numerous electronic devices on the market that are more comprehensive in nature. They have large memories, can operate as environmental controls, and/or can interface with computers. Examples of these devices are the Vanguard (Prentke Romich), the Dynavox (Dynavox Systems), the Palmtop (Enkidu Research), and Gemini and Freestyle (Assistive Technology). VOCAs have static or dynamic displays. A list of resources to locate VOCAs is included in the appendix at the end of this chapter.

Whether electronic or nonelectronic, it is important to remember that these aids are just part of a communication system and that their use will not be automatic. Learning to use an AAC system is challenging, as is finding the right components for an AAC user.

Assessment Strategies

Assessment is an ongoing process that begins with compilation of information about the student's capabilities, her communication needs, and personal preferences. Because AAC systems are multimodal, whether to use aided or unaided components need not be an issue. The initial focus is on the student, not the technology. The goal of the assessment process is to develop an AAC system that will support the student's participation in the school curriculum, at home and in the community, and can be modified for the future. This type of assessment is best accomplished through a collaborative team effort. Team members can include the student, her family, her teachers (both regular and special education), an occupational or physical therapist, and a speech-language pathologist. Other team members might be needed if there are concerns in specific areas such as vision and/or hearing. The assessment process is not quick or easy and is dynamic in nature. It involves assessing both the student and the environments in which she participates.

The Student

Questions that the team will seek to answer regarding the student include:

- How does the student communicate now and for what purposes?
- What are the student's communication needs and goals?
- Where and with whom does the student want and need to communicate?
- What are the student's language, cognitive, sensory and motor skills, and capabilities that will facilitate communication?
- What are the potential barriers to the student communicating in his natural environments?

The first step is assessment of the student's mobility, manipulation abilities, communication, cognitive/linguistic skills, and sensory/perceptual abilities (Mirenda, Iacona, & Williams, 1990).

Mobility Assessment. Mobility assessment considers appropriate seating and positioning and ambulation variables. A physical and/or occupational therapist generally leads this assessment. If the student cannot assume and maintain a stable, well-aligned seated position independently, the therapists determine how much assistance will be required. Because most students with severe physical disabilities spend portions of their day in positions other than sitting, the team must also consider these positions and decide how the AAC system will be integrated for use during those times.

MOTOR ASSESSMENT.   Motor assessment is concerned with evaluating the student's capabilities relative to signing or gesturing for unaided techniques and accessing symbols through direct selection or scanning with aided techniques. The occupational therapist typically takes the lead in assessing hand use to determine whether the student will be able to form signs and/or point with the index finger. Assessment then considers the efficiency of head movement, eye gaze, or other body parts for direct selection. There are a number of easy-to-use formal protocols for fine-motor assessment related to the use of signs (Dunn, 1982), microswitches (York, Hamre-Nietupski, & Nietupski, 1985) and other adaptive communication devices (Goossens' & Crain, 1986).

COMMUNICATION ASSESSMENT.   Generally, two assumptions can be made about the student's communication: (1) that she is already communicating in some way; and (2) that communicative competence is minimal. It is rarely the case that a student does not participate in communicative interactions at some level even though she does not use what we think of as conventional forms of communication. It is also rare to find that a child with severe physical disabilities has acquired communicative competence because, as discussed in Chapter 1, communicative competence is acquired in the context of reciprocal interactions between communication partners. Students with severe physical disabilities have not had the experiences of reciprocal interactions through which communicative competence is acquired.

The speech-language pathologist and other team members may use the ecological inventory procedure (described in Chapter 7), or some modification of that procedure, and direct observations to collect the information they need about how the student presently responds to communicative opportunities and obligations. The goal of observations in the student's natural environments and/or interviews with family members and other caregivers and friends is to determine how the student currently participates in her environment. Specifically, the communication assessment generates information about

- how the student currently communicates in different contexts;
- what the modes and functions of her communication are;
- how effective and functional present communication modes are in different contexts;
- what the student communicates about;
- motivational factors that have the potential to affect the student's communication.

COGNITIVE/LINGUISTIC ASSESSMENT.   Cognitive/linguistic assessment considers receptive language skills and major cognitive attainments related to communication. The focus is on determining (1) how the student presently understands the world, (2) how communication can best be facilitated within this understanding, and (3) the extent to which the student can meet the cognitive demands of the various symbol sets or systems. There are a number of standardized nonverbal tests, such as the Leiter International Performance Scale (Arthur, 1950) and the Columbia Mental Maturity Scale (Burgemeister, 1973), that, when used properly, may yield useful information about the student's cognitive level. These tests are *not* administered to establish a mental age score or to determine "readiness" for an AAC system, but to find out the student's present level of ability relative to such cognitive processes as causality, object permanence, and categorization, and to contribute information for decisions about appropriate symbol systems and vocabulary.

SENSORY/PERCEPTUAL ASSESSMENT.   Sensory/perceptual assessment considers the student's ability to process incoming information. Information about sensory loss and functional use of sensory modalities is critical in the selection of AAC options. Assessment of tactile perception is most challenging, as there are very few reliable assessment procedures.

LITERACY ASSESSMENT.   Literacy assessment is important to decisions about AAC system components and to matriculation through the school curriculum. Beukleman & Mirenda (1998) suggest the inclusion of the following in a literacy assessment:

- print and phoneme recognition;
- word recognition and reading comprehension;
- spelling.

The Environment

The goal of environmental assessment is to develop a comprehensive list of curricular and social activities that the student could access with the support of an AAC system. Identifying potential participation and communicative opportunities during "nonacademic" times is also important. According to the National Joint Committee for the Communicative Needs of Persons with Severe Disabilities (1992), assessment of environments should include identification of the environments that invite, accept, and respond to communicative acts and identify crucial partners.

The preferences and communicative skills of potential communication partners are important to identify. Anyone who has serious reservations about any aspect of the system is not likely to use it. Variables that seem to influence the preferences of the AAC candidate, family, and peers are the appearance of the system, portability, and/or durability. The ages and literacy skills of potential communication partners have to be taken into account; if the output of an AAC system cannot be readily understood by untrained listeners (which is often the case with signs and low-quality synthetic speech), there will be frequent communication breakdowns. The time and skills required to learn the system are another consideration, particularly when manual signs and sophisticated voice-output devices are concerned. If there are no professionals available with the expertise to design and develop a particular "high-tech" AAC system and teach the student how to use it, then that system is not a viable option.

The potential impact of the AAC system on the student's appearance and perception as a competent communicator is also of concern. Among the variables thought to influence perceptions of communicative competence are the intelligibility of the message, the rate and accuracy of message delivery, the pragmatic skills of the user, the grammatical completeness of the message, and the ability of the communication partner to develop effective Reponses strategies (Hoag & Bedrosian, 1992; Kaiser & Goetz, 1993). The team will also want to consider potential barriers in the environment such as attitude, knowledge, policy, skill, or practice (Beukleman & Mirenda, 1998).

The Student and the System

The challenge of the assessment team is to reach consensus on an AAC system that will serve the student today and tomorrow. They do this by matching the features of the systems to the student's capabilities and needs (Wasson, Arvidson, & Lloyd, 1997). Specifically, the team focuses on the selection of (1) device(s) to consider, (2) communication techniques, (3) the symbol systems or sets to be taught, and (4) the communication strategies that need to be developed. The planning guide in Figure 13.3 can guide the decision making process.

Typically, there will be several AAC devices that appear to be a good enough match for the student to be considered. The team will then need to focus on field-testing one or several of the possibilities. Any device the team determines to match the student's capabilities, needs, and preferences should be field-tested. Field-testing allows the potential AAC user, her family, and team the opportunity to try out the equipment. Most manufacturers rent their devices and most states have an assistive technology loan bank from which equipment can be borrowed. Support and instruction is provided during this field-testing period. At the end of the field test, the student's access to the curriculum and participation in communicative interactions are reevaluated and a final decision made.

During the field test, it is important that the vocabulary be carefully chosen because, as Mirenda and colleagues (1990) remind us,

FIGURE 13.3   Suggestions form for team planning meetings

What Are Possible Communication Techniques for This Student?

Aided   *Unaided*

Direct Selection _____   Demonstrative Gesturing _____

Scanning _____   Symbolic Gesturing _____

Encoding _____

What Are Graphic Symbols/Sets This Student Can/Will Use?

Nonelectronic

Board _____   Book _____   Cards _____   Vest _____   Other _____

Electronic (specify)

1.

2.

What Type of Graphic Symbol Characteristics Does This Student Need?

Size? _____   Placement? _____   Number? _____

List an Initial Graphic Symbol Vocabulary for This Student.

List Gestural Symbols or Symbol Sets This Student Can/Will Use.

Describe an Initial Gestural Symbol Vocabulary.

Time and date for the next meeting? _____

Place for the next meeting? _____

"the vocabulary provided through a system will directly determine its functionality for the user as well as the motivation of the user to communicate with the system" (p. 14). In addition to the vocabulary, the communicative functions that the vocabulary serves should also be considered. Mirenda (1999) points to four main purposes of messages: (1) wants and needs, (2) information-sharing, (3) social closeness, and (4) social etiquette. Mirenda (1999) suggests that messages that the student will use on a regular basis, will facilitate educational participation, will enable the student to participate in social interactions with others, and those that are important and cannot be communicated using unaided means be included.

After field-testing is completed and a device has been chosen, funding must be secured. IDEA specifies that assistive technology shall be provided to students who need it to receive a free, appropriate, public education. If the IEP team determines that a student needs assistive technology, the school is obligated to provide the device. Other possible sources of funding are Medicaid and private insurance. Each state has a technology-related program that can assist consumers with funding issues.

INSTRUCTIONAL STRATEGIES

The instructional strategies discussed in this section focus on teaching communication rather than teaching a student to use AAC. AAC is a means to an end, with that end being communication and participation.

Most critical in planning for AAC instruction is to *avoid* these assumptions: (1) that children with severe expressive communication difficulties have had an opportunity or the conditions essential to the acquisition of communicative competence, and (2) that the provision of an AAC system will somehow "automatically" result in the acquisition of communication skills. Therefore, professionals must arrange for the use of carefully planned and supported instructional strategies. Also, they must plan for expanding system use and conversational participation in present and future environments once the student masters initial communication skills.

The very fact that a student has an AAC system and knows how to generate messages will not increase appropriate communication or promote meaningful changes in her daily life unless she has appropriate instruction and support to use it effectively to initiate and participate in conversations (Basil, 1992; Newell, 1992). Research suggests that AAC users tend to be responders, seldom initiating conversations with others (Angelo & Goldstein, 1990). When initiations do occur, they are often limited to object or action requests rather than requests for information that have the potential to initiate conversations. Some possible reasons why students may not use their

AAC system include: (1) inadequate vocabulary or messages needed to initiate and/or participate meaningfully in conversations; (2) lack of conversational/discourse skills; (3) feeling "different" relying on a nonspeech mode; (4) communication partners don't understand the AAC user's symbols; (5) decreased motivation because of failure of past efforts to use communication to affect the environment; and (6) few or no models using the AAC system.

Students learning to use an AAC system have a twofold task. They must learn the symbols/vocabulary and their meanings as well as how to use them in an interactive manner. One of the most serious problems for AAC users is that potential communication partners often fail to see and, therefore, to take advantage of naturally occurring communication opportunities. Potential communication partners must often be cued to notice and respond to initiations and to keep the interaction going. Training peers in the use of the AAC system may be crucial if the system is to be used on a participatory level.

For a student to gain proficiency in using aided and/or unaided AAC systems in the classroom, teachers and peers must begin to use the system(s) (paired with verbal communication) in communication with the student. This kind of use supports both comprehension and production for the AAC user. Several such strategies are reported as successful.

Aided-Language Stimulation

Aided-language stimulation (Elder & Goossens', 1994; Goossens', Crain, & Elder, 1992) was developed to teach AAC users to understand and use graphic symbols for communication. During aided language stimulation, the communication partner points to or highlights the key symbols on the student's communication display while speaking the words. This approach uses a series of least-to-most prompts adapted from milieu teaching strategies. Aided-language stimulation can be used in any ongoing activity as long as the communication partner is familiar enough with the student's display to use it naturally without disturbing the flow of the interaction. Communication display would need to be available for all activities.

System for Augmenting Language

The System for Augmenting Language (Romski & Sevcik, 1992, 1996) is similar to Aided-Language Stimulation except that voice-output communication aids are used. Like aided-language stimulation, partners must be familiar with the displays and willing to use the device. The students are encouraged but not required to use the device in their interactions.

Natural Aided Language

Cafiero (2001) describes natural aided language as a "hybrid strategy (that) incorporates the interactive, generative language basis of aided language stimulation (Goossens', Crain, & Elder, 1992) with the naturalistic strategies of the natural language paradigm (Koegel, O'Dell, & Koegel, 1987) and incidental teaching (Hart & Risley, 1975)" (p. 181). During natural aided language, a visual language is incorporated into the communicative environment. This approach has been used with families (Cafiero, 1995) and in a classroom (Cafiero, 2001).

Aided Input

Aided input incorporates facilitative language intervention strategies (Bunce & Watkins, 1995) in natural settings combined with augmented input (Wegner, 1995). The facilitative language strategies include: event casts, modeling, expansions, and recasts. Aided input was an effective strategy used to increase the initiations and variety of communicative functions of three preschool AAC users during their preschool class activities (Kelpin, 1995).

Milieu Teaching

Milieu teaching is a more structured naturalistic teaching strategy than those already described. (Refer to the discussion of milieu language teaching interactions in Chapters 8 and 10.) Recall that in milieu teaching the teaching takes advantage of the focus or interest of the child, the child's production of language is explicitly prompted, consequences for the child responding are associated with the context, and the teaching episodes are embedded in ongoing interactions (Rogers-Warren & Warren, 1980; Warren & Kaiser, 1986).

Functional Communication Training

Although all behavior has communicative value, it is not necessarily the case that all behavior used for communication is appropriate and socially acceptable. Behaviors such as hitting, pushing, biting, screaming, and pulling someone's arm fall into the category of challenging behaviors. As discussed in Chapter 8, functional communication training is teaching students with severely limited communication skills alternative communicative responses that serve the same function as their problem behaviors. AAC systems have successfully been used to express alternative responses (Durand, 1993).

Conclusion

These guidelines serve as a summary of the major points of the discussion of instructional strategies:

- An AAC system is best learned in a supportive environment in the context of ongoing activities with partners who have knowledge of the system and teaching strategies.
- All components of the student's multimodal AAC system should be taught concurrently in the context of ongoing meaningful, reinforcing, and interactive activities.

- Children must have maximum opportunities to experience receptive use of their AAC system.
- There has to be a plan for ongoing assessment and evaluation of the system.

SUPPORTING AAC LEARNERS

Soto, Muller, Hunt, and Goetz (2001) investigated team members' perceptions of critical issues regarding the inclusive education of students with augmentative and alternative communication needs. The dominant theme was that inclusive education for AAC users is both possible and desirable. Three themes emerged as prerequisites for successful inclusion: administrative support, AAC training, and team collaboration.

A Collaborative Team

Supporting AAC users is a collaborative effort. In addition to the AAC user, her family and/or caregivers and close friends, and present and potential employers, the team includes representatives from general and special education, speech-language pathology, and physical and occupational therapy. Other disciplines that may be involved are psychology, social services, vocational counseling, assistive technology, medicine, and rehabilitation engineering.

Guidelines for collaborative teaming for students who use AAC are basically the same as those for teams concerned with students who use speech as their primary communication mode. The roles and responsibilities of the different disciplines on the team depend on the needs and preferences of the AAC candidate and the family (Beukelman & Mirenda, 1998). However, it is possible to identify a core of basic competency requirements for the primary team members. The roles and responsibilities typically assumed by the speech-language pathologist as suggested by the American Speech-Language-Hearing Association (ASHA, 1989) are shown in Table 13.2.

Similarly, there has been some research considering the competency needs of teachers on AAC teams. Based on a survey of over 200 special education teachers nationwide who serve on school district teams responsible for providing AAC services, Locke and Mirenda (1992) have identified the roles and responsibilities assumed by special education teachers on AAC teams. The roles and responsibilities shown in Table 13.3 were indicated by a majority (at least 70 percent) of the special education teachers who responded to the survey.

The roles of physical and occupational therapists on AAC teams have also been discussed (Stowers, Altheide, & Shea, 1987). Physical

TABLE 13.2 Roles and responsibilities suggested for the language interventionist on the AAC team

- identification of appropriate AAC candidates
- determination of appropriate AAC systems
- development of intervention plans to promote "maximal functional communication"
- implementation of the intervention plans
- evaluation of intervention outcomes
- evaluation and awareness of new AAC technology and strategies
- advocacy in the AAC area
- provision of in-services for professionals and consumers
- coordination of AAC services

TABLE 13.3 Roles and responsibilities suggested for the teacher on the AAC team

- adapting the curriculum for the AAC user
- preparing and maintaining documentation
- writing goals and objectives for AAC users
- assessing cognitive abilities
- acting as liaison between the team and family members
- assessing social capabilities
- providing for ongoing skill development
- identifying vocabulary to be provided in the AAC user's system
- providing information about students' motivation and attitudes toward AAC techniques
- determining students' communication needs

therapists are typically responsible for carrying out gross motor assessments related to the use of AAC techniques, ensuring appropriate positioning and seating, constructing adaptive equipment as needed for positioning and seating, and providing in-service to other team members about positioning and seating. Occupational therapists also assume primary responsibility for remediating functional deficits that impair performance of fine-motor skills, constructing adaptive devices for the arms, hands, and head, and providing in-service to other team members concerning the use of fine-motor abilities (Stowers et al., 1987).

AAC Training

If students using AAC systems are to be successful, they need a well-trained group of supporters and facilitators. These individuals include the AAC user, the regular and special education teachers, peers, related services providers, paraeducators, family members, and other school staff. Training in the area of the AAC system itself is needed. General operation, maintenance, and programming skills need to be shared. In addition, communication partners need to be trained in facilitative, instructional strategies that can be used throughout the day. Training in both of these areas will increase the likelihood that the AAC system will be valued and that communication teaching will go on throughout the day.

Access

In order to learn to use an AAC system, it must be available and accessible. For some students, support is needed to make sure that the system moves with the student, is within reach, and that the appropriate vocabulary is available for the activity that is taking place. The student should have a backup system in the event that her system is unavailable. A paper version of a VOCA display is an example of a backup. Another would be an eye-gaze system.

Vocabulary

To participate both academically and socially, a student will need vocabulary that is specific to the curriculum as well as socially-oriented vocabulary. The vocabulary needed to access the curriculum will be changing frequently, necessitating programming for VOCAs and creation of new displays for communication books. Updating and teaching new vocabulary is critical to academic participation and the responsibility needs to be explicitly assigned within the team.

SUMMARY

The trends of inclusion, the broadened view of communication, the recognition of the multimodal nature of communication, and the advances in technology have contributed to the growth in the number of communication options available to children with severe disabilities. Most important has been the recognition that communication is a right, not something that children must somehow "be ready for." Children are no longer denied communication devices and instruction because they do not demonstrate certain cognitive and/or social behaviors judged to be prerequisite to communication. Once it is determined that communication support is needed, there is now a framework to assist professionals and parents to make the decisions necessary to provide an AAC system that will afford the child maximum participation in a variety of environments with a wide range of communication partners.

Discussion Questions

1. What were the two trends in the 1980s that contributed to the growth in AAC research and applications?
2. What are the three major paradigm shifts that we see currently reflected in the field of AAC?
3. What are the questions that the mobility assessment seeks to answer? What are the questions that the manipulation assessment asks? What questions does the communication assessment seek to answer? What specific questions does the cognitive/linguistic assessment seek to answer? What specifically does the sensory/perceptual assessment consider?
4. What vocabulary would be needed for a kindergartner at circle time? How would you determine what vocabulary to use?
5. Find your state assistive technology center on-line. After you have found the web site, list the services provided by the center.

References

Abrahamsen, A. A., Romski, M. A., & Sevcik, R. A. (1989). Concomitants of success in acquiring an augmentative communication system: Changes in attention, communication, and sociability. *American Journal on Mental Retardation, 93*(5), 475–496.

American Speech-Language-Hearing Association. (1989). Competencies for speech-language pathologists providing services in augmentative communication. *ASHA, 31*, 107–110.

Angelo, D. H., & Goldstein, H. (1990). Effects of a pragmatic teaching strategy for requesting information by communication board users. *Journal of Speech and Hearing Disorders, 55,* 231–243.

Arthur, G. (1950). *The Arthur Adaptation of the Leiter International Performance Scale.* Chicago: C. H. Stoelting.

Basil, C. (1992). Social interaction and learned helplessness in nonvocal severely handicapped children. *Augmentative and Alternative Communication, 2,* 71–72.

Beukelman, D. R., & Mirenda, P. (1992). *Augmentative and alternative communication: Management of severe communication disorders in children and adults.* Baltimore: Brookes.

Beukelman, D. R., & Mirenda, P. (1998). *Augmentative and alternative communication: Management of severe communication disorders in children and adults* (2nd ed.). Baltimore: Brookes.

Bornstein, H., Saulnier, L., & Hamilton, L. (1983). *The comprehensive Signed English dictionary.* Washington, DC: Gallaudet University Press.

Bunce, B. H., & Watkins, R. V. (1995). Language intervention in a preschool classroom: Implementing a language-focused curriculum. In M. Rice & K. Wilcox (Eds.), *Building a language-focused curriculum for the preschool classroom* (pp. 39–72). Baltimore: Brookes.

Burgemeister, B. (1973). *Columbia Mental Maturity Scale, Levels A-H* (3rd ed.). San Antonio, TX: Psychological Corporation.

Cafiero, J. M. (1995). Teaching parents of children with autism Picture Communication Symbols as a natural language to decrease levels of family stress. Doctoral dissertation, University of Toledo, 1990. *UMI Dissertation Services,* UMI Microform 9540360.

Cafiero, J. M. (2001). The effect of an augmentative communication intervention on the communication, behavior, and academic program of an adolescent with autism. *Focus on Autism and Other Developmental Disabilities, 16*(3), 179–189.

Carlson, F. (1985). *Picsyms categorical dictionary.* Lawrence, KS: Baggeboda Press.

Carlson, F. (1994). *Poppin's cut and paste with 1000+ DynaSyms.* Arlington, VA: Poppin.

Daniloff, J., Noll, J., Fristoe, M., & Lloyd, L. (1982). Gesture recognition in patients with aphasia. *Journal of Speech and Hearing Disorders, 47,* 43–49.

Dixon, L. S. (1981). A functional analysis of photo-object matching skills of severely retarded adolescents, *Journal of Applied Behavior Analysis, 14,* 465–478.

Dunn, M. (1982). Pre-sign language motor skills. Tucson, AZ: Communication Skill Builders.

Durand, B. M. (1993). Functional communication training using assistive devices: Effects on challenging behavior and affect. *Augmentative and Alternative Communication, 19,* 168–176.

Elder, P., & Goossens', C. (1994). *Engineering training environments for interactive augmentative communication: Strategies for adolescents and adults who are moderately/severely developmentally delayed.* Birmingham, AL: Southeast Augmentative Communication Conference.

Federal Register. (1992, September 29). Washington, DC: U.S. Government Printing Office.

Goossens', C., & Crain, S. S. (1986). Augmentative communication assessment resource. Wauconda, IL: Don Johnston Developmental Equipment.

Goossens', C., Crain, S. S, & Elder, P. (1992). *Engineering the preschool environment for interactive symbolic communication 18 months to 5 years developmentally.* Birmingham, AL: Southeast Augmentative Communication.

Gustason, G., Pfetzing, D., & Zawolkow, E. (1980). *Signing exact English* (3rd ed.). Los Alamitos, CA: Modern Signs Press.

Hart, B., & Risley, T. R. (1975). Incidental teaching of language in the preschool. *Journal of Applied Behavioral Analysis, 20,* 243–252.

Hoag, L. A., & Bedrosian, J. L. (1992). Effects of speech output type, message length, and reauthorization on perceptions of the communicative competence of an adult AAC user. *Journal of Speech and Hearing Research, 35,* 1363–1366.

Johnson, R. (1985). *The picture communication symbols—Book II.* Solana Beach, CA: Mayer-Johnson.

Kaiser, A. P., & Goetz, L. (1993). Enhancing communication with persons labeled severely disabled. *Journal of the Association for Persons with Severe Handicaps, 18,* 137–142.

Kelpin, V. C. (1995). The outcomes of augmented input and facilitative language strategies with children using augmentative communication devices. Unpublished master's thesis, University of Kansas, Lawrence, KS.

Koegel, R. L., O'Dell, M. C., & Koegel, L. K. (1987). A naturalistic language teaching paradigm for non-verbal autistic children. *Journal of Autism and Developmental Disorders, 17,* 187–200.

Locke, P. I., & Mirenda, P. (1992). Roles and responsibilities of special education teachers serving on teams delivering AAC services. *Augmentative and Alternative Communication, 8,* 200–214.

Millar, D., Light, J., & Schlosser, R. (2000). The impact of AAC on natural speech development: A meta-analysis. Paper presented at Ninth Biennial Conference of the International Society for Augmentative and Alternative Communication, Washington, DC.

Mirenda, P. (1999). Augmentative and alternative communication techniques. In J. Downing (Ed.), *Teaching communication skills to students with severe disabilities* (pp. 119–138). Baltimore: Brookes.

Mirenda, P., Iacona, R., & Williams, R. (1990). Communication options for persons with severe and profound disabilities: State of the art and future directions. *Journal of the Association for Persons with Severe Handicaps, 15*(1), 3–21.

Mirenda, P., & Locke, P. (1989). A comparison of symbol transparency in nonspeaking persons with intellectual disabilities. *Journal of Speech and Hearing Disorders, 54,* 131–140.

National Joint Committee for the Communicative Needs of Persons with Severe Disabilities. (1992). Guidelines for meeting the communication needs of persons with severe disabilities. *ASHA, 34*(3), (Suppl. 7), 1–8.

Newell, A. F. (1992). Today's dream—Tomorrow's reality. *Augmentative and Alternative Communication, 8,* 81–88.

Ratcliff, A. (1994). Comparison of relative demands implicated in direct selection and scanning: Considerations from normal children. *Augmentative and Alternative Communication, 10,* 67–74.

Reichle, J., York, J., & Sigafoos, J. (Eds.). (1991). *Implementing augmentative and alternative communication: Strategies for learners with severe disabilities.* Baltimore: Brookes.

Rogers-Warren, A., & Warren, S. (1980). Mands for verbalization: Facilitating the display of newly trained language in children. *Behavior Modification, 4,* 361–382.

Romski, M., & Sevcik, R. (1992). Augmented language development in children with severe mental retardation. In S. Warren & J. Reichle (Eds.), *Causes and effects in communication and language intervention* (pp. 131–156). Baltimore: Brookes.

Romski, M., & Sevcik, R. (1996). *Breaking the speech barrier.* Baltimore: Brookes.

Romski, M. A., Sevcik, R. A., & Ellis-Joyner, S. E. (1984). Nonspeech communication systems: Implications for language intervention with mentally retarded children. *Topics in Language Disorder, 5,* 66–81.

Rowland, C., & Schweigert, P. (1989). Tangible symbols: Symbolic communication for individuals with multisensory impairments. *Augmentative and Alternative Communication, 6,* 226–234.

Silverman, F. (1980). *Communication for the speechless.* Englewood Cliffs, NJ: Prentice-Hall.

Skelly, M. (1979). *Amer-Ind gestural code based on universal American Indian hand talk.* New York: Elsevier.

Soto, G., Muller, E., Hunt, P., & Goetz, L. (2001). Critical issues in the inclusion of students who use augmentative and alternative communication: An educational team perspective. *Augmentative and Alternative Communication, 17,* 62–72.

Stowers, S., Altheide, M. R., & Shea, V. (1987). Motor assessment for aided and unaided communication. *Physical and Occupational Therapy in Pediatrics, 7,* 61–78.

Warren, S. F., & Kaiser, A. P. (1986). Incidental language teaching: A critical review. *Journal of Speech and Hearing Disorders, 51,* 291–299.

Wasson, C., Arvidson, H., & Lloyd, L. (1997). Low technology. In L. Lloyd, D. Fuller, & H. Arvidson (Eds.), *Augmentative and alternative communication: A handbook of principles and practices* (pp. 127–136). Boston, MA: Allyn and Bacon.

Wegner, J. R. (1995). *A guide to augmented input and language intervention.* Unpublished paper.

Woodcock, R., & Davies, C. (1969). *The Peabody Rebus Reading Program.* Circle Pines, MN: American Guidance Service.

Woodward, J. (1990). Sign English in the education of deaf students. In H. Bornstein (Ed.), *Manual communication: Implications for education* (pp. 67–80). Washington, DC: Gallaudet University.

York, J., Hamre-Nietupski, S., & Nietupski, J. (1985). A decision-making model for using microswitches. *Journal of the Association for Persons with Severe Handicaps, 10,* 214–223.

Zangari, C., Lloyd, L. L., & Vicker, B. (1994). Augmentative and alternative communication: An historical perspective. *Augmentative and Alternative Communication, 10,* 27–59.

Appendix

AAC Resources

IDEAS AND ASSISTIVE TECHNOLOGY

www.fape.org

Chamber, A. (1997). *Has technology been considered?: A guide for IEP Teams.* Reston, VA: Council of Administrators of Special Education; Council for Exceptional Children.

GENERAL AAC REFERENCES:

Augmentative and Alternative Communication. The Journal of the International Society for Augmentative and Alternative Communication.

Augmentative Communication News. www.augcominc.com.

Beukleman, D., & Mirenda, P. (1998). *Augmentative and alternative communication: Management of severe communication disorders in children and adults.* Baltimore: Brookes.

Glennen, S., & DeCoste, D. (1997). *The handbook of augmentative and alternative communication.* San Diego: Singular.

Lloyd, L., Fuller, D., & Arvidson, H. (1997). *Augmentative and alternative communication: A handbook of principles and practices.* Boston, MA: Allyn and Bacon.

http://www.mauigateway.com/~duffy/yaack/ A Web site focused on AAC and young children.

http://www.closingthegap.com

http://www.gustavus.edu/~dkoppenh/

AAC SYSTEMS

http://aac.unl.edu University of Nebraska at Lincoln

http://trace.wisc.edu Trace Center, University of Wisconsin

http://www.aacproducts.org/index.lasso. Communication Aid Manufacturers Association

http://www.ablenetinc.com/company.html AbleNet, Inc.

http://www.communicationaids.com/ Crestwood Company

http://www.prentrom.com/ Prentke Romich Co.

http://www.dynavoxsys.com DynaVox Systems, Inc.

http://www.donjohnston.com/catalog/catalog.htm Don Johnston, Inc.

http://www.saltillo.com Saltillo Corporation

http://www.zygo-usa.com ZYGO Industries, Inc.

http://www.sayitall.com Innocomp

http://www.mayer-johnson.com/ Mayer-Johnson Co.

http://www.words-plus.com/index.htm Words+

http://www.assistivetech.com/ Assistive Technology

http://www.enkidu.net/ Enkidu Research

NAME INDEX

473

Systematic instruction, 277–281
Discrete Trial Training (DTT), 277–278
fading, 280
modeling, 278
prompting, 279–280
reinforcement, 280–281
shaping, 279
task analysis, 278–279
System for Augmenting Language, 450

Tangible symbols, 439
Task analysis, 278–279
Teacher-child interactions, 261–263
Teaming models, 168–180. *See also* Collaborative approach
for augmentative and alternative communication, 452–453
characteristics of effective teams, 177–180
forming teams, 173–174
interdisciplinary teams, 168–169, 172
nature of teams, 172
roles and responsibilities in teams, 174–177
transdisciplinary team model, 168–169, 172
Tech/Four (Advanced Multimedia Devices), 442–443
Tech/Speak (Advanced Multimedia Devices), 443
Television, language development and, 24
Templin-Darley Test of Articulation, 195
Test for Auditory Comprehension of Language, 3rd Edition, 194, 197
Test for Examining Expressive Morphology, 195
Test of Children's Language, 197
Test of Early Language Development-3, 192
Test of Language Development-Intermediate, 3rd Edition, 197
Test of Language Development-Primary, 3rd Edition, 197
Test of Pragmatic Language, 196
Test of Pragmatic Skills, 196
Test of Problem Solving, 197
Test of Relational Concepts, 194

Test of Word Finding, 2nd Edition, 194
Test of Word Finding in Discourse, 194
Test-retest procedures, 388
Theoretical logic, 227
Threshold of hearing, 88
Time delay procedure, 339
described, 348
steps in, 351–352
Time organization, 371–372
Time sampling, 203
Toddler language intervention. *See* Early language intervention
Togetherness, in inclusive classroom, 284
Token Test for Children, 197
Totally blind, 91
Total number of words (TNW), 210
Touch, 10
Tracheostomy, 304, 320
Transdisciplinary play-based assessment (TPBA), 169–170, 223
Transdisciplinary play-based intervention (TPBI), 342
Transdisciplinary team model, 168–169, 172
Transitional programs, 374–375
Traumatic brain injury, 103–105
defined, 103
language characteristics of, 104–105
types of, 103–104
Treatment efficacy
assessment to determine, 227–228
dismissal from intervention, 228–229
Treatment goals, for language intervention, 319–322
Triggering data, Linguistic Theory and, 59, 61–62
Turn-taking skills, 36, 309, 371
Tutors, 381
Two-word utterances, 28–29
Type-token ratio (TTR), 209–210

Unconventional verbal behavior, 98
Underestimation, 199
Under-referral, 190
Universal Grammar (Chomsky), 58–60

Use, informal assessment of, 210–212
Utah Test of Language Development-3, 197

Validity, 193, 198–199, 228, 386
VanGuard (Prentke Romich), 440, 442, 443
Vertical structuring, in early intervention programs, 324–325
Violence, in schools, 122
Visual impairment, 91–93
categories of, 91
defined, 91
language characteristics of, 91–92
referrals for visual assessment, 92–93
Visual perception, 11
Visual structure, in structured teaching, 282
Vocables, 26
Vocabulary, growth of, 27
Vocal stimulation, in early intervention programs, 323
Voice output communication aids (VOCAs), 442–443
Vygotskian theory, 47, 55–58, 65
application to language impairment, 57–58
characteristics of, 55–56

"We" language, 284
Whole-language approach, 167, 380–381
Word meanings, relationship between sentence meanings and, 5
Word order, 60
Words
onomatopoeic, 5
relational, 28
relationship between, 5
relationship between meaning and, 5
substantive, 28
word-finding problems, 210
Words and word combinations, 27–30
Word Test-Elementary, Revised, 194
Writing activities, 381

Zero-to-Three Hawaii Project, 157
Zone of Proximal Development (ZPD), 13, 55–58